WP 660 AZZ

This book is due for return on or before the last date shown below.

| | | |
|---|---|---|
| | | |

*Practical Manual of*
*Operative Laparoscopy and Hysteroscopy*

Ricardo Azziz    Ana Alvarez Murphy

*Editors*

# Practical Manual of Operative Laparoscopy and Hysteroscopy

*Illustrated by Rod W. Powers*

With 110 figures in 121 parts

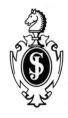

Springer-Verlag

New York Berlin Heidelberg London Paris
Tokyo Hong Kong Barcelona Budapest

Ricardo Azziz
Department of Obstetrics
  and Gynecology
The University of Alabama
Birmingham, AL 35233
USA

Ana Alvarez Murphy
Department of Reproductive Medicine
University of California
San Diego School of Medicine
La Jolla, CA 92093
USA

Library of Congress Cataloging-in-Publication Data
Practical manual of operative laparoscopy and hysteroscopy / Ricardo Azziz,
  Ana Alvarez Murphy, (eds.).
    P.  cm.
  Includes bibliographical references and index.
  ISBN 0-387-97749-X.—ISBN 3-540-97749-X
  1. Generative organs, Female—Endoscopic surgery.　I. Azziz,
Ricardo.　II. Murphy, Ana Alvarez.
  [DNLM: 1. Endoscopy—methods. 2. Genital Diseases, Female—
diagnosis. 3. Genital Diseases, Female—surgery. WP 660 P895]
RG104.7.P73 1992
618.1'059—dc20
DNLM/DLC
for Library of Congress                             91-5209

Printed on acid-free paper.

Production managed by Karen Phillips; manufacturing supervised by Jacqui Ashri.
Typeset by Asco Trade Typesetting Ltd., Hong Kong
Printed and bound by Edwards Brothers, Inc., Ann Arbor, MI.
Printed in the United States of America.

9　8　7　6　5　4　3　2　1

ISBN 0-387-97749-X Springer-Verlag New York Berlin Heidelberg
ISBN 3-540-97749-X Springer-Verlag Berlin Heidelberg New York

# Foreword

In the past decade, the future of gynecologic endoscopic surgery has been largely unpredictable. Now it is obvious that time has changed gynecology in such a way to make many of the procedures that were commonly done obsolete. At no other time in the history of gynecologic surgery has such an explosion occurred thus changing the face of this specialty to such a great degree. But in addition to solving many problems, the past decade has left us with many new and novel dilemmas.

One of the ways in which our field has tremendously evolved is not only have some procedures become obsolete, but to some degree gynecologic surgeons have themselves become obsolete. I write this because those not trained in the new techniques have had to go back and learn these surgical procedures in an unconventional way. This "unconventional way" is attending courses, and being supervised and preceptored by members of one's own hospital staff, then finally transmitted into granting of privileges. It is the young who are the leaders and, paradoxically, bringing experience to the field. In many instances, I have seen the resident who is a better endoscopic surgeon than the Senior Attending.

Not only have new techniques and operations been introduced, such as the use of the resectoscope and electrocautery to remove intrauterine myomas, but a new technology has also arisen. Mastery is imperative. One can not master these techniques by mimicking what other surgeons do, but must understand the principles of the technological advances. Laser physics and properties must be understood and, in addition, optics and television technology are critical to performing excellent endoscopic surgery.

Old timers are playing catch-up ball, but it is the young that are the leaders and pioneers in our field. It is for this reason that this text represents all that is important in endoscopic surgery. It not only is a comprehensive and encyclopedic dissertation on the subject, but it is written by the young leaders in the field. This is a textbook that will go through many editions, passed on from generation to generation of endoscopic surgeons. Not only are the important subjects tackled (i.e. techniques) but also the important principles are covered: adhesion prevention, laser surgery, hemostasis and instrumentation. Such difficult topics as cost effectiveness, risk-benefit ratio and need for randomized clinical studies are attacked with fervor to evaluate results properly.

This is an important text and destined to become a classic. It is comprehensive, principle oriented, and serves a real and tangible need.

I write this foreword with pride as an elder in the field.

Alan H. Decherney, M.D.

# Contents

# Contributors

RICARDO AZZIZ, M.D., Associate Professor, Division of Reproductive Biology and Endocrinology, Department of Obstetrics and Gynecology, The University of Alabama at Birmingham School of Medicine, 619 South 20th St., OHB 549, Birmingham, AL 35233-7333 USA.

RICHARD E. BLACKWELL, M.D., Professor and Director, Division of Reproductive Biology and Professor and Director, Division of Reproductive Biology and Endocrinology, Department of Obstetrics and Gynecology, The University of Alabama at Birmingham School of Medicine, 619 South 20th St., OHB 555, Birmingham, AL 35255-7333 USA.

RICHARD P. BUYALOS, M.D., Assistant Professor, Division of Reproductive Endocrinology, Department of Obstetrics and Gynecology, UCLA School of Medicine, 22-177 CHS, 10833 Le Conte Avenue, Los Angeles, CA 90024 USA.

MARIAN D. DAMEWOOD, M.D., Associate Professor, Division of Reproductive Endocrinology, Department of Gynecology and Obstetrics, The Johns Hopkins School of Medicine, 600 North Wolfe St., Baltimore, MD 21205 USA.

JAMES F. DANIELL, M.D., The Women's Health Group, Clinical Professor, Department of Obstetrics and Gynecology, Vanderbilt University Medical Center, 2222 State St., Nashville, TN 37203 USA.

MICHAEL P. DIAMOND, M.D., Associate Professor, Division of Reproductive Medicine, Department of Obstetrics and Gynecology, Yale University School of Medicine, 339 Farnam Memorial Building, P.O. Box 3333, New Haven, CT 06510-8063 USA.

V. GABRIEL GARZO, M.D., Assistant Clinical Professor, Department of Reproductive Medicine, University of California at San Diego School of Medicine, 510 North Prospect, Suite 202, Redondo Beach, CA 90277 USA.

JACQUELINE N. GUTMANN, M.D., Postdoctoral Associate, Division of Reproductive Medicine, Department of Obstetrics and Gynecology, Yale University School of Medicine, 339 Farnam Memorial Building, P.O. Box 333, New Haven, CT 06510-8063 USA.

JOHN S. HESLA, M.D., Assistant Professor, Division of Reproductive Endocrinology, Department of Gynecology and Obstetrics, The Johns Hopkins School of Medicine, 600 North Wolfe St., Houck 247, Baltimore, MD 21205 USA.

BRADLEY S. HURST, M.D., Assistant Professor, Division of Reproductive Endocrinology, Department of Obstetrics and Gynecology, University of Colorado Health Sciences Center, Campus Box B-198, 4200 East Ninth Avenue, Denver, CO 80262 USA.

EUGENE KATZ, M.D., Assistant Professor, Director, ART Program, Division of Reproductive Endocrinology, Department of Obstetrics and Gynecology, The University of Maryland, 405 West Redwood Street, 3rd Floor, Baltimore, MD, 21201 USA.

DAN C. MARTIN, M.D., Reproductive Surgery, P.C., Clinical Associate Professor, Department of Obstetrics and Gynecology, University of Tennessee, Memphis, 901 Madison, Suite 805, Memphis, TN 38101 USA.

ARLENE MORALES, M.D., Clinical Instructor, Department of Reproductive Medicine, University of California at San Diego, School of Medicine, La Jolla, CA 92093-0802 USA.

ANA ALVAREZ MURPHY, M.D., Assistant Professor, Department of Reproductive Medicine, University of California at San Diego, School of Medicine, La Jolla, CA 92093-0802 USA.

DENISE MURRAY, M.D., Instructor, Division of Reproductive Medicine, Department of Gynecology and Obstetrics, The Johns Hopkins School of Medicine, 600 North Wolfe St., Houch 247, Baltimore, MD 21205 USA.

CHARLES W. NAGER, M.D., Assistant Professor, Department of Reproductive Medicine, University of California at San Diego, School of Medicine, La Jolla, CA 92093-0802 USA.

C. PAUL PERRY, M.D., Assistant Clinical Professor, Department of Obstetrics and Gynecology, The University of Alabama at Birmingham School of Medicine, 1006 First Street North, Alabaster, AL 35007 USA.

HARRY REICH, M.D., Wyoming Valley GYN Associates; Clinical Associate Professor, Department of Obstetrics and Gynecology, Baystate Medical Center; Western Campus: Tufts University School of Medicine, 480 Pierce St., Kingston, PA 18704 USA.

JOHN A. ROCK, M.D., Professor, Department of Gynecology and Obstetrics, The Johns Hopkins School of Medicine; Chairman, Department of Obstetrics and Gynecology, Union Memorial Hospital, 4th Floor, South Building, 201 East University Parkway, Baltimore, MD 21218-2895 USA.

WILLIAM D. SCHLAFF, M.D., Associate Professor and Chief, Division of Reproductive Endocrinology, Department of Obstetrics and Gynecology, University of Colorado Health Sciences Center, Campus Box B-198, 4200 East Ninth Avenue, Denver, CO 80262 USA.

SAMUEL SMITH, M.D., Assistant Clinical Professor, Department of Obstetrics and Gynecology, University of Maryland School of Medicine; Director, Division of Reproductive Endocrinology-Infertility, Sinai Hospital Baltimore, Blaustein Building—2nd Floor, Belvedere at Greenspring Avenue, Baltimore, MD 21215 USA.

MICHAEL P. STEINKAMPF, M.D., Associate Professor, Division of Reproductive Biology and Endocrinology, Department of Obstetrics and Gynecology, The University of Alabama at Birmingham School of Medicine, 619 South 20th Street, OHB 343, Birmingham, AL 35233-7333 USA.

J. BENJAMIN YOUNGER, M.D., Professor and Vice-Chairman, Department of Obstetrics and Gynecology, Division of Reproductive Biology and Endocrinology, The University of Alabama at Birmingham School of Medicine, 619 South 20th Street, OHB 547, Birmingham, AL 35233-7333 USA.

HOWARD A. ZACUR, M.D., Associate Professor and Director, Department of Gynecology and Obstetrics, The Johns Hopkins School of Medicine, 600 North Wolfe St., Houck 247, Baltimore, MD 21205 USA.

# 1

# Advantages and Disadvantages of Operative Endoscopy

*Ricardo Azziz*

## CHAPTER OUTLINE

Gynecologic surgery today may be performed endoscopically in 30% to 80% of patients currently undergoing laparotomy. Gynecologic operative endoscopy, which includes pelviscopic (laparoscopic) and hysteroscopic surgery, uses the techniques of electrosurgery (bipolar or unipolar energy), thermocoagulation, laser ($CO_2$, KTP, Nd:YAG, or Argon), cold-cutting, and extra- and intraabdominal suturing. The ability to perform endoscopy has been possible only with the advent of fiberoptic illumination and intraabdominal insufflation. More recently, with an improvement in our ability to maintain intraabdominal hemostasis, complex surgical procedures are able to be performed laparoscopically. Curiously, the operative instruments used at endoscopy are not significantly different from those used at laparotomy, and have not been the main force behind the development of endoscopic surgery.

There are a number of advantages to using the endoscope for pelvic surgery, not the least of which is economic. These incentives will continue to stimulate the growth, demand, and prevalence of operative endoscopy in gynecology today.

1

# Advantages of Operative Endoscopy

## Combines a Diagnostic and Therapeutic Procedure

The laparoscope or hysteroscope allows the surgeon to perform a diagnostic procedure and, at the same sitting and with the same anesthetic risks, proceed to treat the gynecologic problem encountered. The overall surgical risks to the patient are decreased since the abdomen is entered one time, if at all, and the patient anesthetized only once.

## Improved Cosmesis

Although not frequently considered of major importance, many patients undergoing gynecologic surgery are women of reproductive age to whom cosmesis is important. Laparoscopy, by requiring only a 1-cm incision deep in the umbilicus, and two or three 5-mm incisions in the suprapubic hair line area, maximizes cosmesis. Hysteroscopy, if unaccompanied by laparoscopy, produces no visible scars.

## Reduction in Pelvic Adhesions

Operative laparoscopic procedures have the potential of reducing postoperative adhesion formation when compared to laparotomy. Postoperative adhesions may result from intentional injuries, from unintentional tissue damage (i.e., considered de novo adhesion formation), and from the reformation of lysed adhesions. To study the adhesion formation following an intentional injury, Luciano and colleagues prospectively randomized 20 rabbits to receive a standard $CO_2$ laser injury to the uterus, either by laparoscopy or laparotomy.[1] At the time of the second-look procedure 3 weeks later, these investigators noted that adhesions were absent in laparoscopically treated animals whereas they were present to a significantly greater degree on those uteri injured through laparotomy. Filmar and colleagues used a similar study design with 61 female white rabbits.[2] Instead of a $CO_2$ laser injury they used superficial cuts with scissors

the antimesenteric surface of the left uterine horn. These investigators noted that the extent of adhesions did not differ significantly between laparoscopically and laparotomy treated animals. These two animal studies suggest that laparoscopic surgery may produce the same or fewer postoperative adhesions than an equal injury performed by laparotomy.

In addition to adhesions at sites of organ injury, intraabdominal surgery also leads to the de novo formation of adhesions, an inherent risk of all surgeries. Diamond and colleagues, in a multicenter prospective study of the use of intraabdominal laser versus electrosurgery at laparotomy, reported that at the time of second-look laparoscopy more than 50% of patients demonstrated new adhesions at sites that were previously normal.[3] One should note that this de novo adhesion rate after laparotomy occurred even in the face of the high degree of expertise of the surgeons involved. It is possible that the use of operative laparoscopy leads to a reduction in this de novo adhesion rate. In a multicenter prospective study of 68 patients undergoing operative laparoscopic adhesiolysis, followed by second-look laparoscopy within 90 days of the original surgery, de novo adhesions formed in only 12%.[4]

The reformation of adhesions is more difficult to study due to the many variables involved (location, extent, and type of the initial adhesions; degree of postoperative hemostasis; and adhesiolysis technique). In the study by Luciano and colleagues animals were randomized to have their second-look procedure via laparoscopy or laparotomy, at which time adhesions were lysed. At third look a significant decrease in adhesion score was noted only in the laparoscopically treated rabbits.[1] In the multicenter study of operative laparoscopy, adhesion reformation occurred in 97% of patients, although the overall adhesion score decreased by 52%.[4] This adhesion reformation rate does not appear to be significantly less than that achieved by laparotomy.[5,6] Multicenter prospective and randomized studies with larger numbers of patients are needed to define more closely the adhesion rates after laparoscopic or laparotomy surgery.

There are a number of possible mechanisms

accounting for the reduction in postoperative adhesions after laparoscopic surgery. Dehydration of the peritoneal surfaces in the presence of bleeding is a major factor in the pathogenesis of adhesions.[7] Pelvic dehydration may be reduced somewhat during operative endoscopy because of the closed environment in which surgery is performed. Nevertheless, a large amount of low-humidity $CO_2$ circulates through the abdominal cavity. It remains to be determined whether the insufflating $CO_2$ should be humidified for maximum adhesion-reductive effect. Peritoneal irritation that occurs with the placement of intraabdominal bowel packs is also eliminated. Because the laparoscope continuously magnifies the surgical field up to threefold, excessive peritoneal cauterization or unnecessary pelvic damage is minimized. Finally, the placement of excessive numbers of sutures is discouraged, which would have served as sites for adhesion formation. Adhesion formation and adhesiolysis during operative laparoscopy will be dealt with further in Chapter 7.

## Decreased Hospitalization

No matter how complex the surgical procedure performed, it is rare for the patient to require postoperative hospitalization. Levine noted in 1985 that the average number of inpatient days was 2.0 for salpingectomies, oophorectomies, salpingostomies, and myomectomies performed by laparoscopy, compared to 5.7 days after laparotomy for the same purpose.[8] In this report there was a 69% reduction in postoperative hospitalization time. As greater experience has been acquired with operative laparoscopy, the number of hospitalization days appears to be reduced further. We recently observed that the average inpatient length of stay was only 0.2 days for laparoscopic resective procedures, in which an amount of tissue greater than a biopsy was removed.[9] This yields an effective reduction in postoperative hospitalization of about 96% for these types of procedures, compared to laparotomy. Obviously, hysteroscopic procedures such as metroplasties, which used to require extensive surgery by laparotomy, carry the same advantage. The shorter postoperative hospitalization time leads to significant economic savings and a reduction in patient stress and inconvenience.

## Decreased Postoperative Recovery Time

Although there is a significant association between postoperative recuperation and the extent of intraabdominal laparoscopic surgery, the vast majority of our patients undergoing operative endoscopic procedures are fully recovered and back to work in less than 7 days, regardless of the degree of surgery performed.[9] This compares favorably to the standard 4 to 6 weeks of postoperative rest currently suggested for laparotomy procedures. By allowing the patient to return to work sooner, employee sick pay, the need for additional help to care for children, and the need for the patient's relatives to take time off from work are also reduced.

# Economic Advantage of Operative Endoscopy

The use of operative endoscopy for gynecologic surgery results in direct, significant, and immediate savings to third party payers, employers, and the patient. Because there is minimum postoperative hospitalization time the average cost of the surgical procedure is reduced 50% to 60% when compared to laparotomy, even when taking into account that some laparoscopic procedures may last slightly longer than those performed by laparotomy. This assumes, of course, that the professional fees for laparoscopy or laparotomy are the same for similar gynecologic procedures. Since postoperative recovery time is reduced four-to sixfold, there is a significant decrease in sick pay. Furthermore, unemployment compensation to the patient's spouse or relatives who may require time away from work to care for the patient and/or her children is minimized.

For the purpose of illustration, we will assume that the savings in hospitalization costs approximate $1500 per surgical procedure performed by laparoscopy versus laparotomy.

Furthermore, recovery after laparotomy usually takes 4 to 6 weeks compared to 2 to 7 days for operative laparoscopy, and we will assume a minimum of 20 workings days saved per operative laparoscopic procedure performed. Because most women undergoing operative laparoscopic procedures are of reproductive age, we can safely assume that 50% are employed at an average salary of $7.00 per hour. In calculating the theoretical savings of operative endoscopy we will not include monies saved in child care help or from relatives' work compensation. In 1985 78,400 ectopic pregnancies were diagnosed in the United States alone.[10] If 60% of these ectopics had been treated laparoscopically the total savings in hospitalization costs would have amounted to $70,560,000. The loss of work time would have been reduced by 470,400 days, translating to $26,342,400 in sick pay saved. Salpingo-ovariolysis is 1 of the 20 most common surgical procedures performed in gynecology today. In 1983 approximately 25,000 such procedures were performed in the United States.[11] If 40% of these had been performed laparoscopically the total hospitalization savings would have amounted to approximately $15,000,000. An average of 100,000,000 working days would have been saved or $5,600,000 in sick pay. These figures only serve to illustrate the enormous savings for the patient, her employer, and the insurance carrier inherent in the use of operative laparoscopy.

# Potential Disadvantages of Operative Endoscopy

There are a few potential disadvantages to the use of operative laparoscopy for gynecologic surgeries.

## May Require Surgical Retraining

Many gynecologic surgeons trained before the early 1980s have had limited exposure to laparoscopic or hysteroscopic procedures. Although additional supervised training may be required for many surgeons currently in practice, as residency training programs add operative endoscopy to their surgical curricula, the need for such retraining will decrease significantly.

## Requires More Costly and Complex Equipment

A basic operative laparoscopic set-up, including video imaging, ranges from $30,000 to $40,000 excluding lasers. These expenses are in addition to the cost of a regular laparotomy set-up, since laparotomy back-up should always be available for operative endoscopic procedures. The additional cost of the endoscopic equipment and continuous maintenance and refurbishing must be taken into account when considering the economic advantages of operative laparoscopy. The instrumentation required for the performance of operative laparoscopy is discussed in Chapters 8 and 16.

## Physically More Demanding on the Surgeon

Because operative endoscopy today is performed on surgical tables designed for laparotomy, the surgeon may have to position him or herself in a contorted fashion over the operative site. Furthermore, he or she must become adept in coordinating hand movements while visualizing the pelvic structures through the monocular eye piece of the laparoscope or of the video monitor screen. As improvements are made in endoscopic equipment and surgical training this disadvantage will be reduced.

## Less Able to Plan Operating Time

Many endoscopic procedures initially scheduled as diagnostic result in an operative case, and vice versa. Thus, it is more difficult to plan the operating room and surgeon's schedule. In our institution the mean operating time ($\pm 1$ standard deviation) for diagnostic procedures was $40 \pm 16$ min, that of operative procedures $77 \pm 44$ min, and for resective procedures $104 \pm 65$ min.[9] Thus, the average difference between the duration of a resective or operative procedure and a diagnostic laparoscopy was 64 and 37 min, respectively.

## Operative Time is Greater than Laparotomy

Although the duration of gynecologic procedures is increased during surgical training, in experienced hands operative laparoscopy procedures last about the same as laparotomy,[12] and hysteroscopic surgeries last less.

## Increased Surgical Risks

There are few studies to date that compare the surgical risks of operative laparoscopy versus laparotomy for similar procedures. It is possible that the use of operative laparoscopy actually carries with it a decrease in overall surgical risk since it combines the diagnostic and therapeutic procedure avoiding repeated abdominal entry. Complications during operative laparoscopy may result from insertion of the trocar or Veress needle, or from the operative procedure itself. The risk of requiring a laparotomy for complications arising during operative laparoscopy is approximately 1 to 6 per 1000 procedures.[13–17] The risk of complications and their prevention during operative endoscopy is discussed further in Chapter 21.

## Surgical Results Have Not Been Well Established

The results of some of the laparoscopically performed gynecologic procedures today have yet to be fully established. However, this in and of itself should not deter qualified surgeons from performing these procedures as only the cumulative surgical experience of many centers will produce the necessary information for validating operative endoscopy. Furthermore, there is no reason to believe that operative endoscopy in well selected patients cannot produce the same or better results than surgery through laparotomy. The results of endoscopic surgery will be discussed in many of the forthcoming chapters.

# Patient Selection for Operative Endoscopy

There are relatively few contraindications to performing operative laparoscopy and they generally relate to the laparoscopic portion of the procedure. Absolute contraindications include the presence of bowel obstruction, abdominal hernia, intraperitoneal bleeding in a hemodynamically unstable patient, diaphragmatic hernia, and severe cardiopulmonary compromise. In addition, clear contraindications to performing operative laparoscopy are the unavailability of proper instrumentation, particularly for obtaining adequate hemostasis, or of general anesthesia. Insufficient surgical experience and/or training should be a significant deterrent to performing unsupervised operative endoscopy.

Previous abdominal surgery should not be an absolute contraindication to operative laparoscopy. However, one should consider the appropriateness of laparoscopic surgery in patients with previous bowel surgery on an individual basis. During laparoscopic sterilization previous abdominal surgery increased the overall difficulty of the procedure but not the rate of complications.[18] More recently, two large series studying the direct insertion of the laparoscopic umbilical trocar did not note an increased risk of bowel perforation in patients with previous surgery.[19,20]

Relative contraindications include extremes of body weight and a large intrapelvic mass. Although diffuse peritonitis may be considered a relative contraindication, the laparoscope is useful to diagnose pelvic inflammatory disease and to treat tubo-ovarian abscesses. Furthermore, some patients with ruptured ectopic pregnancies may have signs of peritonitis while remaining cardiovascularly stable and are also candidates for operative laparoscopy. The presence of a bleeding diathesis is also a relative contraindication since it may be much more difficult to control intraabdominal bleeding in these patients.

Very few contraindications to hysteroscopic surgery exist since abdominal distention or general anesthesia and paralysis are not required. Of particular concern are hypoestrogenic patients with marked reduction in uterine volume and elasticity, which may increase the risk of perforation, as well as patients with severe coagulopathies. The need for an accompanying laparoscopy raises the same concerns as before.

# References

1. Luciano AA, Maier DB, Koch EI, et al. A comparative study of postoperative adhesions following laser surgery by laparoscopy versus laparotomy in the rabbit model. *Obstet Gynecol.* 1989;74:220–224.
2. Filmar S, Gomel V, McComb PF. Operative laparoscopy versus open abdominal surgery: a comparative study on postoperative adhesion formation in the rat model. *Fertil Steril.* 1987;48:486–489.
3. Diamond MP, Daniell JF, Feste J, et al. Adhesion reformation and de novo adhesion formation after reproductive pelvic surgery. *Fertil Steril.* 1987;47:864–866.
4. Operative Laparoscopy Study Group: Postoperative adhesion development after operative laparoscopy: evaluation at early second-look procedures. *Fertil Steril.* 1991;55:700–704.
5. Jansen RPS. Early laparoscopy after pelvic operations to prevent adhesions: safety and efficacy. *Fertil Steril* 1988;49:26–31.
6. Trimbos-Kemper TCM, Trimbos JB, Van Hall EV. Adhesion formation after tubal surgery: results of the eighth-day laparoscopy in 188 patients. *Fertil Steril.* 1985;43:395–400.
7. Ryan GB, Grobety J, Majno G. Postoperative peritoneal adhesions: a study of the mechanisms. *Am J Pathol.* 1971;65:117–147.
8. Levine RL. Economic impact of pelviscopic surgery. *J Reprod Med.* 1985;30:655–659.
9. Azziz R, Steinkampf MP, Murphy A. Postoperative recuperation: relation to the extent of endoscopic surgery. *Fertil Steril.* 1989;51:1061–1064.
10. Ectopic Pregnancy—United States, 1984 and 1985. *MMWR.* 1988;37:2637–2640.
11. Rutkow IM. Obstetric and gynecologic operations in the United States, 1979 to 1984. *Obstet Gynecol.* 1986;67:755–759.
12. Goodman MP, Johns DA, Levine RL, et al. Report of the study group: advanced operative laparoscopy (pelviscopy). *J Gynecol Surg.* 1989;5:353–360.
13. Mintz M. Risks and prophylaxis in laparoscopy: a survey of 100,000 cases. *J Reprod Med.* 1977;18:269–272.
14. Hulka JF, Soderstrom RM, Corson SL, et al. Complications Committee of the American Association of Gynecological Laparoscopists: first annual report. *J Reprod Med.* 1973;10:301–306.
15. Cunanan Jr RG, Courey NG, Lippes J. Complications of laparoscopic tubal sterilization. *Obstet Gynecol.* 1980;55:501–506.
16. Yuzpe AA. Pneumoperitoneum needle and trocar injuries in laparoscopy, a survey on possible contributing factors and prevention. *J Reprod Med.* 1990;35:485–490.
17. Riedel HH, Lehmann-Willenbrock E, Mecke, et al. Frequency assessment of different methods of pelviscopical laparoscopy and their rate of complications. *Geburtshilfe Fraunheilkd.* 1988;48:791–799.
18. Chi I, Feldblum PJ, Balogh SA. Previous abdominal surgery as a risk factor in interval laparoscopic sterilization. *Am J Obstet Gynecol.* 1983;145:841–846.
19. Kaali SG, Bartfai G. Direct insertion of the laparoscopic trocar after an earlier laparotomy. *J Reprod Med.* 1988;33:739–740.
20. Byron JW, Fujiyoshi CA, Miyazawa K. Evaluation of the direct trocar insertion technique at laparoscopy. *Obstet Gynecol.* 1989;74:423–425.

# 2

# History of the Development of Gynecologic Endoscopic Surgery

*Marian D. Damewood*

CHAPTER OUTLINE

As early as 500 AD a "siphopherot" or tube made of lead and used to bring the internal female genitalia within range of the physician's eye was described (Fig. 2.1).[1] This ancient accomplishment resulted in visualization of the external cervical os through dilatation of the vagina. In the last two decades developments in the techniques of operative laparoscopy and operative hysteroscopy have had a major impact on the specialty of gynecologic surgery. At present, laparoscopy is the most frequently performed gynecologic procedure in the United States. The development of endoscopic surgery has been primarily stimulated by the worldwide need for permanent sterilization methods. Most importantly, improvements in our ability to achieve intraabdominal hemostasis, primarily through the use of electrocoagulation, has made it possible to perform surgical procedures through the laparoscope.

## Development of Laparoscopy

The first reported observation of the human peritoneal cavity with an optical instrument was by Jacobaeus in Scandinavia in 1910.[2]

However, several developments predated this report. As early as 1805, Bozzani in Germany visualized the urethral orifice with candlelight and a simple tube. This led to Desormeaux's development, in 1843, of the first urethroscope and cystoscope using mirrors to reflect light from a kerosene lamp.[3] After this development Stein, in Germany (1874), developed a photo endoscope. Nitze, also from Germany, added a lens system to the endoscopic tube allowing magnification of the viewed area.[4] The invention of the light bulb in the United States by Thomas Edison had a significant impact on the development of gynecologic endoscopy. Newman in Scotland developed a cystoscope using a small incandescent light bulb at the distal end (1883). Kelling from Germany (1902) first reported peritoneal endoscopy in dogs creating a pneumoperitoneum using a needle and a cystoscope designed by Nitze.[5] Subsequently, Jacobaeus (1910) used a trocar and cannula to induce pneumoperitoneum in women, introducing a Nitze cystoscope through the same cannula to achieve pelviscopy, laparoscopy, or peritoneoscopy.[2]

Several refinements in the technique of peritoneoscopy preceded its application to gyneco-

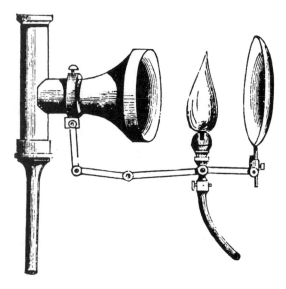

FIGURE 2.1. The "photoendoscope" or siphopherot described in the Talmud.[4]

logic surgery. Orndoff from the United States developed a sharp pyramidal point on the laparoscopic trocar to facilitate puncture.[6] An automatic trocar sheath valve was then introduced to prevent escape of air. Although the

first pneumoperitoneum as created using air, Zollikoffer from Switzerland went on to use carbon dioxide ($CO_2$).[7] A fore-oblique 45° lens system and the use of a second puncture for upper abdominal procedures were introduced by Kalk from Germany (1929).[8] Biopsy instrumentation and cauterization of intra-abdominal adhesions at laparoscopy was re-reported by Fervers from Germany (1933).[9] This report was followed by the introduction of a single puncture operating laparoscope by Ruddock in the United States in 1934,[10] and followed almost immediately by Boesch's utilization of a 40° to 50° pelvic elevation during the procedure. In 1937 Hope (United States) used Ruddock's peritoneoscope to diagnose ectopic pregnancies.[11] In the United States Anderson (1937) and Powers and Barnes (1941) performed endothermal coagulation of the fallopian tube for the purpose of sterilization.[12,13] A laparoscopic uterine suspension was performed in 1942 by Donaldson and colleagues (United States).[14] An alternative approach to peritoneoscopy, the culdoscope, was introduced by Decker in 1944 (Fig. 2.2).

The first gynecologist to use laparoscopy cli-

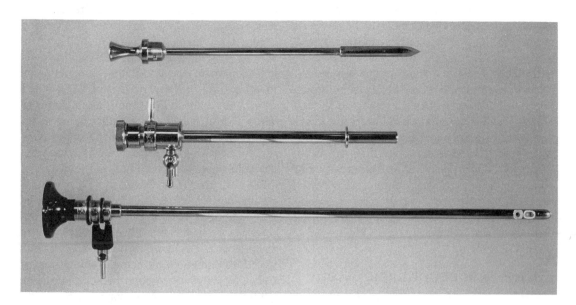

FIGURE 2.2. Decker culdoscope manufactured by American Cystoscope Makers, Inc.. Note incandescent distal lamp and 90° viewing angle. From top to bottom: Pyramidal trocar, sheath with distal stop, and culdoscope (courtesy of Dr. Michael P. Steinkampf).

TABLE 2.1. Chronology of the development of laparoscopy.

| Investigator | Date | Development |
|---|---|---|
| Bozzani | 1805 | Visualization of urethral orifice with candlelight and simple tube |
| Desormeaux | 1843 | Presentation of first urethroscope and cystoscope, using mirrors to reflect kerosene lamplight. First effective endoscope |
| Stein | 1874 | Development of photoendoscope |
| Nitze | 1877 | Addition of lens system to endoscopic tube, thus allowing magnification of area viewed |
| Edison | 1880 | Invention of incandescent lamp bulb |
| Newman | 1883 | Development of a cystoscope using a small incandescent light bulb at distal end |
| Boisseau de Rocher | 1889 | Separation of ocular part from introducing sheath and use of different telescopes through sheath |
| Kelling | 1901 | Creation of air pneumoperitoneum in dogs using a needle, followed by insertion of a Nitze cystoscope |
| Jacobaeus | 1910 | Creation of air pneumoperitoneum in humans using a trocar, followed by introduction of a Nitze cystoscope through the trocar. First recorded observation of a human peritoneal cavity with an optical instrument |
| Orndoff | 1920 | Development of sharp pyramidal point on the trocar to facilitate puncture and automatic trocar sheath valve to prevent escape of air (peritoneoscopy) |
| Zollikoffer | 1924 | Used carbon dioxide instead of air to create pneumoperitoneum |
| Korbsch | 1927 | First textbook with an atlas of laparoscopy |
| Kalk | 1929 | Developed fore-oblique (45°) lens system. Introduced second puncture for upper abdominal procedures |
| Fervers | 1933 | Cauterization of intraabdominal adhesions |
| Ruddock | 1934 | Developed single-puncture operating laparoscope. Published results of 900 peritoneoscopies. 100% diagnostic accuracy in 58 cases of ectopic pregnancy |
| Boesch | 1935 | Utilization of 40–50° of pelvic elevation |
| Anderson | 1937 | Endothermic coagulation of fallopian tube as a method of sterilization |
| Powers & Barnes | 1941 | Sterilization by means of laparoscopy tubal cautery |
| Decker | 1944 | Introduction of culdoscopy |
| Palmer | 1947 | First gynecologist to use gynecologic laparoscopy clinically. Introduced the endouterine cannula for uterine manipulation and tudbal patency testing |
| Hopkins & Kapany | 1952 | Introduction of fiberoptics to endoscopy |
| Palmer | 1962 | Utilization of electrocoagulation for tubal sterilization by laparoscopy |
| Frangenheim | 1963 | Used diathermy for tubal sterilization by laparoscopy |
| Semm | 1963 | Automatic insufflation of the pneumoperitoneum and complete pelviscopy instrumentation set |
| Steptoe | 1967 | First laparoscopy textbook in the English language |
| Steptoe & Edwards | 1970 | Recovery of oocyte with the laparoscope for in vitro fertilization |
| Clarke | 1972 | Introduction of instruments for tubal ligation by laparoscopy |
| Hulka | 1972 | Introduced clips for tubal sterilization by laparoscopy |
| Rioux | 1973 | Development of bipolar cautery for tubal sterilization by laparoscopy |
| Yoon | 1974 | Utilization of silastic rings for tubal sterilization by laparoscopy |

nically on a wide basis was Palmer in France (1947).[15] He was also responsible for the introduction of the endouterine cannula for uterine manipulation and for the development of chromotubation. Further advancements in our ability to perform surgical procedures at laparoscopy occurred with the introduction of fiberoptics in 1952 by Hopkins and Kapany. In the early 1960s Harold Hopkins went on to design the rod lens system used in most endoscopes today. Almost concurrently, Frangenheim[16] in Germany (1963) and Palmer in France continued to develop electrocoagulation for tubal sterilization by laparoscopy. The availability of intraabdominal electrocoagulation was a major impetus to the development of pelviscopy, since this type of surgery would not be possible without the ability to achieve intraperitoneal hemostasis. Additional advancements in pelviscopic techniques and instrumentation have been attributed to Kurt Semm of Germany. In 1963, he introduced the use of an automatic insufflator to maintain pneumoperitoneum.[17] Semm is also credited with the introduction of a complete pelviscopy instrumentation set, which has since been updated and modified.

In the 1970s laparoscopy was increasingly used for intraabdominal surgery. Steptoe and Edwards recovered the first oocyte for in vitro fertilization in 1970 using the laparoscope.[18] Until the introduction of transvaginal ultrasound oocyte retrieval in the late 1980s, laparoscopy has formed an integral part of the in vitro fertilization procedure. Laparoscopic tubal sterilization using clips was introduced by Hulka and colleagues in 1972,[19] Rioux (1973) from Canada developed bipolar cautery for laparoscopic tubal sterilization. Yoon of the United States (1974) laparoscopically applied silastic rings, also for tubal sterilization. The chronology of the development of operative laparoscopy is summarized in Table 2.1.

Concurrent with the development in the technology of laparoscopy, a significant body of information was developed. The first textbook with an atlas of laparoscopy was published by Korbsh from Germany in 1927. Ruddock in the United States in the late 1930s published results of 900 laparoscopies.[20] Specific reference in this publication was given to the diagnostic accuracy of laparoscopy with respect to ectopic pregnancy. Two years later Beling, also from the United States, published a review that listed indications for laparoscopy with specific reference to endometriosis, chronic pelvic inflammatory disease, and the diagnosis of ectopic pregnancy. Palmer in 1947 published results of his case series of 250 procedures. The late 1950s and early 1960s saw the introduction of multiple textbooks of gynecologic laparoscopy. A German textbook was published in 1959 by Frangenheim, followed by Thoyer-Rozat[21] with a French version, and Albano and Cittadini[22] with an Italian text on gynecologic endoscopy. The first textbook of laparoscopy published in the English language was by Steptoe from the United Kingdom, in 1967.[23] Cohen and Fear from the United States presented the first American publication of gynecologic laparoscopy, followed by the first

American textbook of gynecologic laparoscopy in 1970.[24] Additional large case reports concerning outpatient laparoscopic procedures were reported by Wheeless from the United States in 1970.[25]

Standards for laparoscopic surgery have been set and followed in the United States. In 1972 Phillips founded the American Association of Gynecologic Laparoscopists (AAGL), and during the same year Hulka coordinated the first annual report of Complications Committee of the AAGL.

The impact of diagnostic and operative laparoscopy on gynecologic practice has been significant. Laparoscopy has allowed the gynecologist to establish the diagnosis in a large number of clinical situations, and has reduced greatly the need for laparotomy. Additional advances stimulated the laparoscopic treatment of endometriosis, pelvic adhesions, tubal disease, ectopic pregnancies, and ovarian cysts. A significant reduction in cost, postoperative morbidity, and recuperation with respect to laparotomy has also been documented.

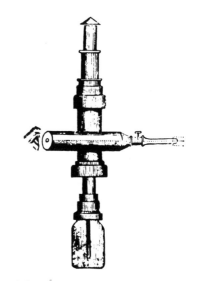

FIGURE 2.3. The first hysteroscope used by Pantaleoni (1868).[27] The alcohol lamp at the bottom provided light for the tapered metal hysteroscope (reproduced with permission from Barbot J. History of hysteroscopy, in Baggish MS, Burbot J, Valle RF [eds]. Diagnostic and Operative Hystaroscopy: A Text and Atlas. Chicago: Year Book Medical Publishers; 1989).

FIGURE 2.4. The hysteroscopic technique of Clado (1898).[29] (reproduced with permission as in Figure 2.3)

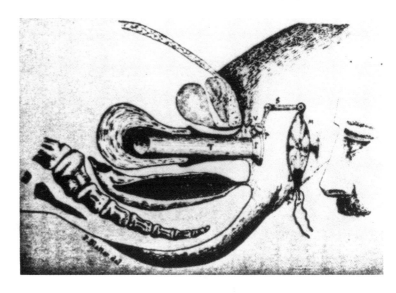

## Development of Hysteroscopy

Attempts at visualization of the uterine cavity preceded the development of peritoneoscopy. As early as 1000 AD, Abulkasim used a mirror to reflect light into the vaginal vault. Desormeaux (1853) in France inspected the interior of the uterus with an early endoscope and reported the first "satisfactory" hysteroscopy. In addition, he identified polyps in the uterus of a postmenopausal patient experiencing vaginal bleeding.[26] Aubinais in 1864[27] inspected the uterine cavity with the naked eye and Pantaleoni[28] from Ireland used a cystoscope (Fig. 2.3) initially designed by Desormeaux to identify uterine polyps (1868). Clado (1898) in France described several models of hysteroscopic instrumentation and published material on the technique of hysteroscopy (Fig. 2.4).[29] This accomplishment was followed by the publication of a treatise on hysteroscopy, with specific reference to contact hysteroscopy (Fig. 2.5), by David in 1908.[30]

Further refinements in hysteroscopy were directed at the development of effective distending media and clear visualization of the uterine cavity. Rubin in 1925 combined the cystoscope with $CO_2$ insufflation of the uterine cavity.[31] In 1928 Gauss used water to flush blood and distend the uterine cavity.[32] The water source in this case was held 50 cm above the patient. Use of a transparent rubber balloon mounted on the endoscope that was subsequently inflated within the uterine cavity was presented by Silander in 1962.[33] Edstrom and Fernstrom in 1970 introduced high-molecular weight dextran as a distension medium.[34] Lindemann in 1970 use $CO_2$ for uterine distension.[35] These developments increased the clinical utility of hysteroscopy. Developments in hysteroscopy are summarized in Table 2.2.

Since the lens systems of earlier hysteroscopes were inferior, inadequate light and image transmission occurred frequently. At present, most hysteroscopes consist of a lens system surrounded by glass fibers carrying light into the uterine cavity. However, Vulmiere in 1952 used a rigid one piece mineral glass guide, which when properly treated could not only illuminate but also magnify the image when in direct contact with the object. In 1963 an optical trocar in an italic sheath was used and perfected in 1973 when Barbot introduced it for clinical use in France.[29] In 1979 Baggish reported the first experience with this instrument in the United States.[29] Contact hysteroscopy optics were combined with the principles of modern panoramic hysteroscopy into a single instrument, the microcolpohysteroscope, introduced by Hamou in 1980.[36] As recently as

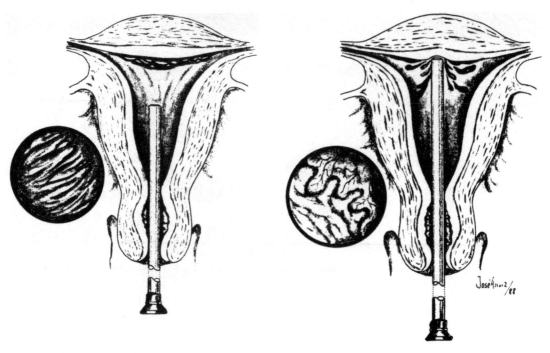

FIGURE 2.5. Early contact hysteroscope (1907).[29,30] **A:** Before contact. **B:** After contact. (reproduced with permission as in Figure 2.3)

TABLE 2.2. Chronology of the development of hysteroscopy.

| Investigator | Date | Development |
|---|---|---|
| Abulkasim | 1000 AD | Utilization of mirror to reflect light into vaginal vault |
| Desormeaux | 1853 | Inspection of interior of uterus with early endoscope, first "satisfactory" endoscope |
| Aubinais | 1864 | Inspection of uterine cavity with the naked eye |
| Pantaleoni | 1868 | Used cystoscope designed by Desormeaux to identify uterine polyps |
| Clado | 1898 | Described several models of hysteroscopic instruments |
| David | 1907 | Treatise on hysteroscopy, with specific reference to contact hysteroscopy |
| Ruben | 1925 | Combination of a cystoscope with $CO_2$ insufflation of the uterine cavity |
| Gauss | 1928 | Use of water to flush blood and distent uterine cavity. Water source held 50 cm above the patient |
| Silander | 1862 | Use of a transparent rubber balloon mounted on the endoscope inflated within the uterine cavity |
| Edstrom & Fernstrom | 1970 | Introduction of high-molecular weight dextran as a distension medium |
| Lindemann | 1970 | Use of $CO_2$ for uterine distension |
| Hamou | 1980 | Introduction of the microcolpohysteroscope |
| Baggish | 1987 | Invention of a focusing panoramic hysteroscope and a four-channel operating sheath particularly advantageous for the Nd:YAG laser |

1987 Baggish introduced a focusing panoramic hysteroscope with a four-channel operating sheath particularly useful for laser procedures.[29]

# References

1. The Talmud.
2. Jacobaeus HC. Uber die Moglichkeit, die Zystoskopie bei Untersuchung seroser Hohlungen anzuwenden. *Munich med Wschr.* 1910;57:2090–2092.
3. Gunning JE. History of laparoscopy. In: Phillips JM, ed. *Laparoscopy.* Baltimore: Williams & Wilkins, 1977:6–16.
4. Nitze M. *Uber eine neue Beleuchtungsmethode der Hoblen des menschlichen Korpers.* Wien: Med. Presse; 1879:V20;851–858.
5. Kelling G. Uber Oesophagoskopie, Gastroskopie und Colioskopie. *Munich med Wschr.* 1902; 49:21–24.
6. Orndoff BH. The peritoneoscope in diagnosis of diseases of the abdomen. *J Radiol.* 1920;1:307–325.
7. Zollikoffer R. Uber Laparoskopie. *Schweiz med Wschr.* 1924;104:264–272.
8. Kalk H. Erfahrungen mit der Laparoskopie (zugleich mit Beschreibung eines neuen Instrumentes). *Z Klin Med.* 1929;111:303–348.
9. Fervers C. Die Laparoskopie mit dem Cystoskop. Ein Beitrag zur Vereinfachung der Technik und zur endoskopischen Strangdurchtrennung in der Bauchhohle. *Med Klin.* 1933; 29:1042–1045.
10. Ruddock JC. Peritoneoscopy. *West J Surg.* 1934;42:392–405.
11. Hope RB. The differential diagnosis of ectopic gestation by peritoneoscopy. *Surg Gynecol Obstet.* 1937;64:229–234.
12. Anderson ET. Peritoneoscopy. *Am J Surg.* 1937;35:36–43.
13. Power FH, Barnes AC. Sterilization by means of peritoneoscopic tubal fulguration. A preliminary report. *Am J Obstet Gynecol.* 1941; 41:1038–1043.
14. Donaldson JK, Sanderlin JH, Harrel jun WB. Method of suspending uterus without open abdominal incision; use of peritoneoscope and special needle. *Am J Surg.* 1942;55:537–543.
15. Palmer R. Instrumentation et technique de la couldoscopie gynecologique. *Gynecol Obstet.* 1947;46:422–429.
16. Frangenheim H. Tubal sterilization under visualization with the laparoscope. *Geburtsch u Frauenheilk.* 1964;24:470–478.
17. Semm K. Das Pneumoperitoneum mit $CO_2$. In: Demling L, Ottenjann R, eds.: *Endoslopie—Methoden, Ergebnisse.* S. Munchen: Banaschewski; 1967:167–169.
18. Steptoe PC. Laparoscopic studies of the ovaries. *Ned Tijdschr Verloskd,* Gynaecol 1970;70:296–300.
19. Hulka JF, Fishburne JI, Mercer JP, et al. Laparoscopic sterilization with a spring clip: a report of the first fifty cases. *Am J Obstet Gynecol.* 1973;116:751–759.
20. Ruddock JC. Peritoneoscopy. *Surg Gynecol Obstet.* 1937;65:623–639.
21. Thoyer-Rozat J. *La Coelioscopie. Technique–Indications.* Paris: Masson; 1962.
22. Albano VE, Cittadini E. *La celioscopia in ginecologia* (monografia). Palermo: Denaro; 1962:I 420.
23. Steptoe PC. *Laparoscopy in Gynaecology.* Edinburgh, London: Livingstone; 1967.
24. Cohen MR: *Laparoscopy Culdoscopy and Gynecography: Technique and Atlas.* Philadelphia: Saunders; 1970.
25. Wheeless CR, Jr. Outpatient sterilization by laparoscopy under local anesthesia in less developed countries. In: Duncan GW, Falb RD, Speidel JJ, eds. *Female sterilization: Prognosis for Simplified Outpatient Procedures.* New York, London: Academic Press; 1972:125–129.
26. Desormeaux A-J. *L'Endoscopie Uterine, Applications au Diagnostic et au Traitement des Affections de l'Urethre de la Vessie.* Paris: Bailliere; 1865.
27. Aubinais: Union Med. 1864; no. 152.
28. Pantaleoni D. On endoscopic examination of the cavity of the womb. *Med Press Circ. London* 1869;8:26–28.
29. Barbot J. *History of hysteroscopy,* in Baggish MS, Burbot J, Valle RF (eds): Diagnostic and Operative Hysteroscopy: A Text and Atlas. Chicago, Year Book Medical Publishers; 1986.
30. David Ch. *L'Endoscopie Uterine, Applications au Diagnostic et au Traitement des Affections Intrauterines.* Paris: Jacques; 1908.
31. Rubin IC. Uterine endoscopy, endometrioscopy with the aid of uterine insufflation. *Am J Obstet Gynecol.* 1925;10:313–319.
32. Gauss CJ. Hysteroskopie. *Arch Gynak.* 1928; 133:18–24.
33. Silander T. Hysteroscopy through a transparent rubber balloon in patients with carcinoma of the uterine endometrium. *Acta Obstet Gynecol Scand.* 1963;42:284–296.
34. Edstrom K, Fernstrom I. The diagnostic possi-

bilities of a modified hysteroscopic technique. *Acta Obstet Gynecol Scand*. 1970;49:327–330.

35. Lindemann J-J. The use of $CO_2$ in the uterine cavity for hysteroscopy. *Int J Fertil*. 1972;17: 221–224.

36. Hamou J. Microhysteroscopy: a new procedure and its original applications in gynecology. J Reprod Med 1981;26:375–382.

# 3

# Principles of Endoscopic Optics and Lighting

*RICHARD P. BUYALOS*

## Light Sources

Illumination of the peritoneal cavity is essential in laparoscopic surgery. There are a variety of light sources with varying spectral emissions and illumination power.[1-3] Light originates from an object when it is heated sufficiently, and the color (wavelength) of the light emitted varies with the temperature of the source. This color property of temperature is measured in degrees Kelvin (K°). Light sources with higher K° contain more high frequency (blue) wavelengths, resulting in a brighter and more accurate image. As light loses heat (lower K°) its spectral emission shifts from blue to red, causing the image to assume a reddish tint.

Until the mid-1960s, endoscopic lighting consisted of the traditional incandescent light bulb. Output was generally between 75 and 250 W, although light sources of less than 150 W were generally avoided in gynecologic endoscopy. An incandescent light bulb transforms approximately 97% of electrical energy into heat, whereas only 2% to 3% is converted into visible light. Ideally, these light sources needed to be equipped with two lamps to facilitate rapid switching should one lamp fail. Preoperatively, both bulbs required inspection to confirm proper functioning. This was particularly crucial to operative endoscopy/pelviscopy where loss of the light source during dissecting or hemostatic procedures would pose a significant risk.

Light sources employed in gynecologic endoscopy today include the 150 to 250 W tungsten/iodine vapor (2800–3200 K°) or halogen-quartz (3200–3400 K°) incandescent lamps. Although these light sources are less expensive, they emit relatively little blue light and are generally insufficient for proper photo-

15

documentation (see Chapter 6). A 150 to 300 W mercury-halide (5600 K°) or 300 watt xenon vapor (6000–6600 K°) arc lamps provide excellent light for visualization and photodocumentation because of their high content of blue spectral light. The bulb life of mercury-halide arc lamps is approximately 250 hr, whereas the xenon vapor lamp may last up to 1000 hr.

Although the light is extremely hot at its source, most of the heat is dissipated along the length of the light cable. It is for this reason that it is called "cold light." Nonetheless, a significant amount of heat is generated at the end of the light cable which may cause thermal injury to the patient or burn paper drapes or clothing with prolonged direct contact.

The brightness of the image transmitted back into the endoscope depends, to a certain degree, on the reflective quality of the peritoneal surface. Pigmented or blood-covered surfaces will reflect relatively little light in contrast to more reflective structures. The light intensity decreases by the square of the distance from the endoscope to the image viewed. Doubling the distance between the endoscope and the tissue being examined (e.g., from 3 to 6 cm) increases the light dispersion fourfold (i.e., from 9 to 36). Consequently, far more light is required for panoramic views.

## Light Transmission Cables

A dramatic improvement in lighting technology occurred with the development of fiberoptic cables, composed of multiple coaxial quartz fibers. These systems absorb and disperse the heat from the light source with relatively little heat being conducted to the end of the cable, while transmitting light of high illuminosity or "lux." Individual fibers are usually 10 to 25 $\mu$m in diameter and consist of an inner core of quartz with a high refractive index fused with an outer sheath of low index material or cladding (Fig. 3.1). Light transmitted through the fiber is reflected inward by the high index/low index intersurface. Visible light (wavelengths of 400–700 nm) enters the proximal end of the fiber and emerges out of the distal end after many internal refractions. Between the fibers,

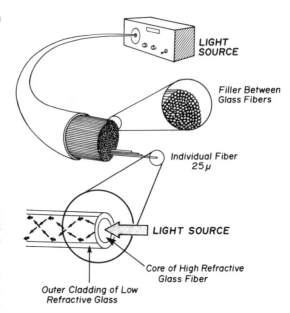

FIGURE 3.1. The structure of fiberoptic cables and individual fibers is depicted. Note that at least 30% of the transverse surface of the cable is occupied by low refractory index cladding and nontransmitting interfiber filler cement.

cementing them together, is a nontransmitting filler material.[1,4]

There are two types of fiber bundles (Fig. 3.2). "Incoherent" bundles are produced by packing multiple fibers together in a random arrangement that transmit high intensity illumination throughout the length of the cable. These systems are usually 1.5 to 2 m in length and transmit light from an external source to the endoscope. In contrast, "coherent" or "oriented" bundles have identical fiber arrangements at both ends of the cable. A "true image" is then transmitted as dots of light through a cable containing as many as 100,000 fibers, each approximately 10 $\mu$m in diameter. The image from the distal end of coherent bundles is fused and focused on the ocular of the endoscope. Coherent bundles are significantly more expensive to manufacture, but permit additional flexion of the endoscope. They are most frequently employed in flexible gastroscopes, colonoscopes, and bronchoscopes. Flexible fiberoptic endoscopes have also been designed for hysteroscopy and falloposcopy,

## Types of Fiber Bundles

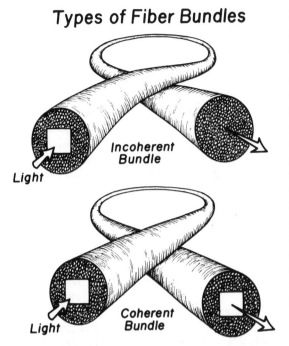

FIGURE 3.2. **Top**: Incoherent bundles have their fibers arranged in random order within the fiberoptic cable. **Bottom**: Coherent bundles demonstrate a uniform fiber arrangement from one end of the cable to the other, and serve to transmit an image.

but currently are not widely used in gynecologic endoscopy.

Because of the presence of low refractory index cladding and filler material in the fiberoptic cable, approximately 30% of the light transmitted from the light source to the origin of the cable is lost in the form of heat. Recently, a new type of light cable without cladding or interfiber filler has been developed. The "fluid light" cable produced by Karl Storz Endoscopy–America Inc., (Culver City, CA) may improve light transmission by approximately 70% compared to fiberoptic cables.

Fiberoptic cables should be frequently inspected for extensive fiber breakage or central burnout, which will rapidly reduce light transmission. If greater than 30% of the fibers are damaged or more than 2 mm of the central area is burned out, the cable should be replaced. To determine if fiber bundles are damaged, the surgeon can shine the end of the cable on a flat surface. Dark spots represent broken fibers. Furthermore, the proximal end of the cable that connects to the light source can burn out with use. High temperatures inevitably will turn even glass surfaces and their synthetic packing materials brown from oxidation. Therefore, this area should be examined frequently.

# Endoscopes

## Lens Chains

Endoscopes are composed of an ocular or eyepiece, a lens chain or optical relay system, and an objective located at the distal end of the endoscope. The lens system employed in contemporary endoscopes may be divided into three classes: classic, Hopkins, and graded index (GRIN) lens systems.[3-6]

In the classic system the width of the lens is far less than the length of the endoscope, and the distance between lenses is relatively large (Fig. 3.3). These endoscopes consisted of a long metal tube containing many thin glass lenses widely spaced within for transmission of a lighted image. The amount of light transmitted by an endoscope is proportional to the

FIGURE 3.3. The classic and Hopkins endoscopic lens systems. In the classic system the width of the lenses is less than the length of the endoscope; in the Hopkins system the lenses occupy the majority of the endoscope.

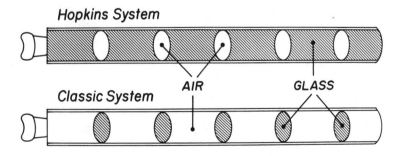

square of the index of refraction of the medium interspersed between the lens. Since air has a refractive index of 1.0, the proportional light transmission is also 1.0. When glass is used as the medium, with a refractive index of approximately 1.5, light transmission more than doubles. Employing these principles, Harold Hopkins reversed the air/glass spaces within the endoscope, substantially improving light transmission (Fig. 3.3). In the Hopkins lens system, most of the length of the endoscope is occupied by the lens. Most laparoscopes and rigid hysteroscopes today employ this lens system.

The GRIN lens system consists of a single rod of glass in which the refractive index decreases gradually from the axis to the periphery (graded). In gynecology this lens system is most often employed in the design of the contact hysteroscope (see Chapter 16).

## Types of Endoscopes

Two types of gynecologic endoscopes are available today (Fig. 3.4). "Straight" endoscopes consist of a central lens chain surrounded by fiberoptic bundles projecting light into the peritoneal cavity. In contrast, "operative endoscopes" contain an additional operating channel through which ancillary instruments are placed. The lens chain is angled in order to bring the eyepiece away from the operating channel. Operating endoscopes contain fewer fiberoptic bundles and therefore transmit less light than straight endoscopes of the same diameter. Additionally, the exaggerated deflection of the returning light in operative endoscopes reduces the brightness of the image.

Laparoscopes are available in different external diameters,[7] but the optical system of operative endoscopes is always smaller than that of straight instruments. For 10 to 12 mm instruments the diameter of the lens system of an operating versus a straight laparoscope is 2.5 to 3 mm compared to 5 to 6 mm, respectively. Laparoscopes usually have a working focus of between 7 and 12 cm, although in most optic systems the true distance for sharp focus is fixed at approximately 5 to 7 cm. The lens within the viewer's eyes can compensate for small deviations from this true focus. When the multiple-puncture technique of operative laparoscopy is employed, straight laparoscopes are usually preferred since they provide maximal light transmission with greater image clarity and field of vision.

Hysteroscopes are of smaller diameter than laparoscopes and consequently transmit less light. Furthermore, they have a greater angle of deflection, in order to maximize their field of vision (see below). Their shorter working distance of approximately 2.5 cm and the smaller size of the uterine cavity compensates for the decreased illumination.

## Viewing Angle

The distal end of the endoscope has been designed with a variety of viewing angles. Most optics have a direct or 0° deflection system that provides the surgeon with a visual field that is collinear with the true field. This angle of vision was previously denoted as 180°, but the classification has now been standardized to the direction of the view from the optic end of the laparoscope, and not toward the viewer. Oblique lenses from 5° to 70° are also available. In general, straight laparoscopes have a viewing angle of 0°, whereas operative laparoscopes have a slight deflection of the viewing field of 5° to 10°. Hysteroscopes are available with viewing angles of 10° to 70°. It should be noted that the greater the deflection the greater the loss in illumination.

The "field of vision" refers to the borders of the field of view. The wider the viewing angle the larger the potential viewing borders, if the instrument is rotated 180° (see Figure 16.1). However, with an increasing field of vision, there may be some distortion at the periphery. Increased magnification of the field is obtained by moving the laparoscope closer to the desired object. Examples of magnification at different working distances for various makes of operative endoscopes are shown in Table 3.1.

## Fogging

The peritoneal cavity has an ambient temperature of 37°C with 100% humidity. When a cold metal instrument such as an endoscope is

FIGURE 3.4. **A:** Straight 0° 10-mm laparoscope (Olympus Corp., Lake Success, NY). **B:** Operating laparoscope with 5-mm operating channel. Stopcock may be removed for placement of $CO_2$ laser coupler (Olympus Corp., Lake Success, NY). **C:** Right angle operating laparoscope with 5-mm operating channel (Richard Wolf Medical Instruments Corp., Rosemont, IL).

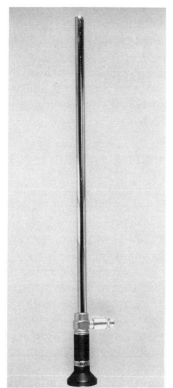

A

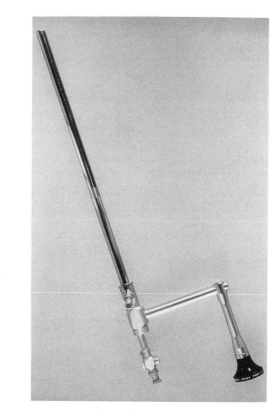

C

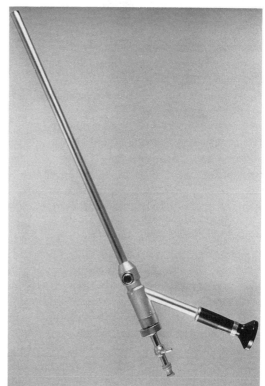

B

TABLE 3.1. 10-mm Hopkins operating laparoscope with 3-mm operating channel: magnification at different working distances.

| Working distance (mm) | Magnification | | |
|---|---|---|---|
| | Wolf[a] | Olympus[a] | Storz[a] |
| 3 | — | 8.2 | 10 |
| 5 | — | 5.7 | 6 |
| 10 | 3.19 | 3.2 | 3 |
| 15 | — | 2.2 | 2 |
| 20 | 1.71 | 1.7 | 1.5 |
| 30 | — | 1.2 | 1 |
| 50 | 0.73 | 0.7 | 0.6 |

[a] Personal communication.
Reproduced with permission from: Murphy AA. Diagnostic and operative laparoscopy. In: Thompson JD, Rock JA, eds. *Telinde's Operative Gynecology*. Baltimore: Lippincott. 1991:361–384.

placed into the abdominal cavity, condensation of water vapor occurs on the glass objective, which results in fogging. This can be prevented by prewarming the endoscope to 40° to 50°C. Fogging can also be reduced by simply soaking the instrument for approximately 3 min in a hot water bath of sterile water or saline at approximately 50°C before insertion into the abdomen. Additionally, a number of manufacturers have designed sterile apparatuses for prewarming endoscopes. Unfortunately, these devices generally require 1 to 2 hr to warm the endoscopes sufficiently because of poor heat conduction in air.

Antifog solutions or detergents such as PhysoHex (Winthrop Laboratories, New York, NY) have been used in the past to minimize fogging by causing moisture droplets to spread themselves rapidly and almost invisibly over the surface of the lens. However, antifogging solutions can distort the lens surface sufficiently to compromise the visual image. The endoscope may also be warmed by placing the objective against the fundus of the uterus or against the large bowel for several seconds. However, this method is generally less satisfactory and may result in some distortion of the object of interest due to moisture droplet accumulation on the lens surface. Fogging that is still present after repeated efforts to clean the lens of the ocular and objective may be evi-

dence of water vapor within the lens chain. This can be detected by holding the endoscope up to an external light source, such as an operating room light, and looking into either end of the instrument to detect water beads inside the lens chain. If this has happened and additional endoscopes are not available, the endoscope may be used temporarily by placing it in a warming oven at approximately 100°C. This converts the water into steam, forcing it to escape from the lens system. After use the endoscope should be returned to the manufacturer for repair to avoid further damage.

# Light Loss

A typical Hopkins endoscope has a dozen or more lenses and many air/glass surfaces. The cumulative light loss from these surfaces (4–7% per interface) can be considerable. Light loss at the air/glass interface is greatly reduced by coating the lens with a thin film of magnesium fluoride, which decreases light reflection to approximately 0.5%. Light intensity is also lost from reflection at light cable–instrument connections. Mismatched, poorly aligned, or loose connections reduce light transmission. Deflection of the field of view or within the lens chain (as in operative endoscopes) further reduces light transmission. A typical system may lose as much as 80% of the light originating at its source as it emerges from the distal end of the endoscope.[1]

# Instrument Sterilization

In general, endoscopes should be gently cleansed, rinsed thoroughly with water, and then sterilized in metal or glass containers. Disinfecting systems with formalin tablets provide the gentlest method of sterilization, but require 24 hr to be completely effective. This method may prove impractical in a busy operating room. Recently, a rapid sterilization method using peracetic acid at low temperatures (55°C) has been developed (Steri-System I, Karl Storz Inc.). This method safely sterilizes all immersible instruments, including endoscopes and light cables, in 20 to 30 min and requires no airing out period. Some manufacturers state that in an emergency sterilization may be accomplished using a gravity displacement steam autoclave at 130°C. High temperature autoclaves will cause the seals between glass and. metal to deteriorate, allowing steam to enter the optic chain, result in fogging of the lens system. Efforts to improve the seals between glass metal interfaces or to reduce the difference in the coefficients of expansion between these surfaces have been relatively unsuccessful. Rapid submersion in cold water after autoclaving, as is done with steel instruments, will quickly destroy these seals and allow introduction of water into the lens chain.

Gas autoclaving with ethylene oxide at 50° to 60°C for 2 to 3 hr can safely sterilize endoscopic equipment. Its chief disadvantage is that it requires a 12-hr airing-out period. Disinfection of endoscopes can be performed at room temperature by soaking in antiseptic solutions such as alkalinized glyceraldehyde (Cydex, Johnson and Johnson Products, New Brunswick, NJ) and is effective in 30 to 60 min.

Maintenance and sterilization instructions for endoscopic equipment is provided by the manufacturers and should be carefully followed.

## References

1. Hulka JF. Biophysics and physiology. In: Hulka J, ed. *Textbook of Laparoscopy*. Orlando: Grune and Stratton; 1985:7–43.
2. Semm K. *Operative Manual for Endoscopic Abdominal Surgery*. Chicago: Year book Medical Publishers; 1987:46–59.
3. Quint R. Physics of light and image transmission. In: Phillips J, ed. *Laparoscopy*. Baltimore: Williams and Wilkins; 1977:18–23.
4. Hopkins HH. Physics of the fiberoptic endoscope. In: Berci G, ed. *Endoscopy*. New York: Appleton-Century-Crofts; 1976:27–63.
5. Hopkins HH. Optical principles of the endoscope. In: Berci G, ed. *Endoscopy*. New York: Appleton-Century-Crofts; 1976:3–26.
6. Prescott R. Optical principles of endoscopy. *J Med Primatol*. 1976;5:133–147.
7. Soderstrom R. Survey of laparoscopes for ob-gyn use. *Contemp Obstet Gynecol*. 1991;36:115–125.

# 4

# Establishing Hemostasis at Laparoscopy

*Ana Alvarez Murphy, V. Gabriel Garzo, and Ricardo Azziz*

The ability to achieve hemostasis is integral to any laparoscopic procedure. This is probably the single most important factor that delayed the evolution of diagnostic and, certainly, operative laparoscopy. The modalities to achieve hemostasis essentially mirror those of laparotomy surgery. Unipolar electrosurgery was first introduced to laparoscopy as a method of sterilization.[1] However, the method came into disrepute because of the high risk of bowel injury or perforation puportedly resulting from arcing of high frequency current. Doubt has been cast on this theory more recently.[2] Histologic evidence suggests that most bowel perforations thought to result from electrosurgical burns were actually secondary to trocar injuries. Electrosurgery is now quite commonly used, as its value and importance once again have been recognized.

Thermocoagulation (endocoagulation) uses direct heat for hemostasis, and was initially proposed by Semm.[3] This was an attempt to circumvent the purported problem of electrocauterization leading to arcing of electrical cur-

rent, with injury to adjacent organs. Its first use was as a method of sterilization using alligator forceps. Since then its use has been extended to include principally myomectomy and conservative surgery for endometriosis.

Basic suturing skills are essential at laparotomy. It is therefore logical that suturing be modified to allow it to be used at laparoscopy. These modifications must account for the altered access to the operative field. Unfortunately, the flexibility with which suturing is carried out at laparotomy is partially lost at laparoscopy. Endoscopic suturing was first demonstrated by Semm who adapted the Roeder loop, previously used for tonsillectomy, for endoscopic use. Since then extracorporeal and intraabdominal suturing has been added to this armamentarium. Laparoscopic clip applicators, both absorbable and nonabsorbable (titanium), have recently become available and added a new dimension to laparoscopic hemostasis. This chapter will discuss electrosurgery, thermocoagulation, suturing and clips. Lasers are discussed in Chapter 5.

# Electrosurgery

American gynecologic laparoscopists use unipolar and bipolar instruments with cutting (undampened) or coagulation (dampened) waveforms more extensively than any other modality to achieve hemostasis. This modality has the ability to fulgurate, desiccate, coagulate, or cut tissue. During electrosurgery a combination of tissue effects, with a preponderance of one type, is usually seen. "Fulguration" refers to the heating of tissue by sparks of current when the electrode is close but not in direct contact with the tissue. This technique requires relatively high voltages and achieves superficial hemostasis with minimal tissue penetration. It can be used to stop diffuse bleeding such as that ocurring after myomectomy. "Coagulation" occurs when the tissue is heated, and protein loses its conformation, subsequently solidifying. Coagulation usually results in tissue blanching. "Desiccation" refers to the evaporation of all liquid until the tissue is completely dry. This occurs at temperatures of 45° to 100°C, while coagulation occurs at lower temperatures (45–60°C).[4] The term "dessication," however, is rarely used and coagulation is used to describe both effects. At temperatures above 100°C, the tissue is essentially vaporized when the intracellular liquid boils, leading to cellular disruption. Depending on the predominant tissue effect, electrosurgery will result in tissue cutting or ablation.

Electrosurgery requires generating units that are able to transform the available low-voltage (110 volts), low-frequency (60 Hz) alternating electrical current into a high-voltage, high-frequency current. Spark gap circuits and triode vacuum tubes have now been replaced by solid-state units, widely employed at laparotomy and laparoscopy.[4,5] The different tissue effects can be achieved by varying the type of current waveform, the power output of the generator, the electric circuit, and the type of electrosurgical instrument tip used.

A significant variable determining the type of tissue damage is the waveform of the alternating electric current. The sine wave may be pure, with continuous regular oscillations (undampened or unmodulated) (Fig. 4.1) or may be released in bursts (dampened or modulated) (Fig. 4.2). The former is usually referred to as "cutting" and the latter as "coagulation" current. The two may be blended to produce a combination that cuts and coagulates (Fig. 4.3). The undampened waveform vaporizes tissue and is ideal for cutting when applied with an instrument of small surface area such as a needle electrode. If an instrument with a large surface area is used, tissue coagulation is the effect principally seen. Dampened current, on the other hand, has a widespread coagulating effect on the surrounding tissue, including blood vessels, and therefore is useful for hemostasis.

Additional variations in tissue effects can be achieved with changes in power density, the

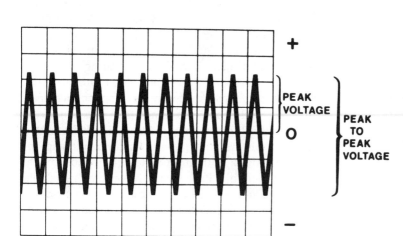

FIGURE 4.1. Undampened (unmodulated) or cutting electric current waveform. (reproduced with permission from Soderstrom RM. Safeguards in laparoscopy: education, equipment care and electron control. Contemp Obstet Gynecol 1978;11:95)

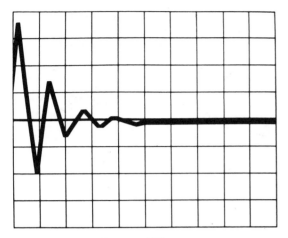

Damped Waves

FIGURE 4.2. Damped (modulated) or coagulating electric current waveform. (reproduced with permission as in Fig. 4.1.)

type of electrosurgical instrument tip, and the electric circuit in use. Generally, higher power densities achieve cutting or ablation whereas lower power densities achieve tissue coagulation. Power density depends on the power output of the electrosurgical unit and the surface area of the tissue being exposed to this current. The latter can be modified by the size of the electrode tip that comes in contact with the tissue. A small surface, such as that seen with a needle electrode or knife edge, will achieve a higher power density than larger instruments. Hence, at the same power output, the former may cut or ablate while the latter may coagulate. For instance, the unipolar knife will cut when the energy is applied with the edge of the blade but may coagulate when the instrument is applied on its side.

Two types of electrical circuits, unipolar and bipolar, can be employed in electrosurgery. In unipolar circuits, the current flows from the generator through the operating electrode, through the patient to the dispersing or "ground" electrode, and finally back to the generator (Fig. 4.4). The unipolar microtip or needle electrode works well for removal of filmy adhesions and for tissue dissection (Fig. 4.5). Cutting current is used in the range of 20 to 80 watts.[4] This minimizes damage to sur-

rounding tissues and is most effective for lysis of adhesions. The needle electrode is available for use with a cannula (Trident or Cohen, Karl Storz, Culver City, CA) that has two ports for irrigation and suction (Fig. 4.6). Additionally, some automatic suction/irrigation devices have a port that allows insertion of the needle electrode. The unipolar knife can be used in much the same way (Fig. 4.5). Scissors can also be obtained with unipolar electrosurgery attachment (Fig. 4.5). These may be used to cut and coagulate simultaneously, as when performing a salpingectomy.

Thermal injuries may occur with the use of unipolar cautery. Faulty contact between the ground electrode and the patient may result in the current dispersing through unwanted pathways of lesser resistance, resulting in undesired thermal injury. The bowel, perhaps because of its high concentration of electrolytes and water, seems to be particularly susceptible to this type of injury. As a safety feature, most electrosurgical units today are unable to operate if the circuit is not properly closed and functioning. Furthermore, when a unipolar cautery instrument is placed down the operating channel of a laparoscope (Fig. 4.7), the endoscope

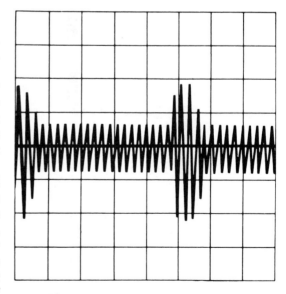

FIGURE 4.3. Blended electric current: combines both damped and undamped waveforms. (reproduced with permission as in Fig. 4.1.)

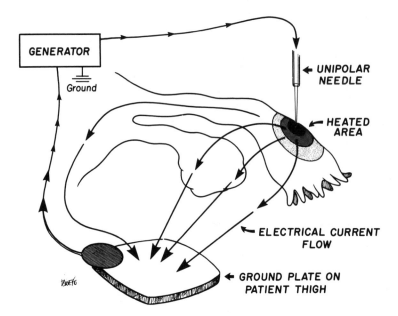

FIGURE 4.4. Scheme of unipolar (monopolar) electric circuit.

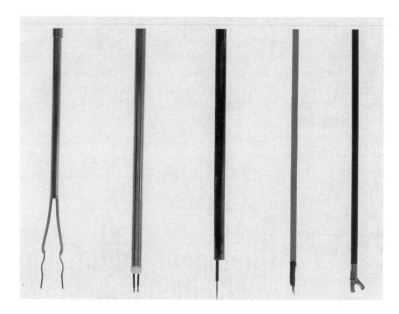

FIGURE 4.5. Electrosurgical laparoscopic instruments **from left to right**: Scissor combined with unipolar capabilities (Richard Wolf Co., Rosemont, IL); Knife electrode (Richard Wolf Co., Rosemont, IL); Needle point or microtip electrode (Karl Storz, Culver City, CA); Vancaillie microtip bipolar forceps (Karl Storz, Culver City, CA); Bipolar (Kleppinger) paddles (Karl Storz Co., Culver City, CA).

itself may become charged, leading to electrothermal injury of surrounding structures. In this situation the interfaces between the insulated metal core of the operative instrument (carrying electric current) and the surrounding operative channel act as a capacitor, resulting in the accumulation of electrons in the metal of the laparoscope. This accumulated electric current can be discharged harmlessly in a dispersed fashion into the surrounding tissues, or in a concentrated manner onto bowel or other organs, with subsequent damage.

In bipolar electrosurgery the circuit is closed by placing the tissue between two electrodes so that the current only goes through the intervening tissue and not the patient's body (Fig. 4.8). Obviously the instrument used to deliver the current must resemble a forcep and

FIGURE 4.6. Cannula **(bottom)** with three ports, two for suction/irrigation and the middle one for placement of the unipolar needle **(top).**

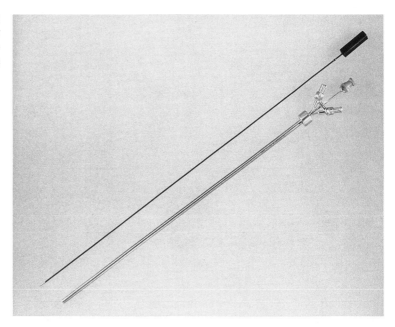

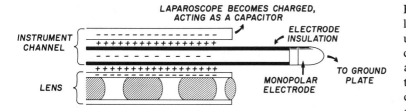

FIGURE 4.7. When an insulated unipolar instrument is used through the operating channel of a laparoscope or via a metallic suprapubic sleeve, the interfaces may act as a capacitor, resulting in electric charge building up in the surrounding metal. This accumulated charge may accidentally discharge in a concentrated fashion, causing tissue damage.

FIGURE 4.8. Scheme of bioplar electric circuit.

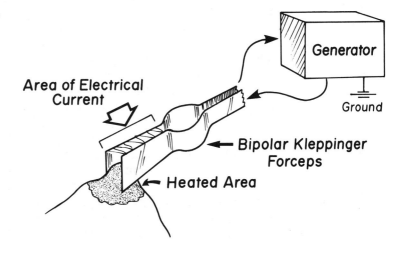

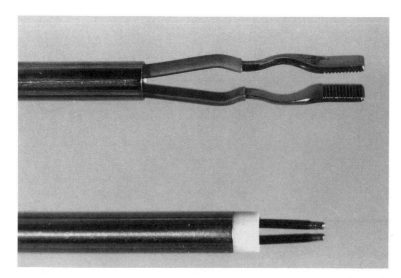

FIGURE 4.9. A close-up view of the paddles of the Kleppinger bipolar forceps **(top)** and the Vancaillie microbipolar unit **(bottom)**.

be insulated so that the current returns to the generator through the second electrode. Bipolar instruments can coagulate and dessicate, but cannot achieve cutting, since power densities high enough to cause vaporization of tissue cannot be achieved.[4] Bipolar instruments are used to coagulate vessels and occlude fallopian tubes.

Bipolar forceps use both modulated and unmodulated current to achieve hemostasis, although most often undampened current is used. Large bipolar paddles (e.g., Keppinger) are used to dessicate large blood vessels, as well as fallopian tubes (Fig. 4.5). Hemostasis can best be achieved by occluding the open vessel with the bipolar paddles before coagulation. The microbipolar forceps (Vancaillie, Storz, Culver City, CA) are not truly forceps since there is a fixed distance between the two electrodes and the tissue to be coagulated cannot be grasped (Fig. 4.9). This instrument has a channel for irrigation that is useful to identify bleeding areas before coagulation. Bipolar instruments, however, do not work well when placed within fluid.

It has been demonstrated that fallopian tubes cannot be fully coagulated unless cutting or unmodulated current is used.[6] As current is applied, tissue resistance increases and the effective power output reduces slowly and then rapidly. The coagulation mode, which has higher peak voltage, will cause desiccation at

the surface, which will impede transmission of electrical energy to the endosalpinx, through increased surface resistance. Cutting or unmodulated current will achieve slower but more effective heat deep in the tissue and coagulate the endosalpinx.

## Thermocoagulation

Thermocoagulation differs from electrosurgery in that the electrical current heats up the electrode itself, and this heat is transmitted to tissue by convection. No electricity comes in direct contact with the tissues. This method is used in the Endocoagulator (Wisap Co., Saurlach, Germany), which is heated from 100° to 120°C for a preset amount of time to achieve coagulation. This method has been popularized by Semm in an attempt to decrease the complications of electrosurgery,[7] although no such benefit has been demonstrated. Three different instrument tips are available for use with the thermocoagulation unit. The point coagulator has a blunt point that heats slowly, but works well if large areas need to be coagulated. However, the point is much too small for microsurgical work (Fig. 4.10). The point coagulator has been used to coagulate stumps, treat endometriosis, or ablate ovarian cyst walls. An alligator forcep was designed for tubal ligation (Fig. 4.10). It has an overhanging

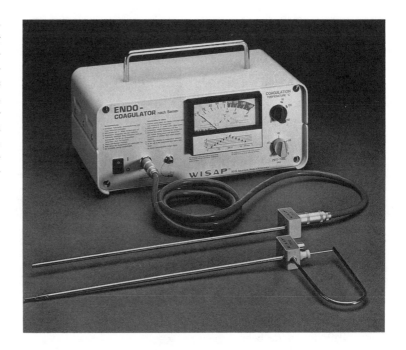

FIGURE 4.10. Thermocoagulator with the point coagulator in the background and the alligator forceps in the foreground. Not shown is the myoma forceps (WISAP Co., Sauerlach, Germany). (reproduced with permission from Garzo VG, Murphy AA. Operative laparoscopic instrumentation. *Sem Reprod Endocrinol.* 1991;9:109–117.)

hook on one paddle. This may facilitate grasping of fallopian tubes, but this paddle cannot be used effectively to grasp bleeding vessels and achieve hemostasis. The myoma paddle has a flat bladelike design that is useful when dissecting myomas from its bed. Because it does not depend on transmission of electrical current, it works well in a wet field. Although not as popular as electrosurgery, thermocoagulation is most often used for laparoscopic myomectomies. Semm has stated that postoperative adhesions are decreased by using endocoagulation rather than electrosurgery[3]; however, no controlled studies are available.

## Suturing

Laparoscopic sutures may be used to obtain hemostasis or approximate tissue. They may be placed such that the knot is tied (or pretied) extracorporeally, or tied intraabdominally.

### Using Extracorporeal Knot Tying

#### Loop Ligatures

The Roeder loop was the first reliable method of laparoscopic suturing, consisting of a suture

loop with a pretied slip knot. A comercially preformed loop, the Endoloop, is available as O-chromic and O-plain catgut, O-Vicryl and O-PDS from Ethicon (Somerville, NJ), or as O-plain Endoschlinge (Fig. 4.11) from WISAP (Sauerlach, Germany). The ligature is formed into a loop using a fisherman's knot and the free end passes up the hollow core of a plastic push guide to be imbedded at its distal tip. Once the loop is placed around the tissue of interest, the plastic guide rod is snapped off from the imbedded tip and used to push the slip knot closed.

The loop is most easily placed into the abdomen by loading into an Endoloop applicator (Fig. 4.12), which is then placed through a suprapubic port. A forceps or ampulla dilator is usually necessary to help place the loop correctly around the tissue to be ligated. The knot is tightened by pushing down on the plastic guide as the suture is pulled up. Tensile strength studies have shown the importance of one or at most two pushes of the plastic guide.[8] More than two pushes significantly decreases knot strength. Depending on the size of bleeding points, only one loop may be necessary. Alternatively, it has been recommended that three ligatures be used when performing

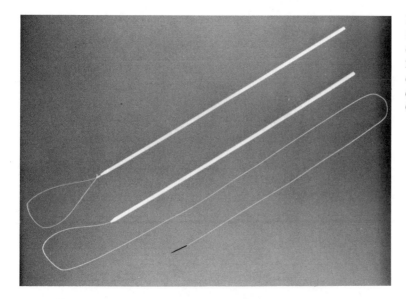

FIGURE 4.11. **Top**: Endoloop (aka Endoschlinge) 0-plain catgut loop ligature. **Bottom**: 2-plain Endosuture (aka Endonaht) on a 3-cm Keith needle (WISAP Co., Sauerlach, Germany).

FIGURE 4.12. Endoloop being loaded into applicator by pushing the plastic push rod up through the distal tip of the applicator and pulling the suture loop up into the shaft of the applicator. The loaded applicator is then placed through a 5-mm suprapubic sleeve.

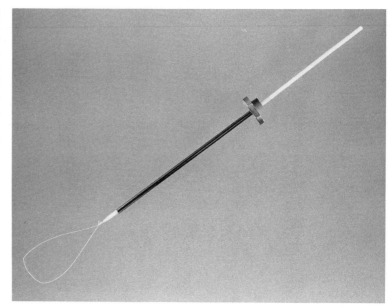

oophorectomy, salpingectomy, and adnexectomy.[9,10]

As an alternative to comercially manufactured loops, sutures of different materials and sizes can be used to make a loop ligature. Either a Roeder knot (Fig. 4.13) or a Duncan loop (Fig. 4.14) can be made and slipped down the ancillary port using a metal knot guide[11]

(Fig. 4.15). This metal knot guide is available commercially or can be made by making a large notch into the end of a laparoscopic probe.[12] If braided suture is used, a Duncan knot is generally easier to use than a Roeder knot. Marrero and Corfman[11] note that the slipping strength of both loops may be increased if a half hitch is added to the knot (Fig. 4.16).

FIGURE 4.13. Diagram of extracorporeal knot tying using the Roeder loop technique.

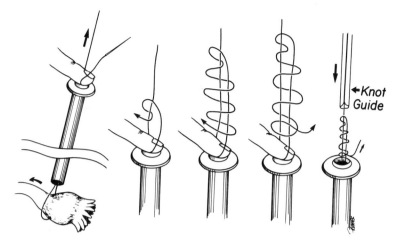

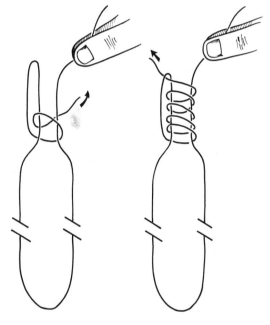

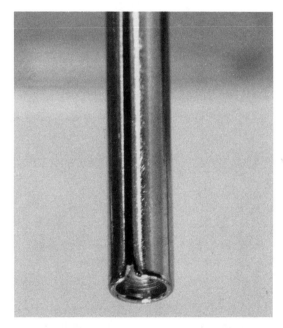

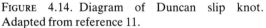

FIGURE 4.14. Diagram of Duncan slip knot. Adapted from reference 11.

FIGURE 4.15. Close-up of tip of metal knot guide (WISAP Co., Sauerlach, Germany).

### Extracorporeal Suturing

The preformed loop ligature is used mainly to secure pedicles and to obtain hemostasis. However, if a tissue needs to be approximated, a suture on a needle may be used and the knot tied extracorporeally (Fig. 4.13). The knot is then pushed into the abdomen with a metal or plastic knot guide. The Endonaht (Wisap Co., Sauerlach, Germany) consists of a 3-cm Keith needle on an 80-cm 2-plain suture with a plastic snap-off push rod (Fig. 4.11). Also available are O-chromic and O-Vicryl Endosutures from Ethicon (Sommerville, NJ). As an alternative to commercially manufactured sutures, one can use a variety of sutures and needles, using

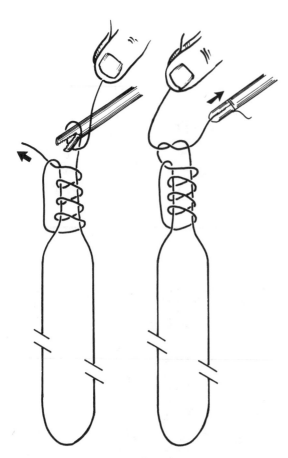

FIGURE 4.16. Diagram of a Duncan loop plus a half hitch. Adapted from reference 11.

rod (with the Endosuture) or the metal knot guide is used to tighten the knot in the abdomen.

## Using Intraabdominal Knot Tying

This technique is usually reserved when the tissue necessitates suturing with 3-0 or finer gauge suture. This is most commonly used to secure a neosalpingostomy or other microsurgical work. Suture of this caliber is too fragile to withstand reintroduction into the cavity with a knot guide. Thus, two techniques of intraabdominal knot tying have been described for use with these sutures. Appropriate microsurgical tech-

the metal knot guide to advance the knot. Some curved needles can be bent slightly to allow introduction into the abdomen through a 3- or 5-mm port.

To suture intraabdominally using an extracorporeal knot, a 3- or 5-mm needle holder (Fig. 4.13) is placed through an Endoloop applicator. The suture is then grasped near the hilt of the needle and drawn up into the shaft of the applicator. The loaded applicator is then introduced into the abdomen through a 5-mm ancillary port. The needle is pushed into the abdomen, regrasped using the needle holder, and the tissue sutured. After passing the needle through the tissues to be aproximated, the suture is then grasped near the needle and brought out of the abdomen through the applicator. A knot, either Roeder or Duncan, is tied extracorporeally, and either the plastic push

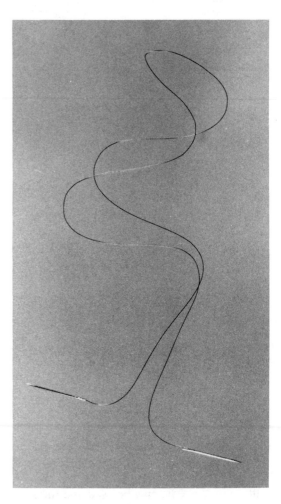

FIGURE 4.17. Double barbed 4-0 PDS suture (Ethicon, Sommerville, NJ) for intraabdominal laparascopic knot tying.

FIGURE 4.18. Close-up of jaws of needle holder. Note deep transverse grooves designed to accommodate the straight needle of the Endosuture.

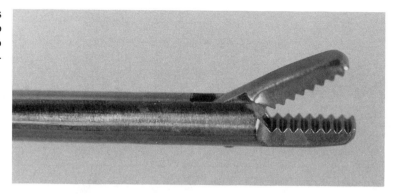

nique should be used at all times (see Chapter 7) and the tissues treated as atraumatically as possible. Although a variety of sutures can be used, a 35-cm 4-0 PDS suture (Z-420, Ethicon, Somerville, NJ) with an ST-4 tapered needle at each end is available (Fig. 4.17). This suture was initially designed for tendon repair but can be used at laparoscopy after the suture is cut in half. Each needle is straight, making it easier to push through tissues.

The first technique for intraabdominal knot tying is essentially the same as for a standard microsurgical knot. The suture is grasped near the hilt of the needle with a needle holder. The suture is then introduced into the abdominal cavity by drawing up into a suture applicator, which is then placed through a 5-mm suprapubic sleeve. Alternatively, the suture can be pushed directly into the abdomen through a 5-mm suprapubic valveless port using a micrograsper (see Fig. 8.11), which allows the needle to slide down alongside its jaws. After being pushed into the abdomen, the needle is regrasped, making sure that it lies in one of the transverse grooves lining the needle holder jaws (Fig. 4.18), and driven through the tissue. A second needle holder or other grasper is used to immobilize the tissue through which the needle is driven. The needle is grasped at right angles to the suture and a surgeon's knot

FIGURE 4.19. Microsurgical intraabdominal knot-tying technique.

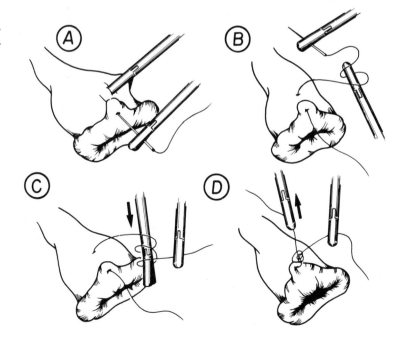

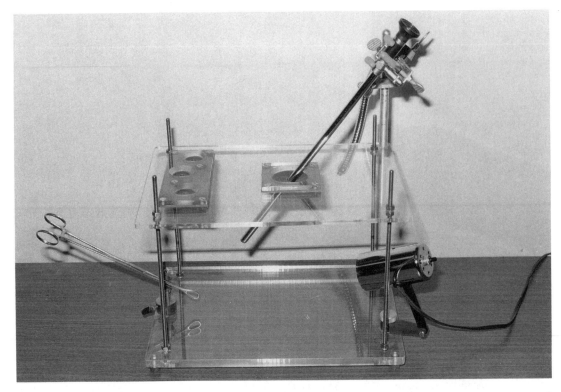

FIGURE 4.20. Pelvic trainer useful to develop the skills necessary for intraabdominal knot tying. This unit was constructed in house.

made (Fig. 4.19). The right angle keeps the suture from slipping off easily. Two other knots are placed using standard microsurgical technique. The needle is cut off and withdrawn from the abdomen by grasping the suture and pulling it out through the applicator. This type of suturing requires a great deal of training as it can be technically demanding and generally frustrating. A pelvic trainer, obtained commercially or manufactured in house (Fig. 4.20), is helpful for developing these skills.

An alternative method of knot tying has been described.[13] It is essentially an intracorporeal technique using a fisherman's knot (Fig. 4.21). A long swagged-on needle is introduced into the abdomen in the same manner as above, and the other end of the suture is held outside the abdomen. The needle is grasped at right angles and rotated around the long end being held. Another needle holder is used to grasp the needle, which is then passed through the loop closest to the tissue. By retracting the long end, which is being held, the knot is formed and tightened. This technique is somewhat easier to perform than the previously described microsurgical knot technique.

## Clips and Automatic Staples

Clips have long been used in general surgery and less frequently in gynecology to obtain hemostasis. Recently, clips for endoscopic use have become available. An endoscopic clip applicator (Fig. 4.22) is available from Karl Storz (Culver City, CA). The PDS ligating clips are available from Ethicon (Somerville, NJ), and are broken down approximately 7 weeks after placement (Fig. 4.23). The clips come in different sizes, which can be placed through a 5- or 10-mm port, and are loaded singly. Unfortunately, because these clips close based on a

FIGURE 4.21. Alternative technique for intraabdominal knot tying using a modification of an intracorporeal fisherman's knot, as described by Thompson and Reich.[13]

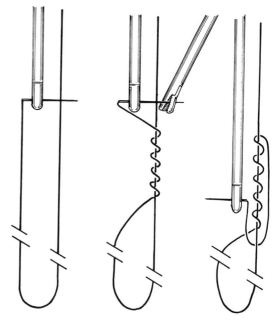

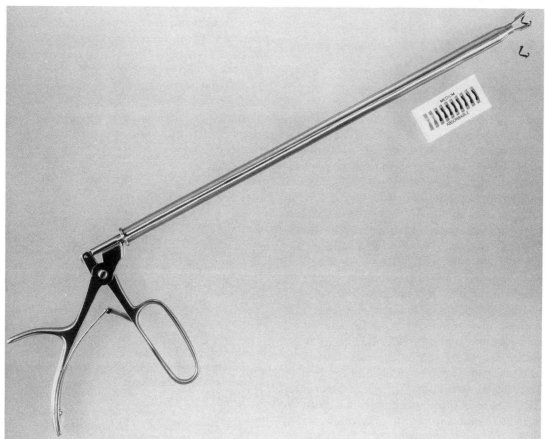

FIGURE 4.22. Laparoscopic clip applier (Karl Storz, Culver City, CA; 11 mm in diameter) and medium PDS ligating clip (AP-200, Ethicon, Sommerville, NJ).

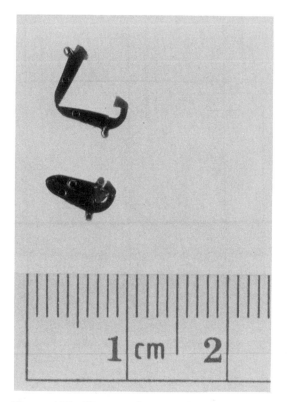

FIGURE 4.23. Close-up of open and closed medium AP-200 ligating clip (Ethicon, Sommerville, NJ).

latch mechanism (Fig. 4.23) they can only be used on small isolated vessels or pedicles. Furthermore, they tend to fall off the applicator when holding the instrument straight down.

Titanium clips are most useful for obtaining hemostasis of moderate size pedicles or vessels. These clips have no latch and are therefore more versatile. A reusable single clip applier is available from Ethicon (Somerville, NJ). The AE-214 uses medium-size clips (TI-200), which are 5.2 mm in length when closed, and the AE-314 uses medium-long clips (TI-314, 8.8 mm in length). A newer disposable multiple-clip applicator (EM-320, Ethicon, Somerville, NJ), comes preloaded with 20 medium-long titanium clips. Similar devices are available from Auto Suture Co., (Norwalk, CT). These are disposable, loaded with 20 medium or medium-large titanium clips, and in either a standard pistol or a bicycle handle grip. Both the multiple- and single-clip applicators fit through a 10-mm trocar. In general,

clips have limited usefulness because the relative lack of maneuverability at laparoscopy may make it difficult to obtain the correct placement angle.

Automatic stapling devices, similar to those used in general surgery for bowel resection, are available from Ethicon (Endo-Cutter) and Auto Suture Co., (Endo-GIA). These devices place two or three rows of titanium clips on either side of the area to be incised. When fired, the instrument automatically staples and then incises. Staple lines are available in 30 and 60 mm lengths. These devices may be useful for laparoscopic hysterectomy and adnexectomy.

## Summary

The ability to achieve hemostasis is key to any endoscopic procedure. The wide variety of methods available for hemostasis makes it imperative that we be aware of them, their uses and their limitations. No method is perfect and surgeons should strive to master a combination of different techniques, for the versatility necessary to achieve our surgical end. The development of new instruments and techniques for achieving hemostasis will greatly advance endoscopic surgery.

## References

1. Boesch PF. Laparoscopie. *Schweis Z Krankenh.* 1936;6:62–67.
2. Levy BS, Soderstrom RM, Dail DH. Bowel injuries during laparoscopy: gross anatomy and histology. *J Reprod Med.* 1985;309:168–170.
3. Semm K. Endocoagulation: a new field of endoscopic surgery. *J Reprod Med.* 1976;31:7–9.
4. Reich H, Vancaille TH, Soderstrom RM. Electrical techniques. In: Martin DC, Holtz GL, Levinson CL, Soderstrom RM, eds. *Manual of Endoscopy.* Santa Fe Springs: American Association of Gynecologic Laparoscopists; 1990: 105–112.
5. Sebben JE. *Cutaneous Electrosurgery.* Chicago: Year Book Medical Publishers; 1989.
6. Soderstrom RN, Levy BS, Engel T. Reducing bipolar sterilization failures. *Obstet Gynecol.* 1989;74:60–64.

7. Semm K. Endocoagulator: new possibilities for tubal surgery via pelviscopy. In: da Paz AC, ed. *Recent Advances in Human Reproduction*. Amsterdam: Excerpta Medica; 1976:242–246.

8. Hay DL, Levine RL, von Fraunhofer JA, Masterson BJ. The effect of the number of pulls on the tensile strength of the chromic gut pelviscopic loop ligature. *J Reprod Med*. 1990;35:260–262.

9. Semm K. New methods of pelviscopy (gynecologic laparoscopy) for myomectomy, ovariectomy, tubectomy, and adnexectomy. *Endoscopy*. 1979;2:85–87.

10. Semm K. Tissue puncher and loop ligation: new aids for surgical–therapeutic pelviscopy (lapa-roscopy)–endoscopic intra-abdominal surgery. *Endoscopy*. 1978;10:110–114.

11. Marrero MA, Corfman RS. Laparoscopic use of sutures. In: Diamond MP, ed. *Clinical Obstetrics and Gynecology–Pelviscopy*. Philadelphia: Lippincott; 1991;34:387–394.

12. Levine RL. Instrumentation. In: Sanfillipo JS, Levine RL, eds. *Operative Gynecologic Endoscopy*. New York: Springer–Verlag; 1989:19–37.

13. Thompson RG, Reich H. Intra-abdominal laparoscopic suturing: a new technique. Abstract (FP-09), 46th Annual Meeting of the American Fertility Society, Washington, DC, 1990.

# 5

# Principles of Endoscopic Laser Surgery

*Richard P. Buyalos*

## Laser Physics

Electrons orbit in the atom at different distances from the nucleus. When an atom is "excited" by external energy (in the form of a photon), electrons are shifted to an orbit farther from the nucleus. The more energy absorbed by the atom, the higher the resulting orbit level of its electrons. This excited state lasts a few millionths of a second, the electron dropping down (decaying) to its usual level, thus achieving thermodynamic equilibrium. During this decay the energy absorbed by the electron is emitted in the form of a photon, a process termed "spontaneous emission." If an atom is in the excited state and is struck with another photon of the same energy as the one already absorbed, the decay process is accelerated. When this happens two photons of identical energy, frequency, and direction are released, in a process termed "stimulated emission." This principle is the basis for the production of laser (*Light Amplification Stimulated Emission of Radiation*) light. The energy released by an atom during spontaneous or stimulated emission represents the difference between the initial and final energy of that atom, which in turn depend on the particular species of atom and its various electron orbits. Thus, different materials will produce lasers of different wavelengths and energy (Fig. 5.1).

Laser energy uses principles of both light and electromagnetic radiation. Light consists of packets of energy (photons) that travel in a sinusoidal (wavelike) motion. Energy (measured in joules) is calculated as $E = h\,f$, where $f$ = frequency and $h$ = Planck's constant or

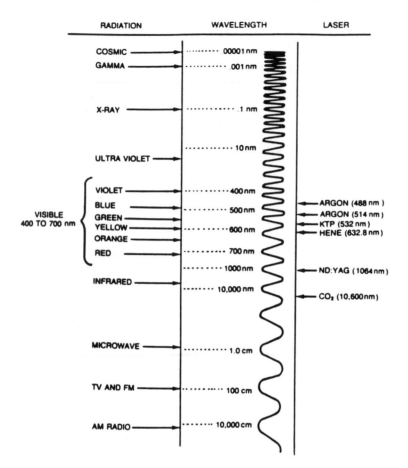

FIGURE 5.1. The electromagnetic spectrum demonstrating various types of lasers and their associated wavelengths. (reproduced with permission from Keye WR Jr. *Laser Surgery in Gynecology and Obstetrics*. Chicago: Year Book Medical Publishers; 1990.)

$6.63 \times 10^{34}$ joule sec. Substituting $c/\lambda$ for $f$, gives $E = h \times c/\lambda$, where $c$ = speed of light (186,000 miles per sec) and $\lambda$ is wavelength of the electromagnetic wave. Therefore, the laser energy emitted is inversely proportional to its wavelength and directly proportional to its frequency. Hence, the smaller the wavelength, the greater the energy.

## Generation of Laser Light

Different atomic species, in the forms of solids, liquids, and gases are used to create lasers (Fig. 5.1). To maintain the laser effect the majority of the atomic population of the laser medium must be in an excited (higher energy level) state. This is referred to as "population inversion." In order to maintain this state of excitability, external energy must be constantly infused into the atom population. For the production of lasers the atom population (or active laser medium) is contained in an optical or resonant cavity. Atoms in the excited state spontaneously emit photons in all directions within the optical cavity. However, most travel along the longitudinal tube axis and are reflected by carefully aligned mirrors at both ends of the resonant cavity. These photons stimulate further emissions from already excited atoms (photon multiplier effect) and generate photon pairs of equal wavelength, frequency, and energy. These photon pairs are reflected within the optical cavity, are further amplified, and finally emerge through a partially transmitting mirror at the end of the tube as the laser beam. The properties of laser light are noted in Table 5.1.

TABLE 5.1. Properties of laser light.

| | |
|---|---|
| Coherent | Laser waves are always precisely in phase with one another, temporally and spatially |
| Collimated | All laser waves are parallel to each other. This facilitates transmission of the laser beam over relatively long distances with minimal scatter |
| Monochromatic | Laser consists of waves of essentially the same wavelength and energy level. This accounts for the reproducible effects on target tissue by a particular laser energy |
| Highest luminosity | It is the brightest existing light |

# Power Density and Exposure Time

Maximal power setting for most surgical laser units range from 20 to 100 W at the exit point of the optical cavity. Despite the relatively low power in watts, the magnitude of the beam energy is amplified immensely by adjusting the focus of the beam with special lenses or controls. The area of the focused beam is referred to as the "spot size." The magnitude of power concentration is usually referred to as the "power density" or power per unit area of beam. Power density is a property of both beam power (wattage) and spot size (determined by the focusing lens), such that:

$$\text{Power density} = \frac{\text{power at the focal spot}}{\text{area of the focal spot}}$$

Power density is therefore directly proportional to beam wattage and inversely proportional to spot size. At a constant beam power, increasing the spot size decreases the beam concentration per surface area, achieving a lower power density. Conversely, a smaller spot size will achieve a significantly higher power density for a given beam power. If we assume an ideal beam with a perfect circular spot shape and uniform energy distribution in this circle, the surface area (A) is: $A = \pi r^2$, where r is the beam radius. Since the radius is half the beam diameter ($r = D/2$), then $A = \pi [D/2]^2$ or $A = \pi D^2/4$. Thus, doubling the beam diameter reduces the power density to $\frac{1}{4}$, while

halving the spot diameter increases the power density by a factor of 4. However, lasers do not have uniform power distribution throughout the beam spot area, and the actual calculation of power density varies depending on the shape of the power distribution of the beam. Nevertheless, the direct relationship of power density to power output and its inverse square relationship to spot size remains of paramount importance in laser use.

Whereas power density is the principal determinant of the effect of a laser beam on target tissue, exposure time is also an important determinant. Ideally, the largest volume of tissue should be exposed for the shortest period of time (i.e., using high power density), without compromising hemostasis. Shortened exposure time reduces thermal conduction, minimizing coagulation of surrounding tissue.

# The Effects of Laser Light on Tissue

Living cells directly exposed to laser light of an appropriate wavelength are generally vaporized through the boiling of intracellular water. As excess photons scatter into the adjacent tissues, some of the surrounding cells are destroyed or damaged by thermal coagulation of intracellular proteins. The zone of thermal or coagulation necrosis is constant at any given power density, but varies with exposure time. The longer the beam is in contact with a particular area, the more heat will be conducted into the tissue adjacent to the vaporization site (Fig. 5.2), resulting in greater surrounding tissue damage and subsequent fibrosis. Many laser-generating units today have the ability to produce beams in a continuous or pulsed fashion. Superpulse mode allows the beam to be delivered in a rapid series of pulses in a controlled repetitive fashion with short pauses between beam pulses. These micropauses reduce exposure time, allowing the tissue to cool between pulses, thus minimizing adjacent thermal damage. The efficacy of the superpulse mode declines when the pulse duration is greater than 10% of the interval between beam micropulses.

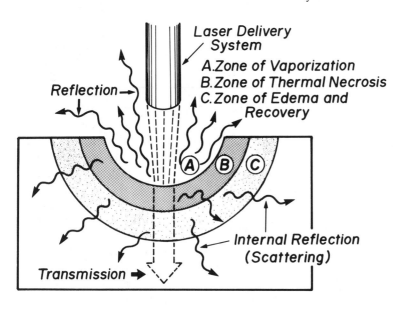

FIGURE 5.2. The cells absorbing the laser beam directly will be vaporized via intracellular boiling. Nonabsorbed photons will be reflected, scatter to surrounding tissues, or transmitted resulting in either cellular necrosis, due to protein coagulation, or reversible cellular injury. The extent of these tissue effects will vary according to the specific type of laser used, the power density and exposure time, and characteristics of the tissue.

TABLE 5.2. Comparisons of the surgical lasers used in gynecologic, endoscopy.

|  | $CO_2$ | Nd:YAG | Argon | KTP |
|---|---|---|---|---|
| Active medium | $CO_2$, nitrogen, helium gases | Neodymium:yttrium-aluminum garnet | Argon gas | Nd:YAG beam frequency doubled by a KTP crystal |
| Wavelength (nm) | 10,600 | 1064 | 418 and 514.5 | 532 |
| Preferential absorbance mm | Water | Dark or black color | Hemoglobin | Hemoglobin, melanin |
| May pass through fluid | No | Yes | Yes | Yes |
| Hemostatic ability | Poor | Excellent | Excellent | Excellent |
| Depth of penetration (mm) | 0.1–0.2 | Contact: 0.3–2; noncontact: 3–7 | 0.3–1 | 0.3–1 |

Modified from Keye WR JR. *Laser Surgery in Gynecology and Obstetrics*. Chicago: Year Book Publishers; 1990, and The Houston Laser Institute. *Laser Surgery Workshop Handbook*, Houston, TX, 1989.

## Types of Lasers in Gynecology

Various media are used to produce laser light for use in gynecology today, including carbon dioxide-nitrogen-helium ($CO_2$) and Argon gases, and neodymium:yittrium-aluminum-garnet (Nd:YAG) and potassium-titanyl-phosphate (KTP) crystals (Table 5.2).

### Carbon Dioxide

Carbon dioxide and other laser energy in the infrared spectrum are preferentially absorbed by tissue that has a high water content (Table

5.2). Approximately 90% of the $CO_2$ laser energy is absorbed and transformed into heat within the initial 30 $\mu$m of exposed tissue. This induces instantaneous boiling of the intracellular water resulting in cell disruption and vaporization. Therefore, the water content of impacted tissue determines its thermal response to the $CO_2$ laser. Since epithelial cells possess a high water content (>90%), $CO_2$ laser energy can vaporize these superficial cells with minimal surrounding tissue damage. Alternatively, in cells with low intracellular water content the energy absorption is poor, resulting in more extensive coagulation. Precise cutting can be achieved with minimal peripheral cellular damage using the $CO_2$ laser.[1,2] However, it has limited hemostatic capacity in comparison to other commonly employed surgical lasers. If coagulation or superficial vaporization is desired, defocusing the beam (increasing the spot size) will decrease the power density while increasing the surface area treated.

Because the $CO_2$ beam wavelength is in the infrared spectrum (10,600 nm) and is invisible to the naked eye, a visible helium-neon (HeNe) laser (633 nm) is used as a parallel aiming beam. It is imperative that the two laser beams be well aligned. This alignment should be ascertained before each use (by firing the beam onto a moist tongue blade). The focusing mirrors and lenses must be inspected regularly through scheduled maintenance to confirm precise alignment.

The $CO_2$ laser and HeNe aiming beam are delivered through an articulated arm that is attached to a coupling device containing mirrors and focusing lenses to deliver the laser energy accurately into the peritoneal cavity. The coupling device can be attached to the head of the laparoscopic channel or to a suprapubic waveguide. The standard $CO_2$ laser laparoscopes use focusing lenses of 300 to 315 mm, with a focal point approximately 2 cm from the end of the delivery port and a focused spot diameter of 0.5 mm. $CO_2$ laser laparoscopes that have focusing lenses of both 250 mm and 300 mm have been introduced and provide greater system adaptability. The 250-mm lens, when used through the shorter probes employed through the suprapubic puncture, can generate smaller spot sizes and higher power densities. However, use of the 250-mm lens through the longer laparoscopic operating channel results in a defocused beam and reduced power densities. Efforts to design flexible fibers for delivery of the $CO_2$ laser beam have been unsuccessful thus far. Rigid hollow wave guides are currently available for $CO_2$ endoscopy. Many of these probes contain a focusing system at the distal end of the probe, allowing beam delivery via the operative channel of the laparoscope or a second puncture.

Power densities of 2500 to 5000 W/cm$^2$ are usually employed in a continuous firing mode.

Lesions in close proximity to vital structures such as ureter, bladder, bowel, or large vessels may be effectively ablated using single-pulse or superpulse modes of 0.05 to 0.1 sec duration. This will provide tissue vaporization of only 100 to 200 $\mu$m in depth. Additional protection of sensitive structures is achieved by injecting saline underneath the peritoneum to elevate it off a ureter or large caliber vessel. Because the $CO_2$ laser light is preferentially absorbed by water, it cannot be transmitted through a fluid medium. Therefore, the $CO_2$ laser cannot be used for operative hysteroscopy, although prototypes are being evaluated for hysteroscopic application.

Additional second puncture instruments are needed to evacuate the plume that forms from tissue vaporization, manipulate pelvic structures, and irrigate the operative field. Ancillary instruments used during $CO_2$ laser surgery must be roughened to diffuse reflection. Instruments that are simply blackened are insufficient to dampen $CO_2$ laser energy, since black objects reflect infrared radiation and expose surrounding tissue to potential damage from a reflected beam. Backstops made of sandblasted or shotpeened titanium metal are preferred. The backstops can be flattened spatulas or rounded probes. When these instruments are moistened the safety margin is enhanced as moisture trapped in the latticework of the instrument absorbs excessive $CO_2$ energy. Quartz rods should be avoided since they can conduct heat to adjacent tissue or absorb heat and potentially shatter in the pelvis. During surgery, additional protection is provided by frequent moistening and irrigation of pelvic surfaces.

## Argon and KTP

The Argon laser beam has combined wavelengths of 488 nm and 514.5 nm. The KTP laser has a wavelength of 532 nm and is produced by doubling the frequency (or halving the wavelength) of a Nd:YAG laser, by passing this beam through a KTP crystal. The physical properties of the Argon and KTP laser are essentially identical.[3–5] Both can be delivered by flexible 0.3- to 0.6-mm fibers that remain cool during use and eliminate the need for focusing devices or lenses. Because the beam diverges as it exits the quartz fiber, maximum power density will be obtained within 2 mm of the fiber tip. The beams are easily visualized (green to blue/green), obviating the need for a tracking beam. Some KTP units can be altered to also produce Nd:YAG laser.

Red pigmented tissues rich in hemoglobin and hemosiderin preferentially absorb these lasers (Table 5.2), which accounts for their hemostatic properties. In addition to their ability both to coagulate and vaporize, the Argon and KTP lasers have the additional advantage of being effective when fired within a clear fluid medium, since the beam is not absorbed. The Argon and KTP lasers are well adapted for use during laparoscopy. There is less plume production and minimal beam scatter compared to $CO_2$ laparoscopy. They have a depth of tissue penetration of 0.3 to 1 mm. In general, they provide a larger margin of safety due to their relatively shallow depth of penetration, short focal lengths, and selective absorption of these wavelengths by vascular tissue and endometrial implants.

The disadvantages of the Argon and KTP lasers include the need for eye filters, possible breakage or damage of quartz fibers, and their higher purchase costs. Although no flowing gases are needed for the production of the laser beams, they require special electrical connections and running water, reducing their portability. Furthermore, these lasers have a limited capacity to incise tissue, but are quite useful for coagulation, particularly of heme-rich tissues.

To coagulate, the fiber is advanced within 1 to 4 mm of the target using a power setting of 2 to 5 W in a continuous mode. Vaporization is usually achieved by using a power setting of 5 to 10 W in continuous mode. Cutting can be achieved in a similar fashion, employing 10 to 15 W of power.

## Nd:YAG

The wavelength of the Nd:YAG laser is 1064 nm (exactly twice that of the KTP laser). Its wavelength is in the infrared spectrum and therefore a HeNe aiming beam is incorporated in these lasers for surgical use. Like the Argon and KTP lasers, flexible fibers are used for delivery of the Nd:YAG laser, which are easily adaptable to laparoscopic and hysteroscopic use. Nd:YAG lasers are less readily absorbed by heme-rich tissue than are the Argon or KTP lasers. In contrast to the Argon or KTP units, there are Nd:YAG devices available that are air cooled and do not require special plumbing and can be moved easily between operating rooms. These units typically generate between 20 and 100 W.

The Nd:YAG laser has been used extensively in thoracic and urologic surgery. Because of its greater depth of penetration, the Nd:YAG laser initially was less popular for intraperitoneal use. Using "bare fiber" noncontact techniques, the depth of tissue penetration of the Nd:YAG laser is 3 to 4 mm (Table 5.2).[6] Because of this penetration, in gynecology the Nd:YAG laser was used initially for hysteroscopic procedures, particularly endometrial ablation. However, many of these devices are air cooled and carry the theoretical risk of embolization. Furthermore, the rollerball and wire loop electrosurgical resectoscopes are probably superior for endometrial ablation (see Chapter 18).

With the development of sapphire tips, both the depth of penetration and the shape of the beam can be controlled more accurately, greatly expanding the applicability of the Nd:YAG laser and increasing its safety margin.[7] The broad beam of a bare fiber can be modified to a variety of chisel and scalpel configurations, providing a superficial depth of tissue penetration. Additionally, the sapphire tips also allow direct "contact" with the target tissue. This provides tactile feedback to the surgeon, unlike the noncontact techniques usually employed with Argon and KTP laser systems, or $CO_2$ laparoscopy, where the focal point of the laser energy is distal to the fiber or wave guide. Disadvantages to the sapphire probes include their relatively high costs, although with proper care they can be used for multiple procedures. Care must be taken to avoid inadvertent contact with surrounding organs because these probes remain hot for several seconds after discontinuing use.

# Laser Safety

The safety of the patient and the operating team is of paramount importance. Trained, experienced assistants are invaluable during laser procedures. Operating theatres must be clearly labeled on the outside door indicating that a laser procedure is in progress. The window in the operating room must be covered. Some facilities have a light that is activated when the laser unit is operating. The type of laser must be specified on the "danger" sign. The optical density for protective eye wear must be appropriate for the wavelength of laser employed. Ideally, protective eye wear appropriate for the given laser should be available outside the operating room. All operating personnel, including the anesthesiologist and assistants, must wear safety goggles or appropriate protective eye wear.

It is absolutely essential that flammable substances or explosive solutions be avoided in the operating room during laser usage. Special care must be taken when using paper drapes. When using $CO_2$ lasers the area surrounding the operative field should be draped with moist laps. The patient's eyes must also be appropriately protected with moist gauze or dressings.

# Laser Plume

The production of smoke after tissue destruction with the lasers has led not only to respiratory complications, but has been implicated as a possible source of mutagenicity. Approximately 75% of the solid particulate matter in laser plume is less than 1 $\mu$m. When inhaled, this small particulate matter is capable of traveling directly to the distal tracheopulmonary tree and being deposited in individual alveoli. Using a dog tongue model it has been shown that 1 g of tissue generates 284 mg of particulate substance. To eliminate 99% of the generated plume, a suction device that can mobilize 28 liters of air/sec when held 1 cm from the origin of the laser plume is needed.

Doubling the distance diminishes the capacity of smoke evacuation by approximately half. The rapid-flow (3–6 liters/min) insufflating devices widely used for pelviscopic procedures are generally adequate for evacuating the laser plume. Although $CO_2$ laser laparoscopy is associated with more plume formation than the Argon, Nd:YAG, or KTP lasers, adequate smoke evacuation systems are still mandatory when using the latter three wavelengths.

# Efficacy

There are no prospective, blinded studies comparing laparoscopic use of lasers with conventional electrosurgery, which have demonstrated an improvement in pregnancy rates or a reduction in adhesion formation. Its use to date is based on the clinical impression primarily of the surgeon. Many surgeons advocate the use of lasers because of their controlled depth of penetration, reduced thermal damage to adjacent tissue, and the reproducibility of the effects of lasers on tissue. These factors must be balanced against the increased equipment costs and operating room fees and the additional training required of the surgeon and supporting staff. Regardless of the availability of lasers, it is extremely important that the endoscopic surgeon master a wide variety of hemostatic and operative techniques.

# References

1. Feste J. Laser laparoscopy: a new modality. *J Reprod Med.* 1985;30:413–417.
2. Martin DC. $CO_2$ laser laparoscopy for endometriosis associated with infertility. *J Reprod Med.* 1986;31:1089–1094.
3. Keye WR Jr, Dixon J. Photocoagulation of endometriosis by the argon laser through the laparoscope. *Obstet Gynecol.* 1983;62:383–386.
4. Keye WR Jr, Hansen LW, Astin M, et al. Argon laser therapy of endometriosis: a review of 92 consecutive patients. *Fertil Steril* 1987;47:208–212.
5. Daniell JF, Meisels S, Miller W, et al. Laparoscopic use of the KTP/532 laser in nonendometriotic pelvic surgery. *Colpo Gynecol Laser Surg.* 1986;2:107–111.

6. Lomano JM. Photocoagulation of early pelvic endometriosis with the Nd:YAG laser through the laparoscope. *J Reprod Med*. 1985;30:77–81.

7. Corson SL, Unger M, Kwa D, et al. Laparoscopic laser treatment of endometriosis with the Nd:YAG sapphire probe. *Am J Obstet Gynecol*. 1989;160:718–723.

# 6

# Photo and Video Documentation in Endoscopic Surgery

*RICARDO AZZIZ*

## CHAPTER OUTLINE

The transmission of an image from the pelvis onto film or video requires that sufficient light be transmitted through the fiberoptic system of the laparoscope, in order to be reflected off the pelvic organs and back up through the endoscopic lens system onto the operator's retina. For still photography, the lighted image is projected through the camera lens onto film within the camera body. In video imaging (and recording), the light reflected off the operative field image must be transmitted through the lens system of the camera head onto the photosensitive chip. The image is then processed electronically for projection onto the monitor screen and/or video cassette recorder.

## Endoscopic Instrumentation

### Endoscope

Most endoscopes used in gynecology today use the Hopkins lens system. In the past, endoscopes consisted of a long metal tube containing a series of glass lenses. Since the refractive index of glass is greater than that of air, Harold Hopkins inverted the air-glass spaces within the endoscopes, resulting in twice the amount of light being transmitted (see Chapter 3). In general, two types of endoscopes are used for gynecologic surgery today. Straight endoscopes consist of a central chain or system of lenses, surrounded by fiber bundles that project light inward onto the pelvic or uterine cavity. Operative endoscopes contain an operating channel through which instruments are placed. The lens chain is angled in order to bring the eyepiece away from the operating port. Operating endoscopes, in comparison to straight endoscopes of the same diameter, transmit significantly less light because they contain fewer glass fiber bundles and have an angulated and smaller diameter lens system.[1] For endoscopic photo/video documentation it is preferable to use a straight endoscope of the greatest diameter possible, since they contain more glass fiber bundles and have a greater diameter lens system. Endoscopes are available in various viewing angles and diameters (see Chapter 3). Straight laparoscopes of greater diameter and 0° or head on viewing angle are best suited for photodocumentation.

Hysteroscopes are of smaller diameter than laparoscopes and have viewing angles of 10° to 70°, which decreases considerably the brightness of the image being transmitted. Furthermore, the reddish, rough endometrial surface reflects less light than the serosa. However, their shorter working distance and the smaller size of the uterine cavity compensates for this decreased illumination, allowing photo documentation to be performed quite satisfactorily through the hysteroscope. Distention of the uterine cavity with $CO_2$ yields a brighter image. Nevertheless, this medium does not satisfactorily prevent blood from obstructing the operative field. Although Hyskon (32% dextran-70) gives a cloudier image, it can tamponade bleeding vessels by virtue of its injection pressure.

## Light Source

There are many different light sources of varying spectral emissions and illumination power (see Chapter 3). The hotter the light source the bluer the light; the colder the more reddish the tint of the image. The 250- to 300-W mercury-halide or 300-W xenon-vapor arc lamps provide excellent light for photo documentation. The type of color film or video system used for recording must be adapted to the light source in order to compensate for the artificial coloration provided to the organs (see below).

The image transmitted back through the endoscope will depend greatly on the reflective quality of the pelvic or uterine surface. Dark or bloody surfaces will reflect relatively less light in comparison to the smooth white surfaces of the ovary. In addition, light is reduced by the square of the distance. If the endoscope were withdrawn twice the distance from the surface of interest, the amount of light required for the same exposure would increase fourfold. Finally, beam splitters, video couplers, and camera lenses all reduce the amount of light transmitted. Thus, the most powerful light source available should be used for photo/video documentation in endoscopy.

## Light-Transmitting Cables

Endoscopic light cables consist of glass fiber bundles, each measuring approximately 25 $\mu$m and consisting of a central core of highly refractive glass with an outer sheath or "cladding" of low refractive glass (see Chapter 3). Since 30% of the fiberoptic light cables are made up of cladding and interfiber filler, the solid liquid light cable by Karl Storz, Inc. may provide more light transmission. Fiberoptic cables should be inspected frequently for breakage or central burnout, as this rapidly reduces the amount of light transmitted. The easiest method is to project the light directly from the laparoscopic end of the cable onto a white surface, from approximately 6 to 12 inches away. If greater than 30% of the fibers are damaged or more than 2 mm of the central area is burned out, the cable should be replaced.

# Instrumentation and Technique of Still Photography

## Camera Body

Practically any single lens reflex (SLR) camera body with through the lens (TTL) viewing can

FIGURE 6.1. Close-up of the Olympus Co. endoscopic still photography system consisting of an OM-1n camera body, SM-EFR 3 combined dedicated lens/light sensor unit, and autowinder.

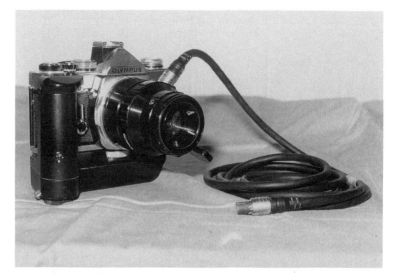

be used. Nevertheless, a camera with interchangeable focusing screens is preferred, since the general purpose ground glass focusing screens should be replaced with a circular clear glass screen used for endoscopic photography. The exception would be the need for a double-cross line focusing screen for use with lenses of longer focal length, requiring more careful focusing.

The camera body should be lightweight. Additional accessories such as remote shutter control, autowinder, and data recorder may be added, although the weight of the camera increases as well. The author's preference is an Olympus OM-1n camera body with a type 1–9 focusing screen, databack recorder, and autowinder (Fig. 6.1).

## Camera Lens

In general, the longer the focal length of the camera lens the greater the amount of film filled by the image. Alternatively, the visual field seen is determined by the endoscopic optics and not by the camera. To fill a standard 35-mm film frame completely ($36 \times 24$ mm), a lens with a focal length of between 120 and 150 mm is required. Unfortunately, increasing the focal length of the lens also increases the demand for light and reduces picture brightness. It also decreases the depth of field and requires more careful focusing.

Fixed or telephoto lenses of 85 to 120 mm in focal length can be used, although telephoto lenses usually require more light. With these lenses a SLR camera will have a film image to actual size ratio of 1:3 to 1:5, depending on the endoscope. SLR refers to cameras that have one mirror showing the focused image to viewer. The F-stop is left wide open (3.5, 2.8, or the lowest possible number) since the size of the aperture is actually determined by the diameter of the endoscopy optic system, which is always smaller than that of the lens. The shutter speed varies with the intensity of the light source and ranges from $\frac{1}{4}$ to $\frac{1}{15}$ sec.

Greater magnification, and thus a larger image on film can be achieved using a "macro"-type lens ("micro" if Nikon brand is used), achieving a 1:1 or 1:2 film image to actual size ratio. Greater degrees of magnification can also be obtained by using zoom lenses of greater focal length, or using special teleconverter adaptors. The Olympus Corp. produces two integrated lens and TTL light sensor systems, the SM-EFR 2 or 3 lens, which have no effective F-stop. The SM-EFR 2 is basically a 105-mm lens, and produces an image of approximately 25 mm in diameter on standard 35 mm film. The focal depth is relatively narrow, which may require a double cross hair focusing screen to improve the sharpness of the image. The author prefers the SM-EFR 3, which is of shorter focal length (82.8 mm) and provides an image 18 mm in diameter on film, but which is brighter and usually in focus throughout (Fig. 6.1).

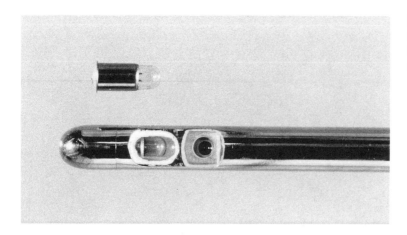

Figure 6.2. Distal incandescent lamp at the tip of a Decker culdoscope. Note replacement bulb alongside shaft.

## Focusing

The longer the lens focal length, the narrower the focal plane. Lenses with shorter focal lengths (SM-EFR 3 or standard 85-mm lens) require minimum focusing and most of the image on film is seen clearly. Focusing can also be accomplished by setting the camera lens focusing ring on infinity and moving the laparoscope back and forth until the desired image is clearly seen. Unfortunately, this focusing technique changes the field's size and illumination. When viewing through the laparoscope, the lens of the human eye (unlike the lens of a camera) will automatically focus images slightly closer or farther than this distance. Therefore, objects that would be slightly out of focus by photography are often not perceived as such by the viewer. The observer's eyesight should be corrected to as close to 20/20 as possible, otherwise he/she may be mislead while focusing.

## Flash Generators

Flash generators can provide extremely potent extra illumination for still photography. There are three types:

1. *Distal flash*: consists of an incandescent light bulb placed at the distal end of the endoscope (Fig. 6.2). Although this system provides extremely good pictures, it emits a large amount of heat with the potential risk of organ burn or intraabdominal bulb breakage. It is not currently in use.

2. *Intermediate or miniflash*: a small flash light source is attached to the light cable directly, and synchronized to the camera via a light meter (Fig. 6.3). It is fairly effective and economical, although somewhat cumbersome. It is available from Eder Co., or as Tiny-Flash from Elmed or Reznick Instruments.

3. *Proximal flash generator*: this consists of an external light source that may form part of the same light source used for diagnostic purposes. The light source is usually a 300-watt mercury-halide or xenon vapor arc lamp. Some of these flash generators can be synchronized to the camera shutter. The Olympus Corp. currently has a dedicated, TTL light sensor unit (SM-EFR 2 or 3) that automatically determines the shutter speed and duration of the flash from a dedicated (either the CLE-F10 or CLV-10) light source. In this system the flash can produce an image in $\frac{1}{100}$ to $\frac{1}{3000}$ sec with a recycling time of 2 to 3 sec (Fig. 6.4).

## Photographic Film

Either Ektachrome or Kodachrome film can be used for slide photography. Kodachrome lasts longer, although it has a reddish hue and is more difficult to develop, since it must be processed directly by Kodak Co. Ektachrome film is easier to process and tends to appear neutral or slightly blue. Both these films are available in "daylight" types, balanced for the blue light ($K^0$ 5000–6000) most frequently emitted by currently available flash systems. A film size of 35 mm is usually prefered. Occasionally 16-mm slide film is used since it requires less light for recording, although the image is relatively grainier.

FIGURE 6.3. Intermediate or mini-flash mounted on OM-1 camera body.

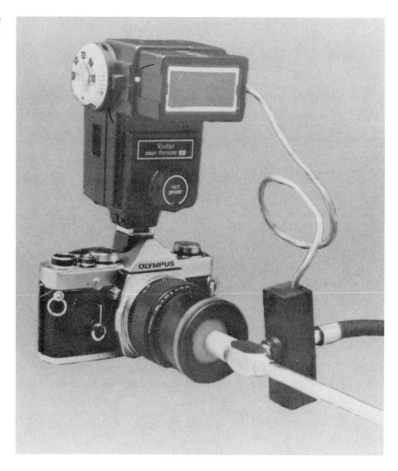

The sensitivity of the film to light is designated by ASA (American Standards Association) or DIN (Deutsche Industrie Norm, primarily in Europe) scores. More recently, the International Standards Organization (ISO) has provided a compilation of these two standards. For most endoscopic photography, film that is 160 to 400 ASA/ISO is preferred.

Slide film is easier to handle and process. However, if there were the possibility of requiring photographs for printing or publishing, it is preferable to use color or black and white print film initially. The quality of the picture is slightly better when slides are made from color print than vice versa.

## Technique of Still Photography in the Operating Room

The equipment for still photography must be present and ready in the operating room at all times, since it is difficult to plan ahead and determine which operative cases may require photo documentation. When taking photographs it is important to maintain a record of the patient's name, date, number of exposures, and any other pertinent information. In addition, a data recording back, which imprints the film with the date or a code number, is extremely useful in later identifying the images. During processing, slides are usually numbered in consecutive exposure order by the developing company. A photo of the patient's nameplate or pertinent information written out can be obtained before beginning endoscopic photography, although this may be difficult to perform well with some lens systems. In order to obtain quality slides or photographs, particularly for teaching or publication, many pictures should be obtained.

The technique preferred by the author for taking photographs in the operating room is to

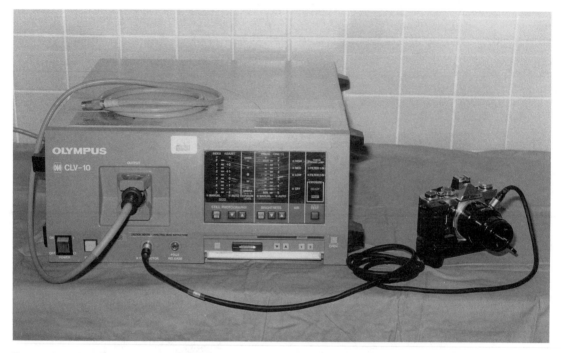

FIGURE 6.4. Olympus still photography and variable video light source, with a xenon vapor arc lamp. Attached is the camera with the dedicated lens and light sensor unit (SM-EFR 3).

double glove, load the camera onto the endoscope, remove the left hand double glove, and position the operative instruments with this hand while controlling the camera with the right. In this manner, contamination of the operative field is minimal and control over the photograph maximum.

For additional information on endoscopic still photography see refs. 2–6.

# Endoscopic Video Imaging and Recording

The video camera, couplers, control unit, TV monitor, and video cassette recorder, along with the light source and endoscope, comprise the video imaging and recording system.

## Light Source

A high intensity light source should be available. Although some systems provide continuous and nonvariable illumination, others can vary their intensity based on the amount of light reaching the camera head (e.g., the Olympus Corp. CLV-10 light source for use with a dedicated camera head). This tends to decrease glaring of the video image.

## Video Camera

Older cameras consist of single or triple television tubes.[7] The single-tube (single frequency, color coded, and phase integrated) cameras electronically split the image transmitted to the color monitor into component colors according to empirical values, and color resolution at times was less than optimal. The triple-tube cameras split the image colors into the three primary colors via a prism that is then processed by three different television tubes. The color resolution of this type of camera is very good, although they are quite bulky, usually requiring a counter-balance suspension system.

More recent video cameras contain a charge-couple device (CCD) chip. Newer CCD chips are composed of approximately 380,000 to 420,000 light-sensitive elements or "pixels." These cameras deliver between 420 and 480 horizontal lines of resolution, which currently is the rate-limiting step in improving image sharpness. Preferably, the camera should be of small size and connecting cables should be fully sterilizable. Some camera heads provide remote controls for the video recorder.

## Camera Couplers

Cameras can attach directly to the endoscope viewpiece through a straight coupler. This has the advantage of allowing all available light to be received by the camera chip. Nevertheless, this forces the surgeon either to perform his operation from the monitor screen or constantly remove the camera.

An alternative has been the use of a beam splitter. This device splits the light received from the endoscope 30%/70%, 20%/80%, or 10%/90%, the lesser portion being transmitted to the surgeon's eye and the remainder to the camera. The beam splitter and straight coupler are usually furnished with a focusing ring and provide a small degree of magnification. For greater convenience the camera head should be able to rotate on the beam splitter without unscrewing, making it possible to change the position of the beam splitter while keeping the video monitor image upright. Many beam splitters were originally designed for arthroscopy or gastroenterology. Compared to gynecology, these applications require a much narrower field of view and a smaller, more light reflective cavity is examined. Thus, each make and type of beam splitter should be tested for use in gynecology.

## Control Unit

The control unit is the power supply and signal processing center. In some control units the hue of the picture can be adjusted manually, adapting the image to the type of light and altering the light sensitivity. More current models are fully automatic, providing a uniform color setting based on a total white image received (i.e., "white balance"). They may also feature a "color bar" setting in order to fine-tune the color appearing on the monitor.

## Color Monitor

The color monitor rarely affects image quality. Most good home television screens today are able to handle 350 horizontal lines of resolution. Video monitors can handle from 450 to 600 lines of resolution. The use of a larger screen size does not increase the brightness or resolution of the image, but may appear more blurred to those observing from a close distance. It is important to fill the monitor screen completely with the projected image, since this will increase the number of scanning lines used and improve the overall resolution. This can be achieved with use of different (20–35 mm) couplers. However, the brightness of the image is reduced by the square of its size on the screen. Assuming the same illumination, a 40% larger image on the television screen will appear half as bright, although with improved resolution.

## Video Recorders

Video recorders are available in many formats. Three-quarter inch tape is used preferentially for producing films for teaching, demonstrations, or exhibits. This tape is more durable and less subject to distortion as it has a greater surface area to signal ratio than standard half-inch format. Furthermore, most editing systems are geared to this format. Nevertheless, Super VHS (half-inch) videotape editing systems are becoming increasingly more sophisticated. Remote controls and character generators are optional equipment.

## Video Printers

Video printers that convert video images to hard copy prints within seconds are available from various manufacturers. Some systems can store up to 50 images on floppy disk (Canon USA, Inc., Lake Success, NY.) for later retrieval and processing. Some printers require that the video image be frozen on the recorder while others automatically do so. In the past some systems used tiny jets to spray each primary colors on paper. Today most systems use a form of color thermal printing. Basically the image is composed of approximately 15 to 20 million dots of cyan, magenta, yellow, and black. Some systems produce black dots by superimposing the three primary colors. A heated printhead is used to melt dots of colored wax or plastic from long ribbons onto the paper. Each color is laid down separately.

One exception is the Polaroid system (Cambridge, MA) which projects the video image onto a miniature internal color television screen. Using a color filter wheel, the image is then photographed three times and printed onto Polaroid paper. Unfortunately, image quality is still nowhere near that obtained with still photography, although it may be useful for clinical documentation and patient education.

## References

1. Taylor HW. A comparative evaluation of the 5 mm laparoscope in gynecologic endoscopy. *J Reprod Med*. 1975;15:65–68.

2. Cohen MR. Photography. In: Phillips JM, ed. *Laparoscopy*. Baltimore: William & Wilkins; 1977:300–305.

3. Marlow J. Endoscopic photography. *Clin Obstet Gynecol*. 1983;26:359–365.

4. Semm K. *Operative Manual for Operative Endoscopic Abdominal Surgery*. Chicago: Yearbook Medical Publishers; 1987:46–53, 57–58, 242–248.

5. Hulka JF. *Textbook of Laparoscopy*. New York: Grune and Stratton; 1985:7–21.

6. Borten M. Laparoscopic complications: prevention and management. Philadelphia: BC Decker; 1986:430–441.

7. Circon. *Circon Micro Video Cameras Operating Manual*. Santa Barbara, CA: Circon Corp; 3.1–3.2.

# 7

# Principles of Laparoscopic Microsurgery and Adhesion Prevention

*Jacqueline N. Gutmann and Michael P. Diamond*

## CHAPTER OUTLINE

Pelvic adhesions are known to play a role in female infertility; additionally, adhesions may lead to complications including bowel obstruction and pelvic pain. Because postoperative pelvic adhesions following laparotomy have been reported in 55% to 95% of cases,[1] the development of strategies to reduce adhesion formation and reformation is of paramount importance to the pelvic surgeon. In this regard, several advances have been made in reproductive surgery over the last quarter of a century. These include the use of microsurgical technique, of adhesion reduction adjuvants, and of endoscopic surgery. This chapter presents our understanding of the pathogenesis of postoperative adhesion development and the surgical techniques and adjuvants currently used in attempts to eliminate their development.

## Pathophysiology of Adhesion Formation

### Normal Peritoneal Healing

Adhesion formation represents an aberrancy of the normal healing process. Hence, in order to understand and subsequently to prevent the formation of adhesions, it is important to re-

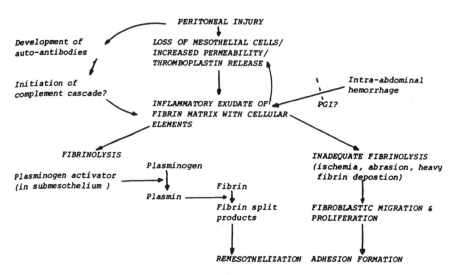

FIGURE 7.1. Scheme of putative mechanism for adhesion formation. (reproduced with permission from Holtz G. Prevention and management of peritoneal adhesions. *Fertil Steril.* 1984;41:497–507.)

view the physiology of normal healing. In response to peritoneal injury, there is a release of histamine and vasoactive kinins, leading to an increase in capillary permeability with the subsequent outpouring of serosanguinous fluid. Within 3 hr, this proteinaceous fluid coagulates, thereby producing fibrinous bands, overlying and between abutting surfaces.[2] These fibrinous adhesions become infiltrated by monocytes, plasma cells, polymorphonuclear cells, and histiocytes. The bulk of the fibrin accumulation is transient and these strands are lysed within 72 hr, as a result of endogenous fibrinolytic activity[3] (Fig. 7.1). The denuded area of the peritoneum is then reepithelialized, with healing becoming complete within 21 days (Fig. 7.2). From studies in animals it appears that the majority of these new mesothelial cells arise from the deposition of pluripotential cells floating in the peritoneal fluid or, more likely, from the development from precursor cells located within the subperitoneal connective layer.[4]

## Adhesion Formations

Disruption of the equilibrium between fibrin deposition and fibrinolysis leads to persistence of the fibrinous strands, which then becomes infiltrated by proliferating fibroblasts (Fig. 7.1). Subsequently, vascularization and cellular ingrowth occur and an adhesion is created.[2] Factors that disrupt this equilibrium are those that suppress fibrinolytic activity and/or those that lead to excessive fibrin deposition.

Tissue ischemia is a major factor in the inhibition of fibrinolysis. Ischemia may result from handling, crushing, ligating, suturing, or stripping of the peritoneum. Several investigators have demonstrated that ischemic injury, regardless of the mechanism, resulted in adhesion formation. Additionally, the relationship between adhesion formation and decreased fibrinolytic activity is well established.[2] Ischemia may also induce adhesion formation by stimulating the growth of blood vessels from a nonischemic to an ischemic site. In addition, desiccation of the peritoneal tissue (particularly during lengthy procedures) leads to mesothelial cell desquamation with a resultant raw basement membrane and fibrin deposition,[5] thus also predisposing to adhesion development.

Excessive formation of the fibrin coagulum, which is most commonly a result of foreign body reaction, also results in the development of an adhesion. Talc, when left in the field from surgical gloves, is absorbed by the peritoneal mesothelial cells. These cells then undergo an inflammatory response with subsequent death

FIGURE 7.2. Change in the relative number of cellular elements and fibrinolysis (fibrin) at the site of peritoneal injury in mature rats during the course of re-epithelization. (reproduced with permission from diZerega GS. The peritoneum and its response to surgical injury. In: diZerega GS, Malinak LR, Diamond MP, Linsky CB, eds. *Treatment of Post Surgical Adhesions.* New York: Wiley-Liss; 1990:1–11.)

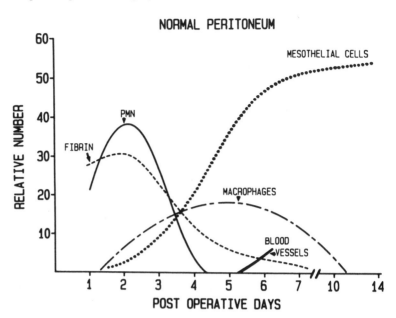

and desquamation. Excessive fibrin disposition occurs and an adhesion is formed. Other common foreign bodies include corn starch powder and lint from drapes, caps, gowns, masks and laparotomy pads, and suture. Suture, in addition to causing tissue ischemia, also acts as a foreign body that instigates adhesion formation.[5]

The presence of intraperitoneal blood has also been proposed to play a role in adhesion formation, although its actual contribution is unclear. The volume of blood, type of blood product used, and the presence or absence of peritoneal injury were demonstrated to influence adhesion formation.[2] Generally free blood in the peritoneal cavity does not lead to adhesions, unless in combination with tissue ischemia.[4]

It is generally believed that the mechanisms responsible for adhesion reformation after surgical adhesiolysis are the same as those responsible for their de novo formation after peritoneal insult, although there are no experimental data to support this theory. Nevertheless, investigators have demonstrated a greater propensity for adhesion reformation than for de novo formation in animals models and clinical trials. This may be due to either a greater extent of tissue damage and hence reduced fibrinolytic activity, or to differences

in the pathogenesis of healing and adhesion formation.[2] Potentially, these differences reflect varying degrees of tissue ischemia, with previously damaged tissue less able to perfuse and fibrinolyse the newly traumatized area.

## Principles of Microsurgery at Laparoscopy

Microsurgical technique was initially applied to the performance of reproductive pelvic surgery by Swolin in 1967.[1] The tenets of operative laparoscopy are similar to those of gynecological microsurgery, and have the objective of preventing or reducing the formation of pelvic adhesions that could compromise the results of the procedure.

The principles of operative laparoscopy are derived from experience at laparotomy. The Trendelenburg position and an adequate pneumoperitoneum displace the bowel from the operating field and aid in proper visualization. A multiple puncture technique is encouraged in order to manipulate pelvic structures properly and maximize the operator's access to the pathology to be treated. Appropriate instruments should be available and adequate surgical assistance, aided by a video monitor or accessory eye piece, is often necessary. The surgical technique should be as atraumatic as possible. Hemostasis is also imperative, and is aided by adequate assistance, visualization, and appropriate instrumentatiOn. Irrigation should be performed continuously, and at the completion of the procedure, in order to remove clots and debris and to detect any persistent bleeding. The use of adhesion reduction adjuvants is also possible. Additionally, the experience of the surgeon is likely to play a role in the successful outcome of operative laparoscopy. This has been demonstrated to be the case at laparotomy, in both an animal model and clinical experience.[2]

A wide variety of procedures performed by the reproductive surgeon at laparotomy can also be performed at laparoscopy. Operative laparoscopy has several undisputed advantages over laparotomy.[6] Procedures performed at laparoscopy are associated with decreased patient morbidity; the patients are often discharged on the day of surgery and return to normal activities within 3 to 5 days, as compared with a 4- to 7-day hospital stay and a 4- to 6-week convalescence period after laparotomy. As a result, there is a concurrent reduction in hospital costs and loss of income secondary to absence from work. In addition, treatment of pathology can be performed at the time of a diagnostic laparoscopy.[7] The issue that remains less clear is the efficacy of procedures performed by operative laparoscopy versus laparotomy.

Intuitively, one would expect that endoscopic surgery is less precise than a formal microsurgical laparotomy; that is, there is a greater chance of injury to adjoining structures and that hemostasis is more difficult to achieve from a distance.[8] On the other hand, during laparoscopic surgery, there is less tissue handling and fewer opportunities for foreign body contamination (i.e., talc, lint, and suture). In addition, desiccation of tissue is far less likely to occur. Animal studies have been performed to assess postoperative adhesion formation subsequent to laparoscopy and laparotomy. In the rat, comparison of postoperative adhesion formation subsequent to standard uterine trauma inflicted at laparoscopy or laparotomy using sharp scissors revealed no significant difference in postoperative adhesion

formation.[9] When a similar study was performed using $CO_2$ laser to inflict a standardized uterine horn incision, Luciano demonstrated that the number of postoperative adhesions was significantly greater in those rabbits who had undergone laparotomy rather than laparoscopy.[8] In addition, Luciano demonstrated that laparotomy, but not laparoscopy, was associated with the formation of de novo adhesions.[8] Diamond and collegueas noted de novo adhesions in greater than 50% of women undergoing laparotomy for microsurgery.[10] Alternatively, in a separate study, Diamond and associates reported that the de novo adhesion formation rate was only 12% following operative laparoscopy.[11] However, the adhesion reformation rate, which occurred to some extent in over 90% of patients, did not differ between laparotomy and operative laparoscopy.[10,11]

One of the tenets of microsurgical techniques is "precise reapproximation of tissue planes."[1] This principle has recently been called into question. Studies in the rat have demonstrated that closure of a laparotomy incision without peritoneal suturing results in fewer adhesions. A large clinical trial has demonstrated no difference in postoperative complications, wound healing, and adhesions to the laparotomy incision, regardless of whether or not the peritoneum was closed.[1] Reduction of adhesions when tissue is not reapproximated may relate to decreased tissue anoxia. Operative laparoscopy is associated with a reduced need and ability to reapproximate peritoneal edges, which may play a factor in reducing postsurgical pelvic adhesions. Clearly, this is an area that requires much future assessment before definite conclusions regarding the value of tissue closure can be determined.

Avoidance of tissue reapproximation by suture has also been applied to pelvic viscera. DeCherney has recommended that the tubal incision after linear salpingostomy for ectopic pregnancy be allowed to close by secondary intention. Meyer and his colleagues examined adhesion formation after ovarian wedge resection with and without reconstruction of the ovary using a polyglactin suture in a rabbit model.[12] Their data support the hypothesis

TABLE 7.1. Classes of adhesion-reduction adjuvants.

Fibrinolytic agents
  Fibrinolysin
  Papain
  Streptokinase
  Urokinase
  Hyaluronidase
  Chymotrysin
  Trypsin
  Pepsin
  Plasminogen activators
Anticoagulants
  Heparin
  Citrates
  Oxalates
Antiinflammatory agents
  Corticosteroids
  Nonsteroidal antiinflammatory agents
  Antihistamines
  Progesterone
  Calcium channel blockers
Antibiotics
  Tetracyclines
  Cephalosporins
Mechanical separation
  Intraabdominal
    Dextran
    Mineral oil
    Silicone
    Povidine
    Vaseline
    Crystalloid solutions
    Carboxymethl cellulose
  Barriers
    Endogenous tissue
      Omental grafts
      Peritoneal grafts
      Bladder strips
      Fetal membranes
    Exogenous material
      Oxidized cellulose
      Oxidized regenerated cellulose
      Polytetrafluoroethylene (PTFE)
      Gelatin
      Rubber sheets
      Metal foils
      Plastic hoods

Modified with permission from Diamond MP, DeCherney AH. Pathogenesis of adhesion formation/reformation: application to reproductive surgery. *Microsurgery*. 1987; 8:103–107.

that the incidence and severity of adhesion formation is increased after suture reapproximation of the ovarian cortex. Given the increased use of endoscopic treatment of ovarian and other adnexal pathology and the inherent difficulty in laparoscopic suture placement, this finding, if confirmed in clinical trials, will have important implications.

The use of the laser has become increasingly popular in reproductive surgery. It has been suggested that the $CO_2$ laser may result in decreased adhesion formation secondary to its ability to make precise incisions, maintain meticulous hemostasis, and reduce tissue handling.[1] Most of the studies using animal models report that postoperative adhesions are formed to the same degree with $CO_2$ laser and electrocautery at laparotomy.[7] Clinical trials performed to date also fail to demonstrate a difference in adhesion formation/reformation at laparotomy using the $CO_2$ laser or electrocautery as assessed by second-look surgery or pregnancy outcome.[1,7] To date, there is little information available on adhesion formation using laser laparoscopy versus other operative laparoscopic techniques.

# Adjuvants for Adhesion Reduction

Despite strict adherence to microsurgical principles, either at laparotomy or laparoscopy, adhesion reformation and de novo adhesion formation commonly occur. This observation, and the need to prevent this occurrence, has led to the development of adjuvants to decrease adhesion formation (Table 7.1). These adjuvants can act at one or more of the stages of adhesion formation: reduction of the initial inflammatory response and subsequent outpouring of sanguinous material, inhibition of the formation of a coagulum from this exudate, stimulation of fibrinolytic activity, mechanical separation of abutting surfaces, and inhibition of fibroblast proliferation.[3]

## Glucocorticoids, Antihistamines, and Nonsteroidal Antiinflammatory Agents

These agents have been used in an attempt to reduce the inflammatory response to peritoneal injury. The corticosteroids are theorized to reduce the inflammatory response by decreasing vascular permeability, stabilizing lysosomes, and inhibiting the synthesis and release of histamines.[2] Additionally, they have been reported to inhibit the proliferation of fibroblasts, although more recent evidence does not support this finding.[3] Small animal studies have demonstrated the efficacy of corticosteroids in adhesion prevention although only when large doses were administered, either before or shortly after the peritoneal injury. Use of steroids in these studies was associated with increased morbidity, including infection and wound disruption. Primate studies failed to confirm the efficacy of corticosteroids in adhesion reduction.[3] Promethazine, an antihistamine, has been reported to inhibit histamine-induced vascular permeability and stabilize lysosomal membranes.[2] Replogle in 1966 described the use of glucocorticoids in conjunction with promethazine as a means to reduce adhesion formation.[13] Other studies have failed to demonstrate a direct benefit of the use of this combination therapy in the prevention of adhesions.[2]

## Nonsteroidal Antiinflammatory Agents

Nonsteroidal antiinflammatory agents (NSAIDs) inhibit prostaglandin synthesis and reportedly decrease vascular permeability and plasmin inhibitors. Oxyphenbutazone has been reported to inhibit adhesion formation in several animal models.[3] Indomethacin has also been demonstrated to reduce intraabdominal adhesions in the rat model. Results of animal investigation using ibuprofen for adhesion prevention are conflicting.[2,3]

## Progesterone

Progesterone has been demonstrated to have antiinflammatory and immunosuppressive activity. It has been reported that adhesion formation is decreased after ovarian wedge resection if the ovary operated on contained a progesterone secreting corpus luteum. Subsequently, it has been shown that intraperitoneal instillation of aqueous progesterone decreased adhesion formation in the guinea pig, although other studies have failed to confirm this finding.[3]

## Calcium Channel Blockers

Calcium channel blocking agents have been demonstrated to protect against cellular injury, inhibit release of vasoactive substances, including histamine and prostaglandins E and F, and prevention of fibroblast penetration into fibrin matrices. In animal studies, Steinleitner and colleagues have demonstrated a reduction of pelvic adhesions after postoperative diltiazem, nifedipine, and verapamil administration.[14] In these studies, administration of the calcium channel antagonist was not associated with any increased morbidity.

## Anticoagulants

Anticoagulants, specifically high-dose heparin given intraperitoneally or systemically, were associated with a decrease in adhesion formation. However, wound disruption and hemorrhage precluded its use. Peritoneal irrigation with heparin solution has not been demonstrated to be effective in adhesion prevention.[2]

## Fibrinolytic Agents

Fibrinolytic agents act to reduce adhesion formation by both a direct effect on the fibrinous mass and by stimulation of plasminogen activator activity.[15] At dosages associated with adhesion reduction, their use has been associated with hemorrhagic complications. At lower dosages, fibrinolytic agents have been proven consistently effective.[2] Plasminogen activator, a serine protease, converts plasminogen to plasmin, which acts as a fibrinolytic agent. Application of plasminogen activator as a gel to abrasions on the rabbit uterine horn decreased the quantity and density of adhesions. In addition, its use after adhesiolysis also resulted in a decrease in adhesions. No wound healing or bleeding complications were noted with any of the dosages used.[16]

## Antibiotic Therapy

Systemic antibiotics, either broad spectrum cephalosporins or tetracyclines, are often given as prophylaxis against postoperative infection and subsequent adhesion formation. There is, however, little to support this practice,[2] which may, in part, be due to the low incidence of postoperative infection during procedures. Peritoneal irrigation with antibiotic-containing solutions (cefazolin and tetracycline) have been shown to result in increased peritoneal adhesion formation in the rat model. Hence, their intraabdominal use is not suggested.

Mechanical separation of pelvic structures is another mechanism by which adhesion formation can be reduced. This class of adjuvants includes abdominal instillates and material barriers.

## High Molecular Weight Dextran [32% Solution of Dextran-70 (Hyskon)]

Dextran-70 is a commonly used adhesion-reducing instillate. It has been suggested that Hyskon acts as a siliconizing agent, coating raw surfaces, and as an osmotic agent, resulting in hydroflotation of pelvic viscera. In addition, there are data that suggest that 32% dextran-70 has immunosuppressive effects in vitro.[3] Much of the literature evaluating the efficacy of 32% dextran in animals demonstrates that its use is associated with a significant decrease in adhesion formation,[3] although it is more efficacious

in preventing adhesion formation than re-formation. The results of large-scale clinical trials evaluating the efficacy of 32% dextran are conflicting.[2] Complications from its use in humans have been reported, including anaphylaxis, pleural effusion, vulvar extravasation, and transient liver function abnormalities.[3]

## Polytetrafluoroethylene

Expanded polytetrafluoroethylene (PTFE or Gore Tex), a mechanical barrier, has been used for several years in vascular and cardiovascular surgery. It has been found to be nonreactive, nontoxic, and antithrombogenic.[16] When formulated as a surgical membrane (0.1 mm thick and < 1 $\mu$m in porosity, which is thinner and less porous than the material used for grafts), it has been shown to reduce adhesion development over a traumatized area. Since PTFE is nonabsorbable it would require removal or to be left in situ permanently.[16]

## Oxidized Regenerated Cellulose Barriers

Oxidized regenerated cellulose was initially developed as a hemostatic material (Surgicel).

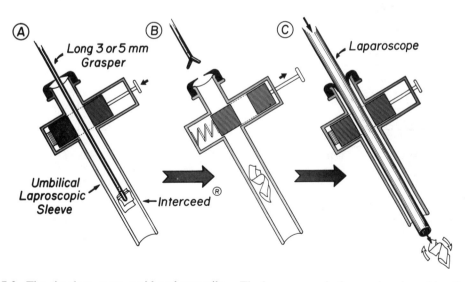

FIGURE 7.3. The simplest, most rapid and versatile technique for the laparoscopic placement of Interceed into the pelvic cavity is illustrated. The laparoscope is withdrawn and the piece (or whole sheet) of fabric is placed directly into the umbilical sleeve, beyond the pressure valve, using a small grasper. The laparoscope is then replaced, pushing the fabric directly into view onto the sigmoid. (reproduced with permission from Azziz R, Murphy AA, Rosenberg SM, Patton Jr GW. Use of an oxidized regenerated cellulose absorbable adhesion barrier at laparoscopy. *J Reprod Med.* 1991;36:479–482.)

Use of this formulation in animals for adhesion prevention was mixed.[16] This prompted modification of the knit, weave, oxidation, and porosity of the fabric to form a new product, Interceed (TC-7), which has been demonstrated to be effective in reducing adhesions in various animal models.[16] Oxidized regenerated cellulose is metabolized into glucose, glucuronic acid, and other oligosaccharides within a short time period (usually 4 days), has not been associated with foreign body reactions, and is easy to handle.[17] It is important to note that the presence of blood diminished the effectiveness of a similar agent, TC-4, in adhesion prevention in the rabbit uterine horn model.[16] Meticulous hemostasis is thus necessary to maximize the efficacy of oxidated regenerated cellulose. In a randomized, multicenter clinical trial of 134 patients, Interceed reduced the incidence, extent, and severity of postsurgical pelvic adhesions, as noted at second-look laparoscopy.[17] Finally, it has been demonstrated that Interceed can easily be placed at the time of laparoscopy[16,18] (Fig. 7.3).

As we can see, there is a wide array of adhesion-reducing adjuvants available to the reproductive surgeon. The results in the literature on the efficacy of these substances are often conflicting. Currently, there is evidence to support the use of Interceed to reduce adhesion formation during gynecological surgery by laparotomy. Other adjuvants, such as plasminogen activator instillation, appear promising but await further evaluation and clinical trials. Nevertheless, the use of adjuvants must not be considered a replacement for meticulous surgical technique.

## Second-Look Laparoscopy

Swolin introduced second-look laparoscopy (SLL) in order to assess the result of certain surgical procedures.[1] As postoperative adhesions are commonly encountered at the time of SLL, the procedure also provides an opportunity to perform adhesiolysis. It is believed that since pelvic adhesive disease plays a role in infertility, lysis of these adhesions may also improve pregnancy rates. Trimbos-Kemper and colleagues performed a "third-look laparoscopy" in patients who had undergone an early second-look procedure with lysis of adhesions at that time. They reported more than half of the adhesions that were separated at the first laparoscopic procedure did not recur.[19] In a smaller group of patients there was a significant reduction in the median adhesion

TABLE 7.2. Pelvic adhesions noted at second-look laparoscopy.

| | Time from inital procedure | Total number of patients | Number with adhesions (%) | Predominant type of adhesion (%) |
|---|---|---|---|---|
| Diamond et al.[20] | 1–12 weeks | 106 | 91 (86) | Filmy (86) |
| DeCherney and Mezer[21] | 4–16 weeks | 20 | 15 (75) | Filmy (80) |
| | 1–3 years | 41 | 31 (76) | Dense (84) |
| Surrey and Friedman[19] | 6–8 weeks | 31 | 22 (71) | Filmy (100) |
| | ≥6 months | 6 | 5 (83) | Dense (100) |
| Pittaway et al.[25] | 4–6 weeks | 23 | 23 (100) | Thick (26) |
| Trimbos-Kemper et al.[18] | 8 days | 188 | 104 (55) | Filmy (NG) |
| Daniell and Pittaway[22] | 4–6 weeks | 25 | 24 (96) | Filmy (76) |
| McLaughlin[23] | 6–12 weeks | 25 | 14 (56) | Filmy (83) |
| Jansen[24] | 1–3 weeks | 73 (no preop adhesion) | 42 (58) | Filmy (NG) |
| | | 183 (preop adhesions present) | 168 (92) | Filmy (NG) |
| Tulandi et al.[26] | 1 year | 36 | 21 (58) | NG |

NG, not given.
Modified with permission from Diamond MP. Surgical aspects of infertility. In: J.J. Sciarra: *Gynecology and Obstetrics.* Philadelphia: Harper and Row; 1988:1–23.

scores at the time of a third-look procedure. Trimbos-Kemper reported a reduction in the incidence of ectopic pregnancies in women who had undergone second-look laparoscopy, although the intrauterine pregnancy rate was unchanged.[19] Surrey and Friedman reported a 52% intrauterine pregnancy rate in 31 patients who had undergone early SLL after reconstructive pelvic surgery. They had no control group, but noted that this pregnancy rate was greater than that in the literature for comparable procedures.[20]

Swolin recommended that the SLL be performed 6 weeks after the initial surgery, to allow treatment of the forming adhesions[1] (Table 7.2). Adhesions found at laparoscopy 1 to 16 weeks after surgery were primarily filmy and avascular,[21-26] when compared with those encountered at laparoscopy 18 months or more after the primary procedure.[22,27] Similarly, it has been noted that bleeding is more commonly encountered if the second-look procedure is performed more than 12 weeks after the initial procedure.[20] Alternatively, it has been suggested that early SLL (i.e., less than 2 weeks after the initial surgery) results in increased bleeding from granulation tissue during adhesiolysis.[1] Other investigators in large series have not encountered this problem.[19] Finally, Diamond et al. have demonstrated that there appears to be no difference in the type of adhesions observed at SLL when laparoscopy is performed within 1 to 12 weeks after the initial procedure.[10] Thus, although it is probable that early SLL reduces postoperative pelvic adhesions, to date no appropriately designed studies to demonstrate its benefit on pregnancy rates in women undergoing infertility surgery have been performed.

# References

1. Diamond MP. Surgical aspects of infertility. In: Sciarra, JJ, ed. *Gynecology and Obstetrics*. Philadelphia: Harper and Row, 1988:1–23.
2. Diamond MP, DeCherney AH. Pathogenesis of adhesion formation/reformation: application to reproductive pelvic surgery. *Microsurgery*. 1987;8:103–107.
3. Holtz G. Prevention and management of peritoneal adhesions. *Fertil Steril*. 1984;41:497–507.
4. diZerega GS. The peritoneum and its response to surgical injury. In; diZerega GS, Malinak LR, Diamond MP, Linsky, CB, eds. *Treatment of Post Surgical Adhesions. Progress in Clinical and Biological Research* Vol. 358. New York: Wiley-Liss, 1989:1–11.
5. Montz FJ, Shimanuki T, DiZerega GS. Postsurgical mesothelial reepithelialization. In: DeCherney AH, Polan ML, eds. *Reproductive Surgery*. Chicago: Year Book Medical Publishers; 1987:31–48.
6. Gomel V. Operative laparoscopy: time for acceptance. *Fertil Steril*. 1989;52:1–11.
7. Diamond MP. Assessment of results of laser surgery. Bailliere's Clin Obstet Gynecol. 1989;3:649–654.
8. Luciano AA, Maier DB, Koch EI, et al. A comparative study of post operative adhesions following laser surgery by laparoscopy versus laparotomy in the rabbit model. *Obstet Gynecol*. 1989;74:220–224.
9. Filmar S, Gomel V, McComb PF. Operative laparoscopy versus open abdominal surgery: a comparative study on post operative adhesion formation in the rat model. *Fertil Steril*. 1987;48:486–489.
10. Diamond MP, Daniell JF, Feste J, et al. Adhesion reformation and de novo adhesion formation after reproductive pelvic surgery. *Fertil steril*. 1987;47:864–866.
11. Diamond MP, Daniell JF, Johns DA, et al. Postoperative adhesion development following operative laparoscopy: evaluation at early second-look procedures. *Fertil Steril*. 1991; 55:700–704.
12. Meyer WR, Grainger DA, DeCherney AH, Lachs MS, Diamond MP. Ovarian surgery in the rabbit: Effect of cortex closure on adhesion formation and ovarian function. *J Reprod Med*. 1991;36:639–643.
13. Reploy le RL, Johnson R, Gross RE. Prevention of postoperative intestinal adhesions with combined promethazine and dexamethasone therapy: experimental and clinical studies. *Ann Surg*. 1996;163:580–588.
14. Steinleitner A, Kazensky C, Lambert H. Calcium channel blockade prevents postsurgical reformation of adnexal adhesions in rabbits. *Obstet Gynecol*. 1989;74:796–798.
15. Doody KJ, Dunn RC, Buttram VC. Recombinant tissue plasminogen activator reduces adhesion formation in a rabbit uterine horn model. *Fertil Steril*. 1989;51:509–512.

16. Seifer DB, Diamond MP, DeCherney AH. An appraisal of barrier agents in the reduction of adhesion formation following surgery. *J Gynecol Surg.* 1990;6:3–9.

17. Diamond MP, Azziz R, Cohen S, et al. Reduction of adhesion reformation following adhesiolysis at laparotomy by Interceed (TC7): final report of the Interceed (TC7) adhesion barrier study group. Abstract, European Society of Human Reproduction and Endocrinology, 1990.

18. Azziz R, Murphy AA, Rosenberg SM, et al. Use of an oxidized, regenerated cellulose absorbable adhesion barrier at laparoscopy. *J Reprod Med.* 1991;36:479–482.

19. Trimbos-Kemper TCM, Trimbos JB, van Hall EV. Adhesion formation after tubal surgery results of the eighth-day laparoscopy in 188 patients. *Fertil Steril.* 1985;43:395–400.

20. Surrey MW, Friedman S. Second-look laparoscopy after reconstructive pelvic surgery for infertility. *J Reprod Med.* 1982;27:658–660.

21. Diamond MP, Daniell JF, Feste J, et al. Pelvic adhesions at early second-look laparoscopy following carbon dioxide laser surgical procedures. *Infertile.* 1984;7:39–44.

22. DeCherney AH, Mezer HC. The nature of post-tuboplasty pelvic adhesions as determined by early and late laparoscopy. *Fertil Steril.* 1984;41:643–646.

23. Daniell JF, Pittaway DE. Short interval second-look laparoscopy after infertility surgery. *J Reprod Med.* 1983;28:281–283.

24. McLaughlin DS. Evaluation of adhesion reformation by early second-look laparoscopy following microlaser ovarian wedge resection. *Fertil Steril.* 1984;42:531–537.

25. Jansen RPS. Early laparoscopy after pelvic operations to prevent adhesions: Safety and efficacy. *Fertil Steril.* 1988;49:26–31.

26. Pittaway DE, Daniell JF, Maxson WS. Ovarian surgery in an infertility patient as an indication for short interval second-look laparoscopy: a preliminary study. *Fertil Steril.* 1986;44:611–614.

27. Tulandi T, Falcone T, Kafka I. Second-look operative laparoscopy 1 year following reproductive surgery. *Fertil Steril.* 1989;52:421–424.

# 8

# Technique and Instrumentation in Operative Laparoscopy

*ANA ALVAREZ MURPHY*

The ability to perform complex operative procedures with the laparoscope is dependent on the skill of the surgeon and the availability of appropriate surgical instruments. In this chapter, we discuss the general instrumentation and technique needed to complete most laparoscopic procedures. Hemostatic techniques (see Chapter 4) and lasers (see Chapter 5) have been discussed. Successful laparoscopy combines the skills of the surgeons, anesthesiologists, and operating room personnel with well chosen and maintained endoscopic instruments and equipment. This team should bring an organized and thought-out approach to the operating room set-up of equipment and instrumentation.

## The Operating Room

Every operating room designed for operative laparoscopy should meet the criteria for a general operating room with full anesthesia, laboratory, blood bank support, and imaging. Major complications are unusual in operative laparoscopy but vascular, urologic, intestinal, and other injuries may occur. Not only must one be skillful enough to recognize the injury, but the capabilities for repair should be available. A sterile laparotomy pack should be available in the operating room before any endoscopic abdominal operation is started.[1]

The laparoscopy cart provides drawers and space for the storage of laparoscopes and instruments as well as the automatic $CO_2$ insufflator, cylinders, electrosurgical unit, cold light source, and suction/irrigation unit. If large enough, the video camera and monitor can also be placed in the cart. Units from the same manufacturer can usually be stacked for more efficient use of space.

## Patient Positioning

The operating table must be able to allow the various patient positions that are essential for gynecologic surgery from supine to lithotomy, including level, Trendelenburg, or reverse and various tilts and heights. It must comfortably and securely support the patient in all these positions. Electrically powered tables meet these requirements best. To optimize the surgeon's mobility and facilitate the positioning of support equipment, the patient's arms are padded and placed at her side rather than extended on lateral arm supports (Fig. 8.1). Leg supports may vary. We prefer stirrups that allow the legs to be in the semiextended position and well supported, such as the Allen's Universal stirrups (Allen Medical Systems Inc., Mayfield, OH) (Fig. 8.2). Additionally, the legs are maintained as flat as possible to maximize the operator's space and mobility of instruments (Fig. 8.1). Careful attention is given to adequate padding to avoid peripheral vascular or nerve injury.[2]

After proper positioning, prepping, and draping, instruments for uterine manipulation and chromotubation are placed. Uterine manipulators are essential to almost all laparoscopic procedures except those in which there is a suspicion of intrauterine pregnancy or gamete intrafallopian transfer is planned.[3] Uterine manipulation facilitates the visualization of pelvic structures and is essential for operative exposure. The most common instruments

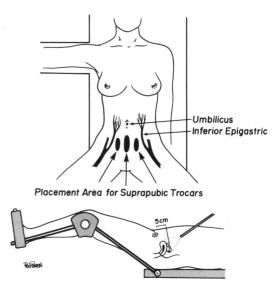

FIGURE 8.1. Proper positioning of the patient for operative laparoscopy includes placing the legs in a frog leg position, with the thighs almost parallel to the longitudinal axis of the body. The left arm (if the operator is right handed) should be tucked alongside the patient's body, since the surgeon usually operates from the patient's left shoulder area. The ancillary sites should be placed as high as possible above the pubis, but no less than 5 cm. Generally, these ports are placed medial to the inferior epigastric artery and vein, taking care to identify these vessels.

available for manipulation and chromotubation include the Cohen olive-tipped cannula, the Hasson balloon uterine elevator, the Harris uterine manipulator-injector, and the Semm vacuum cannula (Fig. 8.3). Many others are available, including the Valtchev, which consists of a head with an intrauterine cannula and a body with a metal bar and tube that pivots on the head.[4] This allows changing the angle of the intrauterine portion of the instruments in relation to the intravaginal portion and anteverts the uterus to a maximum of about 120°. The desired angle can be maintained with a screw.

## Placement of Ancillary Ports

The proper placement of the ancillary ports is of critical importance in reducing the incidence of vascular injuries, in addition to making

FIGURE 8.2. Using the Allen Universal Stirrup (Allen Medical Systems, Inc., Mayfield Heights, OH), the legs are well supported while keeping the knees out of the surgeon's field. (reproduced with permission from Garzo and Murphy.[2])

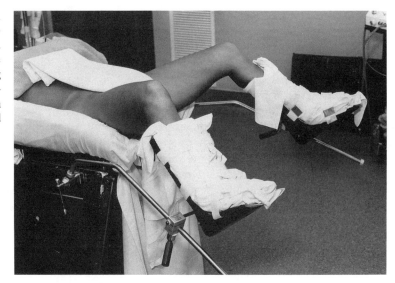

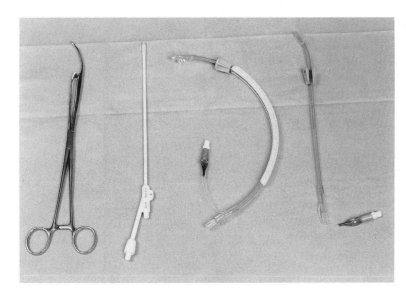

FIGURE 8.3. Uterine elevators and injectors. From left to right: **A:** Hulka tenaculum (Allice tip). **B:** Hasson balloon uterine elevator cannula. **C:** ZSI 4.5-mm uterine manipulator. **D:** ZSI 4.0-mm uterine injector. A and B from Weck-Eder Instrument Co., Chicago IL; C and D from Zinnanti Surgical Instruments, Chatsworth, CA. Gohen olive-tipped or acorn cannula not shown. (reproduced with permission from Garzo and Murphy.[2])

laparoscopic surgery possible. Once the laparoscope has been inserted into the abdominal cavity, the operator must choose the site and number of ancillary ports. Rarely, if ever, should the surgeon attempt to perform a significant operative (even diagnostic) procedure using a single-puncture technique. Usually the first auxiliary site that is placed is a port in the midline suprapubic area. It is extremely important that the surgeon place this puncture as high as cosmetically possible, but never less than 5 cm above the symphysis pubis. This will allow maximum access to the cul de sac and posterior uterus. During placement the bladder should be continuously drained. In the patient who has undergone prior surgery, an attempt should be made to identify the bladder edge laparoscopically, taking care to place the suprapubic puncture cephulad to it. This operator prefers to place a valveless 5-mm sheath at this site in order to facilitate removal of small biopsy specimens.

Once the pelvis has been fully examined, including the appendix and liver edge, a decision must be made as to whether additional suprapubic punctures are needed. Generally it is best to place the next auxiliary port close to the area requiring the greatest amount of surgery. A third puncture site can be added as needed (Fig. 8.1). These additional ports are placed along the suprabic hairline, but there are a few exceptions. The small punctures required for the placement of the laser delivery fiber may be placed slightly more caudally, in order to improve its access to the ovarian fossa and posterior ovarian surface. When performing an appendectomy the third puncture may be placed in the midline, halfway between the umbilicus and the pubis, directed toward the cecum and appendix.

In order to gain the maximum degree of instrument maneuverability, it is important to place the next trocar as far lateral as safely possible, without injuring the inferior epigastric or external iliac vessels (Fig. 8.1). Translumination of the abdomen will occasionally reveal the inferior epigastric vessels, although most often the silhouette seen corresponds to more superficial vessels. To transluminate, the room must be darkened and the laparoscope pressed gently against the abdominal wall. Excessive pressure will decrease vascular perfusion and decrease vessel visibility. An additional method of identifying the inferior epigastric vessels consists of identifying them laparoscopically. The abdominal course of these vessels usually begins just lateral to the insertion of the round ligament, running parallel and lateral to the umbilical ligaments. Generally, the auxiliary ports are placed medial to these vessels, although they may be placed laterally, if needed. In this regard, we recommend that the placement of the suprabic ports always be performed under direct laparoscopic visualization.

# General Laparoscopic Equipment

## Automatic Insufflator

The development of the modern automatic pressure-limited insufflators and the use of $CO_2$ rather than air or $NO_2$ has greatly aided our ability to establish endoscopic access to the peritoneal cavity. The key to safety is our ability to monitor intraabdominal pressure.[5] A useful feature is separate gauges to distinguish true intraabdominal pressure from the total insufflation pressure. Automatic sensors that shut gas off when the intraabdominal pressure reaches 15 to 20 mm Hg can avoid overinflation and compromised venous return. A visual gauge of gas flow is essential at the time of initial insufflation. Most insufflators have a basal flow rate of 1 liter/min with maximum rates of 3 to 9 liters/min. An electronically controlled high-flow mode that maintains the pneumoperitoneum despite gas loss, occurring most frequently during fluid aspiration, instrument changes, and laser plume evacuation, will significantly decrease operating time. The response time to pressure changes should be rapid.

## Light Source

Fiberoptic technology has revolutionized endoscopy. Essentially, it brings in light without the heat generated by the light source. Light is captured from a chamber and carried to the pelvic cavity by a bundle of flexible fibers (see Chapter 3).[6] The amount of light delivered is therefore proportional to the number of intact fibers available for transmission of light. The ability of the surgeon to see is a function of the intensity of the external light source, the quality of the light cord, and the quality of the optics system of the laparoscope. The amount of light required is a function of the object to be viewed. More light is necessary for panoramic views of dark objects, and much less is required for viewing close or light-reflective objects.

A halogen light source (150 W bulb) is sufficient for laparoscopy if video is not used. Light intensity is usually manually adjusted with a rheostat. Light sources for endoscopic photography or video systems provide high intensity light, usually Xenon (300 W), with automatic light intensity control. This is not necessary but very desirable. Additional desirable features in a light source include convenient access to the light bulb and a dual-bulb unit that

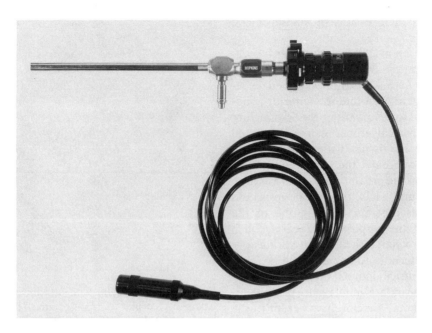

FIGURE 8.4. Video camera attached to 10-mm straight laparoscope (Karl Storz Co., Tutlinger, Germany.)

can switch to a backup in the event of bulb failure.

Cables of different sizes and makes are accommodated by a turret of multiple female couplers. Inspection of fiberoptic light cables should be performed routinely because with use, light-transmitting fibers are lost. The non-functioning cables appear as dark spots when the cable is examined on end. Although more expensive, liquid light cables do not have this problem. See Chapter 3 for additional information.

### Video Imaging

Operative laparoscopy is a team effort. Proper assistance requires that others be able to see what the surgeon is seeing and thereby anticipate his/her needs. The camera used a small, light-weight, high resolution charge-coupled device that is attached to the laparoscope directly or through a beam splitter[3] (Fig. 8.4). A video cassette recorder, preferably with a color hard-copy video printer, should be available. A color monitor of high resolution is necessary, and will permit the surgeon to operate off the screen. This allows for the operator to stand upright, and decreases back strain and eye fatigue. Alternatively, the surgeon may operate by directly visualizing the pelvis through a beam splitter if available. The system will also provide documentation of surgical findings. See Chapter 6 for additional discussion.

## Laparoscopes and Trocars

Pneumoperitoneum is established through insufflation using either a Veress or Touhy needle. The latter is used for epidural anesthesia and is rarely used today. The Veress needle has a blunt inner point that retracts as it penetrates the abdominal wall, springing out to avoid organ puncture when inside the abdominal cavity. A disposable needle is also available.

The umbilical trocar and sheath are inserted after appropriate insufflation has been achieved. Sheaths are available with either a trumpet (piston) or a flapper valve (trap). Trumpet valves decrease the loss of gas with instrument changes but make movement of the instruments up and down the trocar more difficult. Smaller trocar and sleeves are available for the ancillary puncture sites in all the above models.

The trocars are available with either a pyramidal or conical tip. Many surgeons prefer the pyramidal tips because its three sharp edges require less force to perforate the anterior abdominal wall.[7,8] However, using the Z-puncture technique a conical trocar can be inserted through muscular tissues with minimum risk and effort.[9] The greater the force required for trocar insertion the greater the risk of vascular or visceral injury. Thus, the trocar tip should be as sharp as possible. This is one of the advantages of the disposable trocars, which also have a protective sheath that springs out after trocar insertion, to decrease the possibility of further intraabdominal injury. Nevertheless, these trocars are unlikely to prevent injury to organs that are closely adherent to the area of trocar insertion.

Diagnostic and operative laparoscopes are available in a variety of sizes and with different angles (see Chapter 3). Diagnostic or straight laparoscopes are widely used at operative laparoscopy as they provide the most light and field of view for any given size (see Fig. 3.4A). Additionally, many claim insertion of instruments through ancillary sites provides increased depth perception and a wider field of vision.[9]

Operating laparoscopes have a straight channel parallel to the optical axis for the introduction of operating instruments. The most commonly used operating laparoscope is the Jacob-Palmer model, which is offset with two right angles so that the eyepiece is parallel to the axis of the laparoscope (see Fig. 3.4C). The view is identical to that of a straight forward laparoscope. The operating laparoscope can provide a unique angle that at times cannot be achieved with an instrument placed through an ancillary site.[1]

Often, during the course of operative laparoscopic surgery, the surgeon will require both hands to manipulate the suprapubic instruments. In this event an assistant may hold the laparoscope in place, guided by the image on the video monitor. Alternatively, the laparoscopic eyepiece may be attached to a flexible gooseneck device fixed to the operating table.

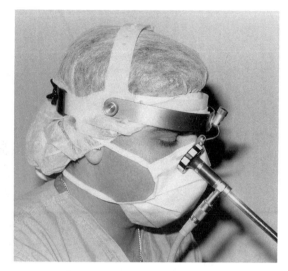

FIGURE 8.5. Headband with attachment for fixing laparoscope ocular to, freeing both of the operators hands (WISAP, Sauerlach, Germany).

A headband with an adapter for the laparoscopic eyepiece, which holds the ocular of the endoscope in the proper position, can also be used (Fig. 8.5).

# Operative Laparoscopic Instruments

In choosing operative laparoscopic equipment the surgeon usually has to select from various vendors. No one company will provide all the instruments needed. Fortunately, despite the number of equipment vendors, the number of manufacturers is limited (and usually located in Europe) so that instruments are usually compatible. Care must be taken not to mix 10-mm and 11-mm or 12-mm instruments, as the 10-mm trocar does not accommodate the larger instruments. Alternatively, the 5-mm suprapubic ports will accommodate 5-mm or 5.5-mm instruments. Following are some of the principal categories of operative laparoscopic instruments.

## For Aspiration and/or Irrigation

Cannulas of different gauges are available for aspiration of cysts and/or injection of saline or

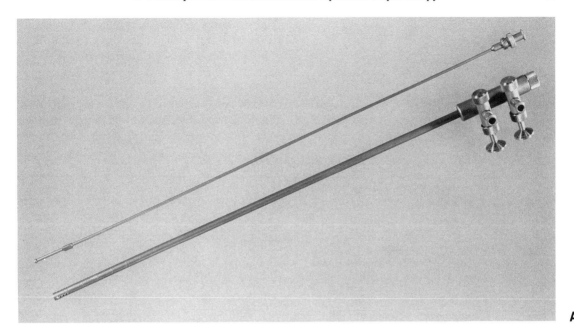

A

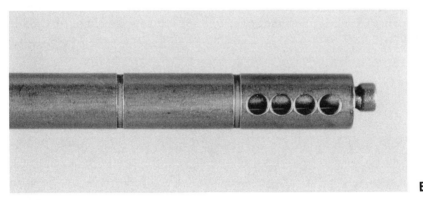

B

FIGURE 8.6. **A:** Nezhat 5-mm suction/irrigation cannula with trumpet valves (*bottom*) and guide for laser fiber placement (*top*). **B:** Tip of aspiration/ irrigation cannula with guide for laser fiber inserted and protruding slightly. (Cabot Medical Corp. Langhorne, PA)

dilute vasopressin. Spinal needles introduced directly through the abdominal wall can serve the same purpose. Small caliber (20- to 22-gauge) needles are preferred for injection of fluid into the pelvic sidewall or adnexa, as there is less leakage from the puncture site.

Large-bore cannulas are used for aspiration and irrigation of the pelvic cavity. Such devices are necessary, for example, to evacuate a hemoperitoneum quickly, remove contents of endometriotic cysts, or remove char during laser surgery. The ability to evacuate a hemo-

peritoneum and identify the source of bleeding during surgery for ectopic pregnancy can make the difference between laparoscopic and laparotomy management of the pregnancy.

Suction cannulas may simply be a valveless tube connected to a 60- or 100-cc syringe. Alternatively, irrigation can be achieved through a similar tube by hooking it up to a bag of intravenous fluid, placed inside a transfusion cuff to increase flow pressure. A Y-connector with a stopcock can regulate which function is performed. The 'Trident' or Cohen cannula

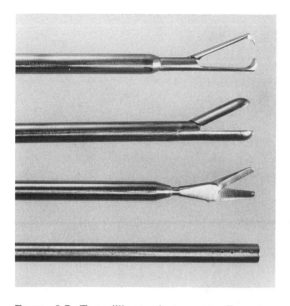

FIGURE 8.7. Ten-millimeter instruments. From top to bottom: **A:** Claw grasper. **B:** Spoon forceps. **C:** Straight scissors, **D:** Suction cannula (all instruments by WISAP, Sauerlach, Germany, with the exception of suction cannula by Reznick Instrument Inc., Skokie, IL).

has a dual valve with stopcocks and a channel for unipolar needle electrode (see Fig. 4.6). This instrument combines irrigation with precise coagulation and is particularly helpful to pinpoint bleeding. Stopcocks, however, can be cumbersome to operate. A variation is the Nezhat suction/irrigation cannula, with an adaptor for the placement of a laser fiber (Fig. 8.6). Because of the 90° angle between the trumpet valve and the shaft of the cannula, blood clots and other debris tend to occlude this device. A straight 10-mm tube connected to wall suction is extremely useful for the evacuation of a hemoperitoneum containing clots (Fig. 8.7).

Automatic units that combine aspiration and irrigation are commercially available and are an essential part of the operative laparoscopy set (Fig. 8.8). Various cannulas are available for use with these automatic aspirator/irrigators, some with interchangeable tips or for use with the unipolar needle or laser fiber (Fig. 8.9). Trumpet valves are easier to use than stopcocks, but their more complex design makes them more vulnerable to malfunction. Cannulas with a single distal opening are more

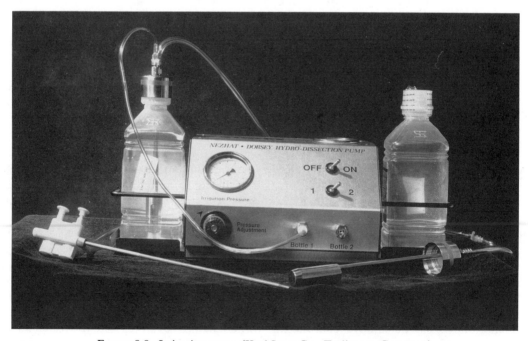

FIGURE 8.8. Irrigation pump (Karl Storz Co., Tutlingen, Germany).

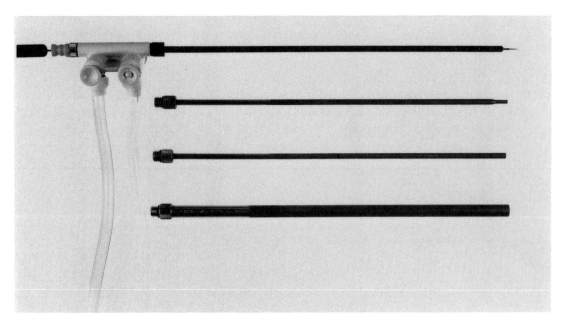

FIGURE 8.9. Different cannulas for aspiration/ irrigation handle. From top to bottom: **A:** Sump tip with microtip unipolar cautery. **B:** Narrow single tip. **C:** Medium single tip. **D:** Large-bore single tip (Karl Storz Co., Tutlingen, Germany).

precise but easily obstructed by clots or tissue. Multiple holes at the suction tip make obstruction and loss of suction less likely. Pneumatic pumps are available that can create dissection planes by instilling fluid at high pressures.

## Probes

Blunt probes are the most often used instruments (Fig. 8.10). They allow adequate visualization of the pelvis and are marked in centimeters in order to estimate size. This is quite useful as the laparoscope may magnify objects, depending on the distance from the object viewed. Some probes are available with tapered ends, in order to examine fallopian tubes with stenotic fimbria (Fig. 8.10). Many other instruments can be used as probes, including closed grasping or biopsy forceps, or an irrigation cannula. However, the blunt probe remains the least traumatic.

## Forceps and Graspers

The ideal graspers hold tissue atraumatically, without significant damage. Such an ideal is

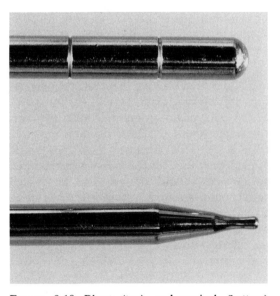

FIGURE 8.10. Blunt (**top**) and conical (**bottom**) probes.

rarely reached. Manipulation of tissue with metal instruments can be very traumatic. One should be careful not to crush tissue by applying excessive force in an attempt to main-

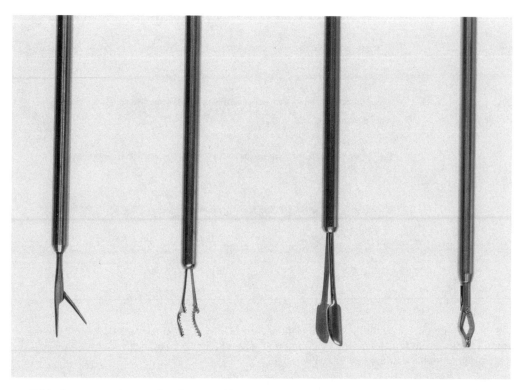

FIGURE 8.11. Laparoscopic grasping forceps. From left to right: **A:** Micrograsping forceps. **B:** Sponge or suturing graspers. **C:** Spatula forceps. **D:** Atraumatic grasper or ampulla dilator. (Karl Storz, Co., Tutlinger, Germany).

tain it in a fixed position. Several grasping forceps are available (Figs. 8.11, 8.12, and 8.13). The ampulla dilator or grasping tongs are most commonly used to dilate phimotic ampulla (Fig. 8.11). The instrument is placed inside the fallopian tube and withdrawn in the open position at various angles. The traditional "atraumatic" grasping forceps is actually quite traumatic (Fig. 8.12) and should not be used, with the possible exception of placement on the utero-ovarian ligament to stabilize the ovary. Thin straight graspers with grooves and no spring are relatively atraumatic yet hold tissue (Fig. 8.11). Particularly useful are the tube and adhesion graspers (Fig. 8.12) manufactured by Karl Storz Co. Hasson has designed a three- and four-pronged grasper with and without teeth (Fig. 8.13).[10] The force applied by the prongs can be controlled and maintained by tightening a screw on the handle.

Large (10-mm or 11-mm diameter) spoon forceps are commonly used to extract tissue from the pelvis (Fig. 8.7), particularly any trophoblast remaining in the cul de sac after ectopic surgery. Large traumatic claw forceps are quite useful to grasp and stabilize tissue that is to be removed, such as myomas or ovaries (Fig. 8.7). The hinged jaws allow large pieces to be grasped. A 5-mm version is available (Fig. 8.12). Biopsy forceps, with a single tooth on each jaw, can be used to remove small biopsies or to fix tissue, such as the cyst wall of an endometrioma during enucleation (Fig. 8.12). The single tooth on each jaw prevents tissue from slipping. If the instrument is to be used to obtain a biopsy, the edges should be kept sharp so that tissue is cut and not avulsed. Hemostasis should be obtained *after* the specimen has been removed to avoid coagulation damage. Often it is easier and more accurate to obtain an incisional biopsy with a scissors or knife.

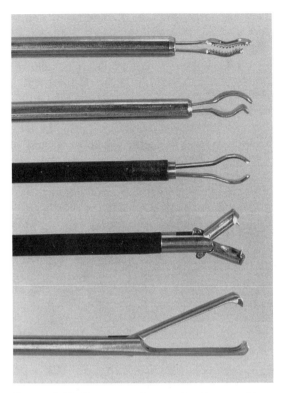

FIGURE 8.12. Laparoscopic grasping forceps. From top to bottom: **A:** Adhesion graspers. **B:** Tube grasper. **C:** "Atraumatic" grasper. **D:** Biopsy forceps. **E:** Claw forceps. (Karl Storz, Co., Tutlinger, Germany).

## Scissors and Scalpels

Scissors are available in many designs that include hook, micro, and serrated (Fig. 8.14). Scissors should be kept sharp or they will avulse rather than cut tissue. Microsurgical dissections may be performed using the microscissors, which are very versatile and quite useful, when sharp. However, they tend to lose their edge quickly and need constant attention. Hook scissors can be used for much the same purpose, as well as for cutting tissue and suture. The serrated scissors (either 5-mm or 10-mm diameter) are not often used as they have little advantage over the above designs and tend to avulse tissue and dull quickly. Disposable scissors have the advantage of being always sharp and for this reason may acquire popularity. Some scissors and scalpels have an insulated shaft, and can be connected to unipolar current for electrocoagulation. The combination of electrocoagulation with cold cutting may be useful for adhesiolysis of vascularized adhesions.

## Morcellator

Removal of large pieces of tissue from the abdomen at laparoscopy can be bothersome and time consuming. Tissue may be cut into

FIGURE 8.13. Hasson three-prong (Bulldog) forceps (Weck-Eder Instrument Co. Chicago, IL). (Reproduced with permission from Garzo and Murphy.[2])

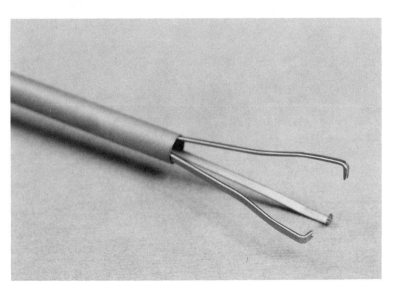

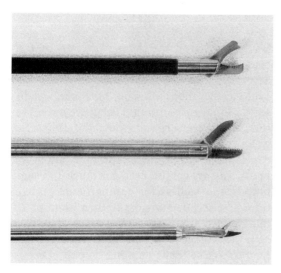

FIGURE 8.14. Laparoscopic scissors. From top to bottom: **A:** Hook, insulated for unipolar cautery. **B:** Straight serrated. **C:** Micro (top by Richard Wolf Medical Instruments Corp., Rosemont, IL; bottom two by WISAP, Sauerlach, Germany).

pieces no larger than the diameter of the puncture site and removed through a 5-mm or 10-mm sleeve with grasping forceps. Alternatively, a suprapubic ancillary puncture site may be enlarged for removal of tissue. If the tissue is difficult to cut or if it should be removed intact, such as an ovary with a possible cancer, a posterior colpotomy incision can be made. This incision may be performed laparoscopically or transvaginally.

A 10- or 11-mm punch biopsy instrument with a storage sheath, the morcellator, may also be useful (Fig. 8.15). When the sheath is full, the instrument is emptied and the morcellation continues. This instrument is particularly effective for the removal of ovaries or small fibroids, although it is much less useful for very fibrotic or calcified fibroids, and for very soft tissues, such as the tube. The manual morcellator is tiring and time consuming. An automated morcellator is now available.

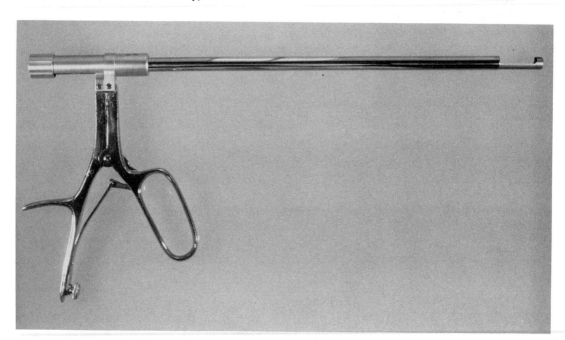

FIGURE 8.15. Morcellator, 10 mm in diameter (WISAP, Sauerlach, Germany).

## Instruments for Enlargement of the Ancillary Site

Enlargement of the size of the ancillary puncture site can be achieved by two methods. The smaller trocar can be withdrawn and a larger one inserted through the previous incision, after enlarging the skin incision. An attempt is made to introduce the trocar through the previous tract to the peritoneum. This can be accomplished only occasionally. Semm has described an alternate method using a dilatation set. A dilator rod is first inserted into the smaller sleeve, which is then withdrawn and replaced with a larger sleeve, which has a screw tip.[9]

## Summary

Although a vast array of equipment is available for gynecologic operative laparoscopy, more innovative instruments need to be designed that more effectively and efficiently allow us to achieve our surgical goals. With proper instrumentation, operative laparoscopy will become less surgical "gymnastics." The recent explosion of operative laparoscopy for the general surgeon will hopefully generate more interest in instrument development.

## References

1. Murphy AA. Operative laparoscopy. *Fertil Steril.* 1987;47:1–18.
2. Garzo VG, Murphy AA. Operative laparoscopy instrumentation. *Semin Reprod Endocrinol.* 1991;9:109–116.
3. Boyers SP. Operating room setup and instrumentation. In: Diamond MP, ed. *Clinical Obstetrics and Gynecology—Pelviscopy.* Philadelphia: Lippincott; 1991:373–386.
4. Valtchev KL, Papsin FR. A new uterine manipulator. *Am J Obstet Gynecol.* 1977;127:738–740.
5. Murphy AA. Diagnostic and operative laparoscopy. In: Thompson JD, Rock JA, eds. *TeLinde's Operative Gynecology.* Baltimore: Lippincott; 1991:361–384.
6. Quint RH. Physics of light and image transmission. In: Phillips JM, ed. *Laparoscopy.* Baltimore: Williams and Wilkins; 1977:18–25.
7. Gomel V, Taylor PJ, Yuzpe AA, Rioux JE. *Laparoscopy and Hysteroscopy in Gynecologic Practice.* Chicago: Year Book Medical Publishers, 1986:1–21.
8. Borten M. *Laparoscopic Complications: Prevention and Management.* Toronto: Decker; 1986:1–414.
9. Semm R. *Operative Manual for Endoscopic Abdominal Surgery.* Chicago: Year Book Medical Publishers; 1984:1–484.
10. Hasson HM. Ovarian surgery. In: Sanfilippo JS, Levine RL, eds. *Operative Gynecologic Endoscopy.* New York: Springer–Verlag; 1989:19–37.

# 9

# Laparoscopic Treatment of Ectopic Pregnancies

*ANA ALVAREZ MURPHY, ARLENE MORALES, and CHARLES W. NAGER*

The incidence of ectopic pregnancies has increased fourfold since 1970.[1] Early diagnosis and treatment has reduced mortality and morbidity, and probably improved subsequent fertility. Advances in ultrasound, particularly transvaginal imaging, and human chorionic gonadotropin (hCG) detection have considerably improved our diagnostic capability. Laparoscopy is an integral part of the diagnostic scheme and recently has become the preferred surgical therapeutic method. Depending on the patient's desire for future fertility and extent of disease, conservative as well as radical surgery may be performed laparoscopically.

## Diagnosis of Ectopic Pregnancies

If an ectopic pregnancy is diagnosed early, it can usually be treated before significant tubal destruction and hemorrhage occur. Those patients with significant risk factors, including previous pelvic inflammatory disease, tubal surgery, or history of ectopic pregnancy, should be screened early in the course of pregnancy with serial serum $\beta$-hCG measurements and transvaginal ultrasounds to confirm the intrauterine location of the gestation. Patients of childbearing age who present with pelvic pain or abnormal vaginal bleeding should be screened with a rapid and sensitive monoclonal antibody urine hCG test. With test sensitivity currently averaging 20 mIU/ml, the false negative rate is about 1%.[2,3] In a hemodynamically unstable and symptomatic patient with a positive urine pregnancy test and a positive culdocentesis for free-flowing nonclotting blood, one should proceed directly to laparotomy or laparoscopy, depending on the skill and experience of the surgeon. In the hemodynamically stable patient with a positive $\beta$-hCG and pelvic pain, a transvaginal sonogram should be performed to evaluate the uterine and adnexal structures initially. If an intrauterine sac is not seen and a complex adnexal mass is noted on sonography, the patient is taken to laparoscopy, since this clinical picture is highly predictive of an ectopic pregnancy.

Alternatively, patients suspected of having an ectopic pregnancy but who are pain free and do not demonstrate a gestational sac or complex adnexal structure by sonogram may be followed carefully with serial quantitated serum $\beta$-hCG measurements. Laparoscopy is usually indicated if the initial $\beta$-hCG is above 2000 mIU/ml and no intrauterine sac is seen on transvaginal sonogram.[4-6] Transvaginal sonography can image a 3-mm intrauterine gestational sac, generally correlated to serum $\beta$-hCG levels as low as 1000 to 2000 mIU/ml (by the IRP standard). If the initial $\beta$-hCG is below 2000 mIU/ml, the differential diagnosis includes an early intrauterine or ectopic pregnancy, and the $\beta$-hCG level is repeated in 48 hr. Normally, at least a 66% rise in $\beta$-hCG levels is observed if a normal intrauterine pregnancy is present. An abnormal increase, plateau, or decrease in the quantitated pregnancy test denotes an abnormal gestation—either a spontaneous abortion or an ectopic pregnancy. A dilatation and curettage (D&C) may be performed to detect the presence of intrauterine chorionic villi, either grossly (e.g., by flotation of the specimen in sterile water) or on frozen/permanent section. If no villi are found at D&C, laparoscopy is recommended unless the clinical setting is highly suggestive of a complete spontaneous abortion or the $\beta$-hCG levels continue to fall toward negative. With this algorithm most ectopic pregnancies can be diagnosed early, minimizing tubal damage and patient morbidity. The most common initial differential diagnosis that may be mistaken for an ectopic pregnancy is a threatened abortion. The most common differential diagnosis when the ultrasound shows an adnexal mass is an intrauterine pregnancy with a bleeding corpus luteum cyst(s).

# Patient Selection and Prerequisites for Laparoscopic Surgery

In order to perform laparoscopic surgery safely for ectopic pregnancy, one must have a skilled surgeon, an appropriately selected patient, and the appropriate instrumentation. The most important requirement for the laparoscopic treatment of ectopics is surgical experience. As laparoscopic surgery involving small ectopic pregnancies are relatively easy to perform, many surgeons begin their training treating these pregnancies, which is quite appropriate in the stable patient as long as an experienced surgeon is on hand to supervise. However, it is inappropriate for a novice to operate on a hemodynamically unstable patient.

Contraindications to laparoscopic treatment, particularly in regard to size and location of the ectopic, are relative depending on the experience and skill of the surgeon. Nevertheless, an intramural ectopic may be more difficult to manage than an isthmic or ampullary tubal pregnancy. Although excessive size of the pregnancy has been mentioned as a relative contraindication, this depends more on the surgeon's ability to identify the pelvic anatomy clearly. Furthermore, the extent of the preoperative intraabdominal bleeding does not usually offer much of a problem, unless the patient is hemodynamically unstable. Reich and colleagues reported on the laparoscopic treatment of 109 ectopic pregnancies.[7] Sixteen were ruptured, three had unstable vital signs, and three were interstitial. There were no intraoperative complications and no laparotomies were performed.

# Instrumentation

Many operative laparoscopic instruments are available for the treatment of ectopic pregnancies.[8] However, a few specific instruments are key. An aspirator/irrigator is helpful in evacuating a hemoperitoneum quickly and effectively. The aspirator may also be attached directly to wall suction. It must also be able to irrigate large volumes of fluid rapidly to assure good visualization and to remove any remaining trophoblast from the pelvis. In addition, a 10-mm suction cannula, connected to wall suction, may be helpful in evacuating clotted blood.

Hemostasis of the operative site may be achieved using various modalities including ligature, electrocautery, thermocoagulation, or laser energy.[9] However, it is a good precaution always to have a bipolar coagulator available, as this instrument can achieve hemostasis quickly, safely, and effectively. In general, lasers, particularly $CO_2$, provide precise cutting but poor coagulation. Both traumatic and atraumatic forceps should be available. Additionally, methods of removing the resected tissue should be considered before surgery and the appropriate instruments obtained.

# Surgical Technique

The patient should have general anesthesia with good muscle relaxation and be placed in the dorsal lithotomy position with the buttocks protruding from the table. As outlined in the Diagnosis section, a D&C may be performed first, and the tissue examined grossly or sent for frozen section. Otherwise the uterus should not be instrumented if there is the possibility of a viable intrauterine gestation, and the patient desires preservation of the pregnancy. Once the diagnosis of an ectopic pregnancy is made at laparoscopy, a rigid metal or plastic cannula may be placed in the cervical so for manipulation. Video monitoring of the procedure is helpful for teaching purposes and to maximize assistant involvement. A straight 10- or 11-mm laparoscope is preferred, although an operating laparoscope can be used. Ancillary puncture sites are placed cephalad to the uterus, and generally in the midline and lateral on the side of the ectopic pregnancy. Most often only two ancillary sites are needed, although occasionally a third puncture site may be required.[5]

# Total Salpingectomy

The treatment of choice for an ectopic pregnancy when preservation of fertility is not an issue, is a total salpingectomy. Additionally, if the tube has been markedly destroyed by the ectopic or prior tubal disease, a conservative procedure may not be possible or advisable.[9]

A salpingectomy may be performed by successive coagulation and cutting of the mesosalpinx. Cautery can be achieved with unipolar and bipolar electrocoagulation or thermocoagulation. Cutting is usually performed using hook scissors (Fig. 9.1). The tubal isthmus proximal to the ectopic is coagulated before transection. Serial cautery of the mesosalpinx can begin either at the fimbriated end of the tube or proximal to the ectopic pregnancy. Surgical ease determines in which direction dissection proceeds. Right-handed surgeons usually find it easier to operate from right to left. Care must be taken to coagulate and cut the mesosalpinx as close to the fallopian tube as possible to avoid excessive damage to the ovary and its blood supply. The excised portion of the tube can then be removed through an enlarged ancillary puncture site using a 10-mm claw forceps or through the channel of an operating laparoscope with a 5-mm grasping forceps. As in all laparoscopic procedures for ectopics, care must be taken not to leave trophoblastic tissue behind, since peritoneal implantation and persistent hCG activity may be observed. Extensive irrigation and aspiration are useful in removing any remaining gestational tissue.

Salpingectomy may also be performed using loop ligatures (Endoloop, Ethicon Co., Somerville, NJ). Three loops are placed proximal to the ectopic pregnancy and the tube transected (Fig. 9.2). However, the distal mesosalpinx may need to be coagulated partially and cut to minimize the amount of tube left behind.

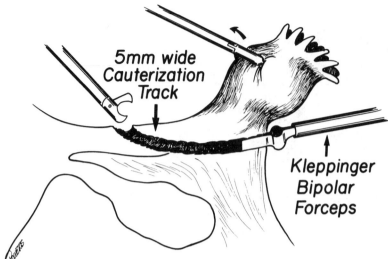

5mm wide
Cauterization
Track

Kleppinger
Bipolar
Forceps

FIGURE 9.1. Salpingectomy can be performed by successive coagulation (with either electrocautery or thermocoagulation) and cutting of the mesosalpinx. The proximal tube is coagulated and transected.

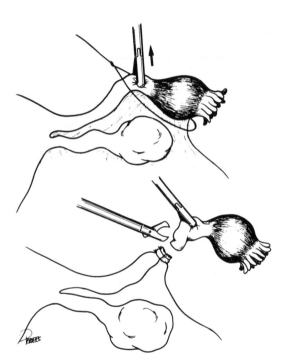

FIGURE 9.2. Salpingectomy can be performed using loop ligation. Three loops are placed proximal to the ectopic pregnancy and the tube is transected. Occasionally, the distal mesosalpinx needs to be dissected to allow sufficiently proximal placement of the loop.

## Conservative Procedures

For patients desirous of further childbearing, it is appropriate to offer a conservative procedure. Sherman et al. suggest that conservation of a tube with an ectopic pregnancy, when coexistent sterility factors are present, is associated with an increased subsequent pregnancy rate (76% vs. 44%).[10] The risk of recurrent ectopic pregnancy appears to be minimally increased in patients undergoing a conservative procedure. Tulandi and Guralnick have noted that the repeat ectopic pregnancy rate approximately doubles in patients after conservative surgery for an ectopic pregnancy, and the patient must be carefully counselled in this regard.[11] Furthermore, before surgery patients must be advised about the possibility of persistent trophoblast, which may require additional surgical or medical therapy. All patients undergoing a conservative surgical procedure must have a quantitated β-hCG level checked postoperatively on a weekly basis, until negative. Patients undergoing conservative tubal surgery for an ectopic pregnancy must be reliable and able to return for their serial β-hCG measurements.

## Linear Salpingostomy/Salpingotomy

Unruptured and selected ruptured isthmic and ampullary ectopic pregnancies may be treated with linear salpingostomy. In the study by Pauerstein and colleagues,[12] 67% of ectopics were located within the tubal lumen while the remaining were extraluminal or mixed (Fig. 9.3). Thus, in approximately one-third of cases the tubal lumen may be intact at the time of salpingostomy/salpingotomy.

In the past, all isthmic ectopic pregnancies were treated by segmental resection rather than linear salpingostomy. However, we believe that in those patients with an unruptured isthmic ectopic pregnancy desiring conservative surgery, a linear salpingostomy should be attempted first. If bleeding is significant a segmental resection (see below) is then performed. It is quite possible that the treatment of isthmic ectopics with methotrexate therapy may eventually prove to result in the least morbidity and the highest tubal conservation and patency rates.

A linear incision is made with either a unipolar needle cautery or laser along the antimesenteric side of the tube dilated by the ectopic (Fig. 9.4). Alternatively, the ectopic can be opened using a knife or scissors. The incision site can be coagulated with electrocautery or thermocoagulation before incision if desired. One method of coagulating the antimesenteric aspect of the ectopic is to glide the slightly separated paddles of a Kleppinger bipolar forceps over the surface of the tube (Fig. 9.5). Heat generated by current arcing between the paddles coagulates the surface of the tube. The mesosalpingeal vessels beneath the site of the ectopic can be gently coagulated before performing the linear salpingostomy/salpingotomy.

Some surgeons use dilute vasopressin solution to minimize bleeding from the operative site. Concentrations of vasopressin (Pitressin) ranging from 0.05[13] to 2.0[14] units/ml can be injected into the mesosalpinx just below the ectopic, using a 20- or 22-gauge spinal needle placed through the abdominal wall. This may decrease bleeding not only from the incision but from the bed of the ectopic as well. Alternatively, the vasopressin solution may be injected directly over the area to be incised.

Upon incision, the ectopic usually extrudes and can be gently removed with forceps or aspiration. Care must be taken not to damage normal tubal mucosa unnecessarily, in an overzealous attempt to remove any remaining trophoblast. Occasionally it is helpful to irrigate the lumen forcefully through the antimesenteric incision, as this may dissect the ectopic gestation from the tubal wall and facilitate removal. The implantation site is observed closely for bleeding and any remaining trophoblastic tissue. With small early ectopic pregnancies one may encounter deep infiltration of trophoblast into the tubal wall resulting in persistent bleeding. Irrigation and coagulation with needle-point cautery or bipolar may be necessary. Coagulation of mesosalpingeal vessels supplying that portion of fallopian tube may also be necessary. More simply, pressure on the surgical site can be applied using a grasper. If the blood loss cannot be stopped with these maneuvers a segmental resection or partial salpingectomy may need to be performed.

The tubal incision is usually not closed. Fistula formation at the incision site is a possible complication, but does not appear to be common. If the defect appears to be very large or marked eversion of the mucosa is seen, an interrupted suture of 4-0 PDS may be placed using the intraabdominal tying techniques previously described. After conservative surgery by laparotomy, Tulandi and Guralnick[11] observed that pregnancies occur sooner after salpingostomy without tubal suturing than those where tubal suturing is performed.

### Segmental Resection

In the patient with a ruptured isthmic or ampullary ectopic pregnancy who desires conservative surgery, segmental resection with subsequent reanastomosis may be the only choice. Segmental resection is reserved for ruptured ectopic pregnancies depending on the extent of tubal damage and, rarely, a failed isthmic or ampullary salpingostomy.

Segmental resection may be accomplished with electrocautery, thermocoagulation, laser, or loop ligature. Coagulation of the tube both proximal and distal to the ectopic is accom-

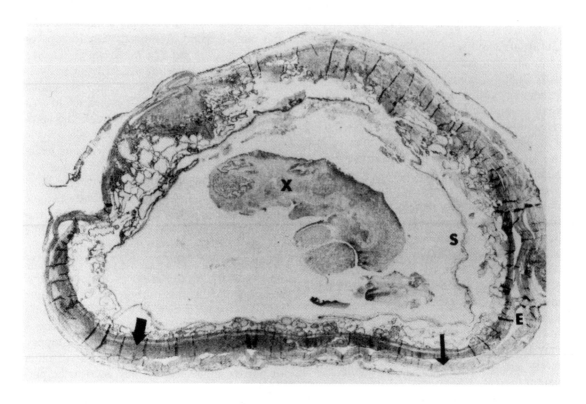

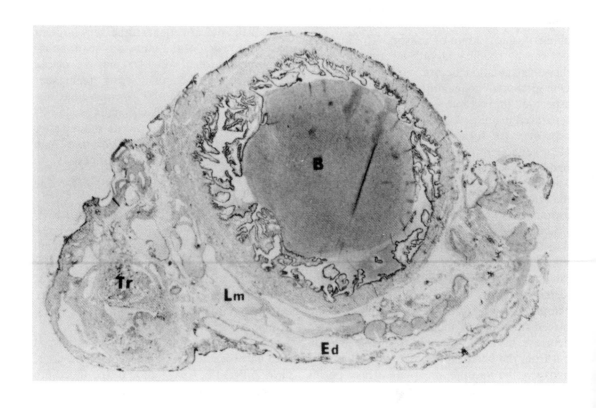

FIGURE 9.4. Laparoscopic linear salpingostomy. A linear incision is made along the antimesenteric border of the tube over the ectopic pregnancy, using KTP, Argon or $CO_2$ laser, or unipolar needle cautery. The ectopic usually extrudes from the tube and is gently removed with adhesion or biopsy forceps.

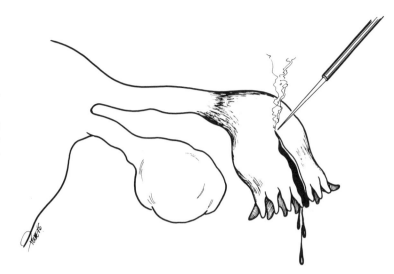

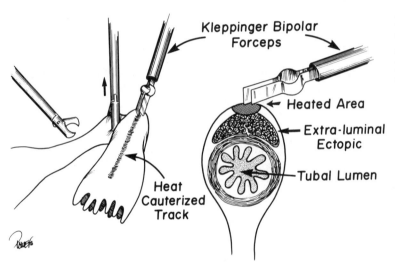

FIGURE 9.5. Laparoscopic linear salpingostomy using bipolar cautery. The slightly separated paddles of the Kleppinger forceps are run over the antimesenteric aspect of the ectopic pregnancy. Cauterization of a narrow track of tubal surface is obtained by the heat generated by the electricity arching between the paddles, and minimally by the electron flow through the tissue, thus reducing peripheral damage.

plished and the tube is then transected. The mesosalpinx just below the ectopic is successively coagulated and cut (Fig. 9.6). The procedure is facilitated by applying gentle traction to the segment of ectopic-containing tube to be removed. Upon complete transection, the mesosalpinx is inspected carefully and all bleeding points coagulated.

A variation of the Pomeroy technique for tubal sterilization may be used. The site of the ectopic pregnancy is placed under traction and an Endoloop is placed around its base. The ligated tubal segment containing the ectopic pregnancy is then transected and removed. Unfortunately, this technique results in a large amount of tubal destruction. Nevertheless, it is

FIGURE 9.3. **Top:** Intraluminal ectopic pregnancy (X, embryo; S, gestational sac; E, endosalpinx; thick arrow, maternal blood within lumen interspersed with chorionic villi; thin arrow, myosalpinx). **Bottom:** Extraluminal ectopic pregnancy. (B, maternal blood in lumen; Lm, lymphatic dilatation; Ed, stromal edema; Tr, trophoblastic tissue). (Reprinted with permission from Pauerstein CJ. Anatomy and pathology of tubal pregnancy. *Obstet Gynecol.* 1986;67:301–308.)

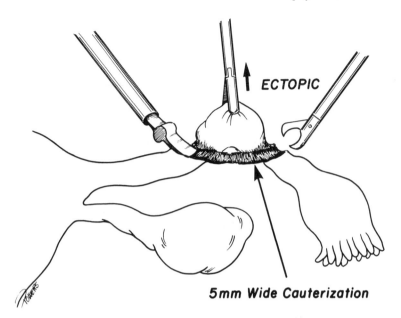

ECTOPIC

5mm Wide Cauterization

FIGURE 9.6. Laparoscopic segmental resection. The normal fallopian tube on either side of the ectopic pregnancy is coagulated and transected. The mesosalpinx below the ectopic is coagulated and cut.

quick and easy to perform, particularly when tubal bleeding is brisk.

A variation of the cautery method of sterilization has also been used. The segment of tube containing the ectopic pregnancy is thoroughly coagulated with electrocautery or thermocoagulation. Obviously, the segment of tube is destroyed and no specimen can be sent to pathology. Furthermore, a significant portion of tube may be damaged. The potential for fertility remains after anastomosis at a later date. Nevertheless, this technique is rarely used and can hardly be recommended.

## Ovarian Ectopic Pregnancy

Although ovarian pregnancies are rare, most can be treated through the laparoscope. An attempt should be made to excise the ectopic with either lasers or unipolar needle cautery if normal ovary can be discerned. After dissection, the ovary is carefully inspected to assure good hemostasis and complete removal of trophoblastic tissue. The ovarian defect is not closed. If the ectopic gestation encompasses the entire ovary and normal ovary cannot be discerned, an oophorectomy is performed (see Chapter 12). Since the ovarian vascularity is increased, this type of laparoscopic surgery should be performed only by an experienced surgeon.

## Interstitial Ectopic Pregnancy

Interstitial or cornual ectopic pregnancies may be attempted through the laparoscope, depending on size and experience of the surgeon. The fallopian tube is transected distal to the ectopic pregnancy and dissection of the mesosalpinx is extended toward the uterus. Dissection into the myometrium is performed with cautery or fiber laser. The myometrium may be infiltrated with Pitressin before dissection.

## Removal of Resected Tissue

Removal of the products of conception or resected fallopian tube can, on occasion, be extremely tedious. Small pieces of tissue can be removed through the ancillary 5-mm puncture sites. Larger pieces of tissue may be removed through an ancillary 10-mm site. Alternatively, forceps may be introduced through the instrument channel of an operating laparoscope, and the tissue grasped and brought out through the sleeve. Holding the trumpet valve open, the laparoscope and grasped tissue is completely removed. If the fallopian tube or gestational products are larger than 10 mm in diameter, relaxing incisions may be made into the specimen with scissors to decrease its size and allow removal through the 10- to 12-mm trocar in one piece. Alternatively, the tissue may be cut into pieces no larger than 10 mm in diameter. Removal may also be achieved by mincing the tissue using a 10-mm morcellator or by extracting intact tissue using a uterine polyp forceps introduced directly through the suprapubic site. Rarely is it necessary to perform a posterior colpotomy to remove a fallopian tube. When removing the specimen containing the ectopic great care must be taken not to spill trophoblast. After removal, thorough aspiration and irrigation or forceps may be used to remove any remaining tissue.

## Medical Therapy

Medical or nonsurgical treatment of ectopic pregnancies is acquiring increasing importance. Unfortunately, the need for laparoscopic diagnosis encourages a surgical solution to the problem. Nevertheless, methotrexate therapy may be considered in the following circumstances:

1. in a patient whose D&C does not reveal trophoblasts, but with persistent or rising $\beta$-hCG levels
2. when an ectopic is present in a tube that is severely adhered and difficult to dissect free
3. when an unruptured isthmic ectopic pregnancy is encountered
4. in patients who are poor surgical candidates and are at high risk for having an ectopic
5. in patients with persistent ectopics after surgical treatment (see below)

One of the regimens for the treatment of an ectopic pregnancy is the administration of 1 mg/kg methotrexate intramuscularly (IM) alternating with citrovorum (0.1 mg/kg).[15] This is continued until there is a 15% or greater decrease in two consecutive daily $\beta$-hCG titers. No more than four cycles are given without a drug-free interval of 1 week. An alternative protocol advises a single dose of 50 mg/m$^2$ methotrexate IM without citrovorum rescue injections.[16] Another regimen is the administration of oral methotrexate 0.3 mg/kg for 4 days, in a single daily dose that should not exceed 25 mg per 24 hr.[17] Side effects are minimal and the treatment is outpatient. A quantitative $\beta$-hCG, liver functions, blood urea nitrogen (BUN), creatinine, complete blood count (CBC) and differential, are obtained before and 1 week after treatment. Ectopics containing an embryo with fetal heart tones or with $\beta$-hCG levels greater than 10,000 mIU/mL do not appear to respond as well to these protocols as smaller gestations.

## Complications

The most common complication specific to the laparoscopic treatment of ectopic pregnancy is hemorrhage. Pregnancy increases the vascularity of these tissues and blood loss may be significant. If excessive intraoperative bleeding is encountered, coagulation can be performed with electrocautery, laser, thermocoagulation, vasopressin injection, or application of direct pressure. If the hemorrhage becomes uncontrollable by laparoscopic methods, a laparotomy should be performed. Other complications include damage to adjacent structures, particularly when there are dense adhesions present.

As previously discussed, trophoblastic tissue may persist as the result of any conservative procedure for ectopic pregnancy. All patients undergoing a conservative procedure should be followed with $\beta$-hCG levels until the titer is negative. Patients with persistent ectopics tend to have an initial decline in $\beta$-hCG and progesterone levels 3 to 6 days after surgery, with a subsequent rise or plateau in these levels.[18] Persistent trophoblastic tissue may be treated surgically with either a repeat laparoscopy or laparotomy. Nevertheless, persistent $\beta$-hCG levels do not mandate a total salpingectomy, and a segmental resection usually suffices.

However, the treatment of choice today for patients with persistent ectopic pregnancy is methotrexate therapy. Rarely do these patients require more than one course of therapy.

## Results

Shapiro and Adler performed the first surgery for ectopic pregnancy through the laparoscope in 1973.[19] Since then multiple studies have attested to the feasibility and safety of laparoscopic surgery for ectopic pregnancy. In the 1980s, large series by Pouly and colleagues,[20]

Mecke and colleagues,[13] and Reich and colleagues[7] found that subsequent pregnancy rates were historically comparable to laparotomy. Pouly and colleagues[20] in a series of 321 patients treated laparoscopically reported a 57% intrauterine pregnancy rate, a 22% recurrent ectopic pregnancy rate, and a 4.8% persistence rate. DiMarchi and colleagues[21] also reported a persistent ectopic pregnancy rate of 4.8%, however, a 20% persistence rate has been reported in a small series.[13] Most studies note postoperative intrauterine pregnancy rates between 45% and 65%.[5] Overall, repeat ectopic rates range from 5% to 30%, with an average of approximately 15%.

The benefits of laparoscopy versus laparotomy are evident (see Chapter 1). Case control studies by Brumsted and colleagues[22] and randomized prospective studies by Vermesh and colleagues[23] and Nager and colleagues[24] demonstrated that laparoscopic therapy for the treatment of ectopic pregnancies has significantly reduced the hospital stay and cost, and delay to normal activity. In most cases, laparoscopy should replace laparotomy for the surgical treatment of ectopic pregnancies.

# References

1. Centers for Disease Control. Ectopic pregnancy: United States, 1987. *MMWR*. 1990;39:24–25.

2. Norman RJ, Buck RH, Rom L, Joubert S. Blood and urine measurement of human chorionic gonadotropin for detection of ectopic pregnancy? A comparative study of quantitative methods in both fluids. *Obstet Gynecol*. 1988;71:315–318.

3. Romero R, Kadar N, Copel JA, Jeanty P, DeCherney AH, Hobbins JC. The effect of different human chorionic gonadotropin assay sensitivity on screening for ectopic pregnancy. *Am J Obstet Gynecol*. 1985;153:72–78.

4. Fossum GT, Davajan V, Kletzky OA. Early detection of pregnancy with transvaginal ultrasound. *Fertil Steril*. 1988;49:788–790.

5. Bateman BG, Nunley Jr WC, Kolp LA, Kitchen III JD, Felder R. Vaginal sonography findings and hCG dynamics of early intrauterine and tubal pregnancies. *Obstet Gynecol*. 1990; 75:421–426.

6. Bree RL, Edwards M, Bohm-Velez M, Beyler S, Roberts J, Mendelson EB. Transvaginal sonography in the evaluation of normal early pregnancy: correlation with hCG level. *Am J Radiol*. 1989;153:75–82.

7. Reich H, Johns DA, DeCaprio J, McGlynn F, Reich F. Laparoscopic treatment of 109 consecutive ectopic pregnancies. *J Reprod Med*. 1988;33:885–889.

8. Nager, CW, Murphy AA. Ectopic pregnancy. *Clin Obstet Gynecol*. 1991;34:403–411.

9. Murphy AA. Diagnostic and operative laparoscopy. In: Thompson JD, Rock JA, eds. *TeLinde's Operative Gynecology*. 7th ed. Philadelphia: Williams and Wilkins; 1991:361–384.

10. Sherman D, Langer R, Sadovsky G, et al. Improved fertility following ectopic pregnancy. *Fertil Steril*. 1982;37:497–502.

11. Tulandi T, Guralnick M. Treatment of tubal ectopic pregnancy by salpingotomy with or without tubal suturing and salpingectomy. *Fertil Steril*. 1991;51:53–58.

12. Pauerstein CJ, Croxatto HB, Eddy CA, Ramay I, Walters MD. Anatomy and pathology of tubal pregnancy. *Obstet Gynecol*. 1986;67:301–308.

13. Mecke H, Semm K, Lehmann-Weillenbrock E. Results of operative pelviscopy in 202 cases of ectopic pregnancy. *Int J Fertil*. 1989;34:93–100.

14. Henderson SR. Ectopic tubal pregnancy treated by operative laparoscopy. *Am J Obstet Gynecol*. 1989;160:1462–1464.

15. Stovall TG, Ling FW, Gray LA, Carson SA, Buster JE. Methotrexate treatment of unruptured ectopic pregnancy: a report of 100 cases. *Obstet Gynecol*. 1991;77:749–753.

16. Stovall TG, Ling FW, Gray LA. Single dose methotrexate for treatment of ectopic pregnancy. *Obstet Gynecol*. 1991;77:754–757.

17. Horne LA, Younger JB. Low dose oral methotrexate therapy of presumed ectopic pregnancy. 45th Annual Meeting of the American Fertility Society, 1989, San Francisco, CA. Abstract #0-02.

18. Vermesh M, Silva PD, Sauer MV, Vargyas JM, Lobo RA. Persistent tubal ectopic gestation: patterns of circulating $\beta$-hCG and progesterone, and management options. *Fertil Steril*. 1988; 50:584–588.

19. Shapiro HI, Adler DH. Excision of an ectopic pregnancy through the laparoscope. *Am J Obstet Gynecol*. 1973;117:290–293.

20. Pouly MA, Mahnes H, Mage G, Canis M, Bruhat MA. Conservative laparoscopic treatment of 321 ectopic pregnancies. *Fertil Steril*. 1988;46:1093–1097.

21. DiMarchi JM, Kosasa TS, Kobara TY, Hale

RW. Persistent ectopic pregnancy. *Obstet Gynecol.* 1987;70:555–561.

22. Brumsted J, Kessler C, Gibson M. A comparison of laparoscopy and laparotomy for the treatment of ectopic pregnancy. *Obstet Gynecol.* 1988;71:889–893.

23. Vermesh M, Silva PD, Rosen GF, Stein AL, Fossum GT, Sauer MV. Management of unruptured ectopic gestation by linear salpingostomy: a prospective randomized clinical trial of laparoscopy vs. laparotomy. *Obstet Gynecol.* 1989; 73:400–408.

24. Nager CW, Wujek JJ, Kettel LM, Chin HG, Murphy AA. Operative laparoscopy vs. laparotomy in the management of ectopic pregnancy: a prospective trial. American Fertility Society 46th Annual Meeting, 1990, Washington, DC. Abstract 0–099.

# 10

# Laparoscopic Tubal Surgery and Adhesiolysis

*JOHN S. HESLA and JOHN A. ROCK*

CHAPTER OUTLINE

Major advances in instrument design over the past two decades have allowed the development of endoscopic techniques for correction of pelvic pathology. These reconstructive procedures have in many circumstances supplanted traditional open abdominal microsurgery due to equivalence in outcome and lower patient morbidity and expense. When performed properly, operative laparoscopy fulfills the major tenets of microsurgery. Major endoscopic fertility-promoting procedures for the treatment of tubal disease are described in this chapter.

## Salpingo-ovariolysis

Adnexal adhesions may lead to infertility by preventing ovum capture by the fimbria and in-hibiting normal tubal motility. Common patterns of adhesion development include immobilization of the ovary against the posterior leaf of the broad ligament or pelvic sidewall, fixation of the distal oviduct of the ovary and broad ligament, envelopment of the ovarian cortex by avascular adhesions, scarring of the fimbria ovarica and encapsulation of the distal end of the fallopian tube, and obliteration of the posterior cul de sac.

An inverse relationship exists between the grade of adhesions and conception rate, independent of the condition of the adnexae.[1] The surgical prognosis is dependent on the type, location, and extent of adhesions. Both fine, avascular adhesions and thick, poorly vascularized adhesions are amenable to laparoscopic dissection. Intimate adherence of one organ to another may arise from prior pelvic surgery and recurrent, severe infection. Such confluent adhesions and thick, highly vascularized fibrous bands may require laparotomy for effective therapy; nevertheless, surgical separation of these tissue planes is likely to lead to denudation of the peritoneal surface and extensive adhesion reformation. Hence, prognosis is poor for this category of disease regardless of technique employed.

## Technique

Careful identification of the intraabdominal structures is necessary before commencing dissection. Any adhesion bands extending from the omentum to the anterior abdominal wall should be freed before proceeding with salpingo-ovariolysis. These adhesions are often well vascularized and should be coagulated before division with bipolar or endothermic crocodile forceps. Persistent bleeding of the omental pedicle may be secured with repeat thermocoagulation, electrocoagulation, or by placement of an endoloop ligature.

Inspection of the anatomic landmarks of the oviduct and ovary is necessary before undertaking endoscopic adhesiolysis to avoid inadvertent incision of the fimbria ovarica, ovarian vasculature, and tubal serosa. The adhesion band should be stretched by one or two 5-mm grasping forceps or blunt probes in order to demarcate the adhesion from the adjoining organ. Multilayer adhesions should be divided one layer at a time for prevention of trauma to underlying structures that may not be immediately recognized. Wide tubo-ovarian adhesions are first incised with hook scissors, microscissors, or a 3-mm knife electrode near their attachment to the tubal serosa (Fig. 10.1). Adhesions to the ovarian surface may be grasped with a biopsy forceps and removed, taking care to apply traction against the direction of the fibers (Fig. 10.2). Ovariolysis is facilitated by applying traction to the utero-ovarian ligament with grasping forceps. This technique is particularly helpful when adhesions are present to the posterior leaf of the broad ligament. The scissors, needle electrode, or laser must be used at a perpendicular angle

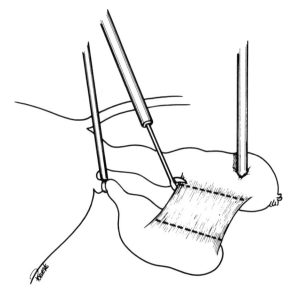

FIGURE 10.1. Lysis of avascular adnexal adhesions. Structures are manipulated with an aspiration cannula and traumatic forceps, placing the adhesive band on traction. It is important to attempt to excise the adhesive band at its insertions, rather than performing a simple incision.

to the adhesion being lysed. Adnexal hemostasis may be achieved with the microbipolar cautery, thermocoagulator, or via initial injection of a dilute vasopressin solution (20 U in 20 ml Ringer's lactate) into the tissue layer being dissected. Posterior cul de sac adhesions must also be excised because of the possibility that ovum capture may occur in this region.

The postoperative inflammatory response and extent of tissue destruction is lessened by use of a sharp dissection with the scissors or scalpel as compared to laser and electrosurgery. Nevertheless, laser laparoscopy has been shown to be associated with a low rate of postoperative adhesion recurrence and may avoid the formation of de novo adhesions.[2] The laser beam with small spot size in the enhanced super pulse mode is applied to the edge of the adherent surface in a sweeping motion in order to vaporize the tissue fibers. Care must be taken to avoid tearing the adhesion at its attachment by applying too much traction, since bleeding leads to a reduction of absorption of the laser beam. The tip of a nonreflec-

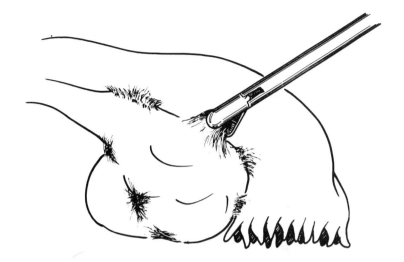

FIGURE 10.2. Removal of superficial ovarian adhesions. The adhesions are grasped with a biopsy forceps and gently removed, taking care to apply traction against the direction of the fibers, not peeling the ovarian cortex.

tive titanium suction aspiration cannula, a manipulation wand, the platform of the wave guide sheath, or a pool of irrigant may serve as the backstop to the $CO_2$ laser beam. Adhesions that cover large surface areas of the ovary may not be amenable to standard excision techniques and instead may be vaporized using a laser beam with a large spot size (greater than 2 mm) and lower power density (500–1000 W/$cm^2$). Copious irrigation of the site of adhesion vaporization should be performed with warm, heparinized Ringer's lactate to remove carbonized debris and blood.

An alternative technique in adhesiolysis involves the application of irrigant at pressures as high as 800 mg Hg in order to develop cleavage planes between the pelvic sidewalls, fallopian tube, ovary, and bowel.[3] This is particularly effective when the adhesions are filmy or gelatinous in nature as may exist during the early resolution phase of an infection or shortly after a primary surgical procedure. The suction tip of the aspiration-irrigation system also may be used to grasp and manipulate the pelvic organs during adnexal surgery.

## Results

The intrauterine pregnancy rates after salpingo-ovariolysis via laparotomy range from 32% to 66% in the literature.[4,5] Several laparoscopic series have equalled these rates (range 29.5–81%).[3,4,6–10] In Gomel's report of 92 patients with moderate to severe adnexal adhesions, 46% of all intrauterine pregnancies occurred within 6 months of operative intervention.[4] Pregnancy rates are generally lower when adhesions involve both the fallopian tube and ovary, presumably due to a greater likelihood of concurrent fimbrial involvement and impairment of oocyte recovery.

## Fimbrioplasty

Postinflammatory fimbrial damage may take the form of fimbrial agglutination, fimbrial encapsulation by fibrous tissue, and stenosis of the apex of the tubal infundibulum (prefimbrial phimosis). These conditions are amenable to laparoscopic treatment using techniques that have been derived from laparotomy procedures.

### Technique

The fallopian tube is distended via transcervical instillation of indigo carmine dye. Periadnexal adhesions are lysed and removed before fimbrial reconstruction. Any fibrous tissue covering the terminal end of the tube is excised with the pointed unipolar electrode, the laser, or with fine scissors. The fallopian tube is stabilized by grasping the serosa of distal ampulla with atraumatic forceps. The closed 3-mm alligator forceps are introduced through

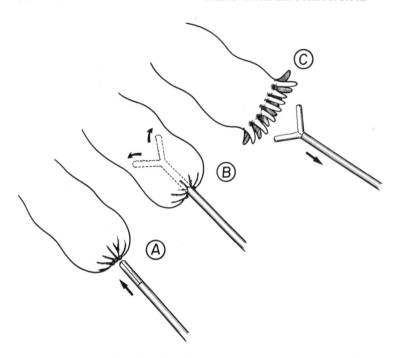

FIGURE 10.3. Fimbrioplasty. Blunt deagglutination of fimbria with alligator forceps. The fallopian tube is stabilized with atraumatic forceps.

the small tubal ostium. The jaws of the instrument are then opened within the lumen, and the forceps are gently withdrawn to deagglutinate the fimbria (Fig. 10.3).[4] This may be repeated several times in different directions in order to achieve maximal dilation of the fimbriated end. The tubal ostium also may be entered with a conical tube probe and/or traumatic grasping forceps to achieve the desired separation.[9] The latter instrument may be particularly useful in cases of severe stenosis of the ostium.

Fimbrial bridges are freed with the point unipolar electrode or with laser. Bipolar cautery may be necessary for hemostasis. Particular care must be taken in cases of severe agglutination, since forced insertion of the forceps into the stenosed tubal lumen may traumatize the fragile mucosa. Such damage may lead to complete fimbrial occlusion postoperatively.

Prefimbrial phimosis is overcome by incising the fibrous bands that constrict the infundibulum with the laser or a pointed electrode and blended current. The shallow radial incision should be made along avascular points, commencing at the fimbriated end and extending beyond the region of the phimosis. A greater degree of eversion of the tubal mucosa may be achieved by application of defocused laser or low power cautery to the infundibular serosal surface. This desiccates and constricts the superficial tissue layer.

## Results

Recent series of microsurgical fimbrioplasty via laparotomy report intrauterine pregnancy rates of 49% and 68%.[5,11] The success achieved by laparoscopic fimbrioplasty has ranged from 21.5% to 50% in the literature.[4,9,10] In addition, the ectopic pregnancy rate from this procedure is approximately 5% whether it is performed through the endoscope or laparotomy.

## Salpingoneostomy

The introduction of microsurgical techniques has resulted in great improvements in pregnancy rates for many infertility surgical procedures. Although the application of these principles to the repair of distal tubal occlusion has resulted in a significant increase in postoperative tubal patency over conventional macrosurgery, the pregnancy rates after microsurgical tuboplasty remain poor.[12] This is due to irreversible damage of ciliary function and muscular peristalsis or inadequate restoration of normal tubo-ovarian anatomic relationships.

Laparoscopic salpingoneostomy has been proposed as an alternative method of therapy.[3,7,9,13,14] Endoscopic reconstructive procedures fulfill the microsurgical principles of gentle tissue handling, constant irrigation of the operating field, careful hemostasis, avoidance of reactive sutures, and precise tissue dissection. Benefits of laparoscopic surgery include minimal physical impairment, shortened hospital stay, and reduced economic cost. In addition, the procedure can be performed as part of the initial diagnostic laparoscopy. These factors as well as the continued advances in *in vitro* fertilization therapy necessitate a reassessment of the utility of tuboplasty via the conventional laparotomy approach. Nevertheless, laparoscopic salpingoneostomy is difficult to master and should be reserved for experienced endoscopic surgeons.

Tubal function and hence pregnancy rates subsequent to salpingoneostomy are primarily dependent on the status of the fallopian tube at the time of surgical intervention. Partial or complete destruction of the endosalpinx and multifocal luminal occlusion are usually the consequence of chlamydial and gonococcal salpingitis, whereas extrinsic tubal damage in association with fimbrial occlusion may arise from appendicitis, previous adnexal surgery, and rarely endometriosis. The sequelae of nongynecologic pelvic infection represent the best response category for tubal repair due to the lack of extensive involvement of the tubal wall.

Hysterosalpingography with water-soluble contrast media should be performed before laparoscopy in order to identify abnormalities of the cornua and distal tubal occlusion and to assess intratubal architecture.[15] The prognosis is worsened by an absence of ampullary mucosal folds or the presence of a "honeycomb" pattern of the ampulla, irregular reticular images that suggest intraluminal adhesions. Conversely, increased pregnancy rates are seen when rugae are present on a preoperative hysterosalpingogram, even when the tubal obstruction is complete.

Several classification systems have been proposed to characterize prognosis after surgical repair of the hydrosalpinx.[15–17] These incorporate the findings of hysterosalpingography and diagnostic laparoscopy, including the size of the sactosalpinx, condition of fimbria and tubal mucosa, associated adnexal adhesions, and rugal pattern seen at the time of hysterosalpingography.[15] Postoperative pregnancy rates are typically less than 10% in patients with severe disease. The hydrosalpinx with a rigid, thickened wall may show little evidence of dilation but nevertheless has an exceedingly poor prognosis. Fibrosis of the muscularis layer interferes with tubal transport. Multiloculated cystic changes in the endosalpinx and severe associated peritubal and periovarian adhesive disease also adversely affect surgical outcome. Thin walled hydrosalpinges allow better surgical dissection of the fimbria and eversion of the mucosa.

## Technique

The surgical technique requires meticulous attention to details that must not be sacrificed when operating with laparoscopic instruments. Visualization may be augmented, if desired, by loupe magnification attached to the laparoscope or via video camera monitoring. Intraumbilical and two to three suprapubic/lower abdominal incisions are necessary for placement of instruments. The fallopian tube is immobilized with grasping forceps placed through the operating channel of the laparoscope or through a midline or lateral suprapubic sheath. A favored approach to tubal dissection involves insertion of the laser or scissors through a 5- to 7-mm trocar sleeve located at a medial site 3 to 5 mm superior to the suprapubic line. The shorter focal length of the laser beam introduced through an ancillary port provides a greater power density than that obtained through the operating channel of the laparoscope.

Infundibular tubal occlusion is frequently accompanied by perisalpingeal and periovarian adhesions. These must be freed before proceeding with the salpingoneostomy. Transcervical installation of dilute indigo carmine dye distends the hydrosalpinx and aides in the identification of the scarred ostium, fimbria ovar-

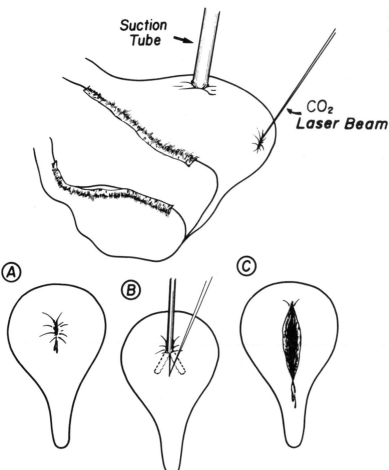

FIGURE 10.4. Salpingoneostomy. Linear salpingoneostomy with release of minimally damaged fimbria.

ica, and adjacent structures. Inspection of the distal tube may demonstrate streaks of radial scarring, which should be used as guides for the tubal incisions with the laser, scissors, or the needle electrode. If laser is employed, a superpulse beam of 25 W or continuous mode beam of 30 to 40 W with a 1.0-mm spot size is applied to the stellate scar of the occluded infundibulum after immobilizing the tube with atraumatic forceps. Rather than perforating the full thickness of the wall and thereby promoting immediate collapse of the hydrosalpinx, the tube should be superficially scored with the laser from the ostium toward the ovary and fimbria ovarica following the old scar line. The incision is then carried down until dye is encountered. The atraumatic forceps may then be repositioned to stabilize the margins of the incision, carefully avoiding the delicate mucosa that has been everted by the out-rushing indigo carmine dye. In cases where normal fimbria are released, a single linear incision is usually adequate for eversion of the ampulla (Fig. 10.4). In the majority of cases, however, two additional radial incisions are necessary to achieve sufficient exposure of the residual fimbria; this results in a "Y"-shaped incision of the terminal tube (Fig. 10.5). The platform of the wave guide sheath may be used as a backstop so that the beam does not penetrate the tubal wall and damage the endothelium of the other side of the oviduct. Ringer's lactate irrigant placed in the posterior cul de sac may also be used as a backstop for the laser beam. Bipolar cautery or a lower power defocused laser beam may be employed for hemostasis. If the

FIGURE 10.5. Salpingoneostomy. Site of inverted "y" incision. Hydrosalpinx is stabilized with laparoscopic and suprapubic atraumatic forceps.

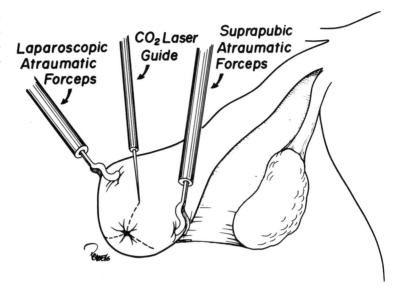

**Laparoscopic Atraumatic Forceps**

**$CO_2$ Laser Guide**

**Suprapubic Atraumatic Forceps**

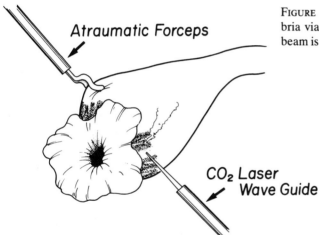

**Atraumatic Forceps**

**$CO_2$ Laser Wave Guide**

FIGURE 10.6. Salpingoneostomy. Eversion of fimbria via desiccation of serosal edge. The $CO_2$ laser beam is defocused and set at 3 to 5 W of power.

tube is very vascular, 1 to 2 cc of a dilute vasopressin solution (20 U in 20 ml normal saline) may be injected directly into the tube with a laparoscopic needle to minimize bleeding. Upon completion of the incision(s), the serosal edge of the distal tube is everted with the 3- to 5-W power, defocused $CO_2$ laser (Fig. 10.6). This desiccation causes a contraction of the serosa. The degree of eversion should be exaggerated to prevent postoperative closure. A single suture of 4-0 PDS may be placed to secure the fimbrial margin to the ampullary serosa in those cases in which the chance for reobstruction appears high.

An alternative technique involves the application of mechanical and electrocautery dissection. Adhesiolysis is performed as above to mobilize the distal tube. After distending the hydrosalpinx by chromopertubation, the avascular lines are traced with fine monopolar cautery or point thermocoagulation. The tube is then opened with laparoscopic microscissors or fine-point electrode. After the initial incision is made that allows access to the tubal lumen, additional dissection of the tubal wall may be approached from the interior, following the pattern of the fimbria and luminal folds. Hemostasis is secured with microbipolar cautery. The mucosal flaps are mobilized with atraumatic forceps. The neostomy edges may be everted with light electrocoagulation or thermocoagulation. Low current must be used to avoid damage to the muscularis. Suturing is usually avoided due to its propensity for adhesion formation. In cases of a thickened, sclerotic tubal wall, an adequate eversion may not be achieved with the above technique of serosal coagulation. In such instances, 4-0 PDS suture is used to fix the distal flaps to the ampullary serosa via an intraabdominal instrument tie or an extracorporeal tie as described by Reich.[3] An alternative technique involves application of one or two Hulka clips or newly developed absorbable clips to everted edges of the tube.[7] The Hulka clips are removed 2 to 3 months later by second-look laparoscopy.

The peritoneal cavity is copiously irrigated with Ringer's lactate solution containing 5000 U heparin per liter during and at the completion of the tuboplasty. Meticulous hemostasis is necessary to optimize outcome. Doxycycline antibiotic prophylaxis is administered the day before surgery and for 3 days postoperatively. Ancillary modalities employed to impede adhesion formation include the placement of an absorbable adhesion barrier (Interceed) between the fallopian tube and pelvic sidewall as well as the intraperitoneal instillation of 200 ml of 32% dextran-70 (Hyskon), or 1 to 2 L of Ringer's lactate at the conclusion of the procedure to achieve hydroflotation.

If available, intraoperative salpingoscopy is recommended to visualize the entire length of the ampullary lumen.[16] The salpingoscope is introduced immediately after the opening of the ostium to identify intratubal adhesions. If luminal damage is extensive, the laparoscopic tuboplasty may be abandoned for in vitro fertilization therapy.

## Results

The number of published reports on endoscopic salpingostomy and the sample size per series are rather small. Although the success rates have ranged from 0% to 44%,[3,7,9,10,13,14] the mean outcome of these series generally approximates the overall intrauterine preg-

nancy rate of 19% to 35% achieved via laparotomy.[16] This confirms the premise that the results of tubal surgery are mainly related to the severity of tubal damage and type and extent of adhesions rather than the surgical technique employed. Nevertheless, the lower success rate noted in some reports illustrates that successful endoscopic repair of the hydrosalpinx is a tedious and technically difficult undertaking.[10] In 1989, Nezhat et al. reported a pregnancy rate of 48% after laparoscopic salpingoneostomy in those patients who had well preserved cilia and fimbrial folds noted at salpingoscopy.[7] This contrasts with a 6% conception rate in their 16 patients with severely damaged tubal lumens. Furthermore, the conception rate is lower when the hydrosalpinx is accompanied by dense adhesions as compared to a lesser degree of adhesions.[17]

An attempt at laparoscopic salpingostomy is not contraindicated when the patient has poor prognostic variables for a successful conception. However, if the tubal wall is thin, there is little distal dilatation, the endosalpinx appears normal, and there are few fixed adhesions, exploratory laparotomy is recommended for reconstruction unless the surgeon has demonstrated mastery of this laparoscopic technique.

## Uterine Suspension

Endoscopic plication of the round ligaments may be performed in those circumstances in which a greater degree of uterine anteflexion is desired to impede postoperative adhesion formation of the adnexal structures and posterior cul de sac. The round ligament is grasped with traumatic forceps and an Endoloop, Silastic band, or laparoscopic clip is applied to the looped ligament, thereby shortening it. This operation is rarely performed.

## Second-look Laparoscopy

The term "second-look laparoscopy" generally refers to laparoscopy after a primary reconstructive procedure via laparotomy. The interval between the initial reproductive surgery and the laparoscopy may vary from 3 days to 2 or more years. Fibrosis of unlysed fibrin begins 3 days after serosal trauma and is completed by 21 days.[18] Endoscopic adhesiolysis is performed in an attempt to restore a greater degree of normality to the pelvic structures and hopefully improve intrauterine pregnancy rates. The success of such procedures is widely debated. A few studies have suggested that second-look laparoscopies effectively reduce peritoneal adhesions[18,19]. However, the impact on conception rates is less certain whether the second-look laparoscopy was performed within 8 days of the initial laparotomy[19], or after one year.[20] The interval from surgery to conception appears reduced although the cumulative pregnancy rate may not be significantly improved. Hence, the value of a second-look laparoscopy after a primary endoscopic reconstructive procedure seems modest.

## Conclusion

The efficacy of laparoscopic tubal reconstructive procedures has been established over the past decade. Nevertheless, treatment of extensive adnexal disease requires meticulous technique and should not be attempted by the inexperienced endoscopist.

## References

1. Caspi E, Halperin Y, Bukovsky I. The importance of periadnexal adhesions in tubal reconstructive surgery for infertility. *Fertil Steril.* 1979;31:296–300.
2. Nezhat CR, Nezhat FR, Metzger DA, Luciano AA. Adhesion reformation after reproductive surgery by videolaseroscopy. *Fertil Steril.* 1990;53:1008–1011.
3. Reich H. Laparoscopic treatment of extensive pelvic adhesions, including hydrosalpinx. *J Reprod Med.* 1987;32:736–742.
4. Gomel V. Salpingo-ovariolysis by laparoscopy in infertility. *Fertil Steril.* 1983;40:607–611.
5. Schoysman R. Tubal microsurgery versus in vitro fertilization. *Acta Eur Fertil.* 1984;15:5–13.
6. Bruhat MA, Mage G, Manhes H, et al. Laparoscopic procedures to promote fertility. Ovar-

iolysis and salpingolysis. Results of 93 selected cases. *Acta Eur Fertil.* 1983;113–115.
7. Nezhat C, Winer WK, Cooper JD, et al. Endoscopic infertility surgery. *J Reprod Med.* 1989;34:127–134.
8. Donnez J. $CO_2$ laser laparoscopy in infertile women with endometriosis and women with adnexal adhesions. *Fertil Steril.* 1987;48:390–394.
9. Mettler L, Giesel H, Semm K. Treatment of female infertility due to tubal obstruction by operative laparoscopy. *Fertil Steril.* 1979;32:384–390.
10. Fayez JA. An assessment of the role of operative laparoscopy in tuboplasty. *Fertil Steril.* 1983;39:476–479.
11. Patton GW. Pregnancy outcome following microsurgical fimbrioplasty. *Fertil Steril.* 1982;37:150–155.
12. Cholst IN. Surgery on the fimbrial portion of the fallopian tube. *Sem Reprod Endocrinol.* 1984;2:160–167.
13. Gomel V. Salpingostomy by laparoscopy. *J Reprod Med.* 1977;18:265–268.
14. Daniell JF, Herbert CM. Laparoscopic salpingostomy utilizing the $CO_2$ laser. *Fertil Steril.* 1984;41:558–563.
15. Rock JA, Katayama P, Martin EJ, et al. Factors influencing the success of salpingostomy techniques for distal fimbrial obstruction. *Obstet Gynecol.* 1978;52:591–596.
16. The American Fertility Society. The American Fertility Society classifications of adnexal adhesions, distal tubal occlusion, tubal occlusion secondary to tubal ligation, tubal pregnancies, Müllerian anomalies and intrauterine adhesions. *Fertil Steril.* 1988;49:944–955.
17. Mage G, Pouly JL, Bouquet de Joliniere J, et al. A preoperative classification to predict the intrauterine and ectopic pregnancy rates after distal tubal microsurgery. *Fertil Steril.* 1986;46:807–810.
18. Jansen RPS. Early laparoscopy after pelvic operations to prevent adhesions: safety and efficacy. *Fertil Steril.* 1988;49:26–31.
19. Trimbos-Kemper TCM, Trimbos JB, van Hall EV. Adhesion formation after tubal surgery: results of the eight-day laparoscopy in 188 patients. *Fertil Steril.* 1985;43:395–400.
20. Tulandi T, Falcone T, Kafka I. Second-look operative laparoscopy 1 year following reproductive surgery. *Fertil Steril.* 1989;52:421–424.

# 11

# Laparoscopic Treatment of Endometriosis

*Dan C. Martin*

## CHAPTER OUTLINE

Laparoscopy has enabled the gynecologist to make the diagnosis of endometriosis with relative ease. In addition, laparoscopy has been acquiring increasing importance as a treatment modality. No longer is laparoscopy used only to treat minimal and mild disease, since advanced disease is being safely and effectively treated endoscopically. The laparoscopic approach to surgical treatment of endometriosis has many advantages over laparotomy (see Chapter 1). The decrease in morbidity and cost has been well established. Additionally, laparoscopy may decrease the incidence of de novo adhesion formation when compared to laparotomy.[1]

The surgical approach to the treatment of endometriosis is determined in part by the therapeutic goals. When fertility is to be preserved, the techniques must balance endometriosis removal versus residual tissue trauma. An overly aggressive excisional approach may result in excessive postoperative adhesion formation, which will become more of a factor in the infertility than endometriosis itself. On the other hand, pain secondary to fibrotic endometriosis requires aggressive resection of all palpable and visible abnormalities. When a tissue diagnosis is needed, biopsy or excisional technique is used.

## Diagnosis

Morphologically different forms of endometriosis have been described.[2] The ability to recognize the various forms of endometriosis may be more important than the specific surgical technique used, particularly in young women and patients with pelvic pain. Near-contact laparoscopy followed by $CO_2$ laser excisional techniques has been used to identify and confirm lesions as small as 180 $\mu$m.[2] However, not all lesions can be recognized at laparoscopy or laparotomy. Small lesions can be missed because of their size[3] whereas larger lesions may be missed because of their depth of penetration.[4] Deep lesions may be more easily palpated than visualized.[5] Video monitoring provides increased magnification and resolution by using large monitors,[6] and can improve the coordination of surgical assistants and other operating room personnel. However, video imaging also decreases the degree of image resolution at the usual operating distance and impairs the ability to detect atypical or small endometriotic implants, a factor that must be taken into consideration when operating directly off the monitor screen. It is extremely important for all surgeons to become familiar with all the morphologic appearances of endometriosis before undertaking its diagnosis and treatment.

## Indications and Patient Selection

Patients with endometriosis generally present with abdominopelvic pain/dysmenorrhea/dyspareunia, infertility, or pelvic mass. Some may already carry the diagnosis of endometriosis, based on a previous surgical intervention. Alternatively, some patients are diagnosed at the time of the initial operative laparoscopy.

## Pelvic Pain

Patients undergoing diagnostic laparoscopy for pelvic pain generally have failed therapy with nonsteroidal anti-inflammatory agents and/or oral contraceptives. Before surgical intervention a careful history should be obtained exploring other causes of pelvic pain such as chronic pelvic infection, bowel disease such as irritable bowel, or urinary tract disorders including bladder dysfunction or nephrolithiasis. Gastrointestinal or urologic evaluation and consultation may be considered. The clinical presentation depends to a certain degree on the location and the extent of disease, although the severity of symptoms does not correlate directly with the extent of disease.

## Infertility

Infertile patients undergoing diagnostic laparoscopy should have completed a basic evaluation, including semen analysis, documentation of ovulation (e.g., basal body temperature plotting with a luteal phase progesterone serum level or endometrial biopsy), hysterosalpingography, and a timed postcoital (Sims-Huhner) test. In these patients laparoscopy should be both diagnostic and operative. At the time the consent is obtained the patients should be counseled regarding the possibility of operative laparoscopy if endometriosis or other pathology is found.

## Pelvic Mass

Pelvic masses secondary to endometriosis are usually symptomatic, although not invariably. If bowel symptoms are present sigmoid/colonoscopy should be performed before or at the time of laparoscopy. In all patients with a pelvic mass suggestive of endometriosis, particularly if cul de sac involvement is extensive, consideration should be given to the possibility of requiring an intraoperative surgical or oncologic consult. Moreover, all of these patients should probably undergo bowel preparation before surgery.

# Techniques and Instrumentation

The laparoscopic techniques used to destroy endometriosis are coagulation (desiccation), vaporization, and excision. The term "coagulation" is used to encompass concepts that include, but are not limited to, heating, desiccation, denaturation, protein coagulation, cauterization, and carbonization of tissue. Coagulation can be produced by unipolar and bipolar electrocautery, thermocoagulation, and fiber-propagated lasers. Vaporization is accomplished by converting high power density laser or electrical energy into heat, which vaporizes or "boils" intracellular water. Excision of endometriosis can use any of these techniques, in addition to scissors and other mechanical hemostatic devices such as loops, sutures, or clips. Bipolar coagulators, unipolar knives, thermocoagulators, and lasers have been used to ablate (coagulate, vaporize, or excise) endometriosis. The surgeon should be trained in all these techniques, since a combination of approaches is superior to a single modality. Careful attention to the clinical presentation, the goals of the patient, and extent of disease will be helpful in choosing the most useful technique in a specific clinical situation.

Although coagulation and vaporization are adequate for most cases, the $CO_2$ laser has been used to resect lesions as deep as 14 mm and to dissect the ureter and bowel away from endometriosis and adhesions.[7–9] Scissors, bipolar coagulation, thermocoagulation, and unipolar knives are more generally available and appear adequate for most, but not all, cases. Operative laparoscopists should have mastered the use of endoscopic scissors and electro- or thermocoagulation before using the laser.

## Treatment of Peritoneal and Soft Tissue Endometriosis

It is extremely important that the peritoneal surfaces of the pelvis be examined carefully and all lesions treated before manipulation or surgery of the adnexa is undertaken. Excessive pelvic manipulation leads to bleeding and peritoneal abrasion, which may obscure the pres-

TABLE 11.1. Advantages of excision of endometriotic lesions over vaporization or coagulation.

| |
|---|
| Creates less thermal distortion |
| Creates less smoke |
| Leaves less carbon |
| Provides tissue for diagnosis |

ence of endometriotic implants. Small implants (2 mm or less) can be treated effectively in any fashion. However, some lesions are sampled by biopsy or random excision for diagnostic purposes before vaporization or coagulation. Bipolar cautery is effective on lesions that are small or that can be held within the cautery paddles. However, initial dissection may be needed so that the lesions can be properly grasped and controlled. Thermocoagulation may also be used, although the area of cautery cannot be any less than the diameter of the coagulation tip (approximately 5 mm). Furthermore, peritoneal lesions should be grasped and dissected away from underlying organs. Argon, KTP, or Nd:YAG fiber lasers are also useful for treating these small lesions.

Vaporization or excision down to the level of healthy tissue is more useful for larger lesions, although deep lesions are more accurately excised than vaporized (Table 11.1).[9] Excision is begun by cutting through the peritoneum into the loose connective tissue below with either scissors, knife, or fiber lasers, although this author prefers to use the $CO_2$ laser. The lesion is outlined and the loose connective tissue and fat noted. A blunt probe, forceful irrigation (aquadissection), or spreading of the scissor blades is then used to dissect these layers. Injection of normal saline or lactated Ringer's subperitoneally, using a 20- to 22-gauge spinal needle placed transabdominally, can be used to push the peritoneum away from vessels, bowel, bladder, or ureter. This technique may be particularly useful in conjunction with $CO_2$ laser excision/vaporization, since this energy wavelength is readily absorbed by water, impeding damage to underlying organs. Although this technique may be useful to protect subperitoneal structures, it should be avoided when direct visualization and dissection of the

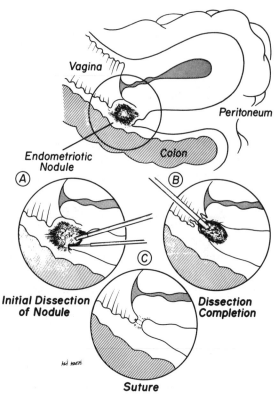

FIGURE 11.1. Deep laparoscopic dissection of the rectovaginal space, in combination with colpotomy, for the treatment of a large endometriotic nodule of the rectovaginal septum. **A:** Initial laparoscopic dissection of nodule. **B:** Completion of dissection via colpotomy incision. **C:** Suturing the rectovaginal septum.

ureter and bladder appear to be more advantageous. Once the peritoneum is dissected from the underlying connective tissue, the lesion is excised and removed. Specimens that are too large to be removed through the trocar can be cut or morcellated into smaller pieces.

Deep dissection into the rectovaginal septum combined with colpotomy has been used for excision of large cul de sac lesions extending to the vagina (Fig. 11.1).[8]

After laser vaporization, carbon may accumulate within the peritoneal surface and be confused with or conceal endometriosis, both at the time of surgery and at subsequent laparoscopy. In addition, carbon sublimates at 3652°C, increasing the secondary thermal burn when the laser is applied again. High power density lasers in superpulse mode may decrease carbonization by facilitating rapid vaporization with a decrease in lateral tissue desiccation or coagulation. Superficial carbon can be removed by lavage or by using pusher sponges.

## Treatment of Ovarian Endometriosis

Ovarian endometriotic lesions are managed according to size. Those less than 5 mm in size are biopsied and coagulated, vaporized, or excised. The infiltration of these small lesions into the ovarian cortex can be irregular and vaporization should extend 2 to 4 mm into healthy-appearing ovary. Endometriomas between 5 mm and 2 cm are generally decapitated and the base vaporized. However, some of these lesions may be more appropriately managed as described below (see also Chapter 12).

The technique used to manage endometriomas greater than 2 cm depends on its general characteristics at the time of surgery. Two- to 5-cm endometriomas are managed by drainage, incision, and dissection of the cyst wall. It is extremely important to free the ovary completely from surrounding adhesions and completely restore its mobility before enucleating the endometriotic cyst. If the endometriomas drain before surgery or open at the time of ovarian manipulation dissection is more difficult. Usually these openings are located on the posterior aspect of the ovary, at the site of its adherence to the broad ligament. Dissection of the cyst should begin at the site of the spontaneous rupture. If the cyst has not spontaneously drained, a small incision is made parallel to the long axis of the ovary. This incision is made at the cyst's most dependent (lower) portion, in closest proximity to the pelvic side wall, to decrease the possibility of bowel adhesions (Fig. 11.2). The lining of the cyst wall is then thoroughly irrigated. A circumferential relaxing incision may be performed over the thinned surface of the cyst to facilitate definition of the plane between normal ovarian cortex and cyst wall. The cyst wall is then stripped out of the ovary with either blunt or sharp dissection. A twisting technique may be used to remove the cyst wall. If the base of

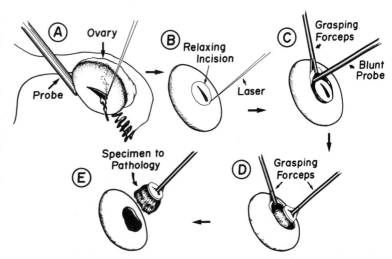

FIGURE 11.2. Resection of an endometrioma. **A:** An incision is made in the most dependent portion of the ovary. **B:** A relaxing incision is made circumferentially through the thinned and damaged cortex overlying the endometrioma, after drainage and irrigation of the cyst wall lining. **C:** A plane of dissection is established with either a blunt probe or forceps. **D:** Dissection is carried out bluntly or sharply. **E:** The entire cyst wall is sent to pathology.

the capsule is adherent to the hilar vessels, coagulation of any remaining cyst wall is used instead of stripping to avoid tearing these vessels. Ovarian suturing is generally unnecessary.

When the endometriomas exceed 5 cm, laparoscopic stripping techniques may increase operating time from 2 to 5 hr, and laparotomy may ultimately be necessary 3 to 5 hr into the operation. In addition, removing these large cysts may increase the chance of sacrificing the ovary when compared to performing a staged procedure. A staged procedure may be preferable for these large cysts, in order to increase preservation of healthy ovary (see page 107). Alternatively, the cyst wall may be vaporized.

Grossly, the appearance most commonly associated with a histologically confirmed endometrioma is an irregular brown or red mottling on a white cyst-lining capsule. A uniform brown appearance of the cyst wall is equally likely to be an old hemorrhagic corpus luteum or an endometrioma. Thus, on occasion an old corpus luteum may be mistaken for an endometrioma.[10]

## Treatment of Bowel Endometriosis

Bowel involvement is suggested by the presence of palpable tumor near the bowel, rectovaginal tenderness, a rectovaginal shelf, rectal bleeding at the time of menses, or persistent pain after laparoscopic removal of recognized lesions. In general, resection of infiltrating bowel lesions requires laparotomy. Furthermore, infiltrating bowel lesions smaller than 1 cm, and approximately 50% of appendiceal lesions, are more readily recognized by palpation than visualization. Large endometriotic implants of the bowel wall may protrude extensively into the lumen with minimal serosal manifestation (Fig. 11.3).[5] Unfortunately, few lesions are detected by preoperative barium enema, colonoscopy, sonography, computed tomography (CT) scanning or imaging magnetic resonance (MRI). Patients suspected of having a bowel lesion need to undergo a preoperative colonoscopy to rule out adenocarcinoma of the bowel. If the mucosa is fixed, full thickness penetration by endometriosis is often present. Before surgery the bowel is prepped, as the most common indication for laparotomy is suspected bowel involvement. In addition, autologous blood donation is discussed with these patients, since these procedures frequently can be associated with significant blood loss and subsequent transfusion.

An initial attempt at partial thickness resection of infiltrating bowel endometriosis with anatomic distortion and associated pain was attempted at laparoscopy in five patients. Immediate laparotomy for bowel resection was performed in two of these patients because of the extent of disease. Although the other three had apparent resection of their bowel endometriosis, persistent pain and tenderness resulted in a delayed laparotomy in all three. All

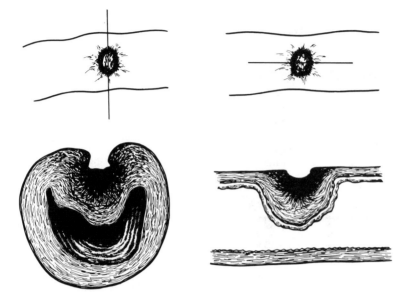

FIGURE 11.3. Endometriosis lesions of the bowel. Lesions may present with the majority of the mass protruding into the bowel lumen, while superficially the lesion appears small. (Transverse view on left, longitudinal on right.)

five had deep muscularis involvement.[5] This agrees with previous conclusions on the need for laparotomy in patients with pelvic pain and bowel endometriosis.

Treatment of lesions in the rectovaginal septum generally requires a gynecologist or general surgeon experienced with bowel surgery in this area (Fig. 11.1). Deep rectosigmoid resection and reanastomosis by laparotomy is a distinct possibility when endometriosis is located deep in the pelvis,[11] and these procedures are generally avoided in infertility patients who do not have symptoms attributable to bowel infiltration. Furthermore, the uterosacral ligaments can become infiltrated with endometriosis, the disease extending toward the sacrum or pelvic floor. Low-lying lesions of the uterosacrals or perirectal tissue are best palpated at the time of rectovaginal examination. If these lesions are not noted preoperatively they are easy to miss at surgery.

Although most infiltrating bowel lesions are best detected and treated by laparotomy, laparoscopic vaporization will be adequate for 50% to 90% of superficial endometriotic implants and adhesions on bowel. Dissection of superficial lesions can be performed by defocusing the $CO_2$ laser in a repeat pulse or superpulse mode. This avoids the distortion and damage associated with coagulation and vaporization. Patients who have persistent pain after laparoscopic ablation may require medical suppression and/or laparotomy.[11]

## Treatment of Bladder Endometriosis

Bladder implants up to 5 mm are handled in a manner similar to the peritoneal lesions discussed above. Deep penetration into muscularis should be anticipated as the lesions become larger. Lesions 2 cm and greater generally require resection of the bladder wall at laparotomy, when the indication is pelvic pain or when there is ureteral distortion.

## Treatment of Ureteral Endometriosis

When endometriosis lies over the ureter, two techniques may be used to resect the lesions. Injection of physiologic solutions subperitoneally can be used to push the ureter away and to provide a protective barrier between the ureter and the surgical destruction. An alternate technique is to make an incision in the peritoneum above and away from the ureter. The peritoneum is then grasped and pulled toward the midline. A blunt probe is used to dissect and gently push the ureter laterally and away. The laser may be used to incise into the surrounding loose connective tissue, avoiding the ureter. Care must be taken not to disturb the periureteral vessels, since further cauterization in this area may result in a delayed ureteroperitoneal fistula. The endometriotic lesion is then resected in its entirety. When the ureter cannot be pushed away from the peritoneum, it is possible that the ureter has become infiltrated with endometriosis.

If the ureter is transected or damaged in the process of resecting endometriosis, some urologists feel that a reanastomosis in a diseased area should not be performed and that an implantation is indicated. However, Gomel has treated ureteral laceration by repair at laparoscopy. An unpublished case of a delayed ureteroperitoneal fistula was managed by ureteral catheter placement for 8 weeks. If not prepared for ureteral surgery, avoid dissection near the ureter, especially when it is adherent to endometriosis.

## Staged Procedures

It is not possible to treat all endometriosis cases at the time of the initial diagnostic laparoscopy. Semm's "three-phase therapy" involves debulking as much endometriosis as possible at the initial surgery, avoiding tubal surgery at this time.[12] The patient is then placed on 3 to 9 months of hormonal suppression, and a repeat pelviscopy performed to remove any remaining endometriosis and treat any additional adhesions and tubal disease.

Koninckx (personal communication) has suggested a staged procedure for the treatment of ovarian endometriomas, which involves drainage, irrigation, examination, biopsy, and coagulation of the inner lining of large endometriomas at an initial laparoscopy. This appears to decrease the removal of healthy ovarian tissue.[10] Serial sonography, with or without medical suppression, is used to monitor for persistence or recurrence of the cysts. A subsequent operative laparoscopy is performed if the endometrioma recurs.

Endometriosis, particularly around the ure-ter, bowel, or major blood vessels, is often left behind intentionally during operative endoscopy. Partial treatment by pelviscopy may provide sufficient relief, making laparotomy or medical therapy unnecessary. If symptoms persist despite medical therapy, a repeat laparoscopy or laparotomy is considered. Repeat laparoscopy for recurrent endometriosis is particularly useful in younger patients. Nevertheless, laparotomy may reveal palpable bowel or rectovaginal lesions not seen at laparoscopy. Intentionally avoiding dissection of these areas has not completely avoided damage to them. Delayed rectal perforation and delayed ureteroperitoneal fistula have occurred in patients in whom endometriosis was intentionally left on the ureter and rectum. Furthermore, diaphragmatic endometriosis has been associated with subsequent recognition of pulmonary endometriosis that may have represented direct extension.

## Results

### Pregnancy Rates

A 92% pregnancy rate after resection of ovarian endometriomas (12 of 13 patients) was reported by Reich and McGlynn using electrocoagulation and dissection with scissors.[13] Using $CO_2$ laser techniques, Martin reported an 80% pregnancy rate in patients with severe endometriosis as their only infertility factor.[14] These represent among the highest pregnancy rates after the treatment of extensive endometriosis. Pregnancy rates after coagulation (both electrosurgical and thermal) vary from 24% to 74% with an average rate of 46% among 417 patients in eight series.[15] In 12 studies following $CO_2$ laser ablation with a total of 1536 patients there was a range of 47% to 69%, with an average pregnancy rate of 56%.[14–16] Kojima and colleagues found similar results using the Nd:YAG laser.[17] The argon and $CO_2$ lasers had similar pregnancy rates, which decreased with the greater duration of infertility.[14,18] These findings suggest that young patients delaying childbearing and patients who have short-term infertility should be optimistic about their prognosis. On the other hand, patients with long-term and male factor infertility should not be inappropriately encouraged. Three separate studies using life table analysis indicate that laparoscopic treatment provides equal results to medication therapy or laparotomy in patients with mild or moderate disease, and is equal to or better than laparotomy for severe cases.[6,15,16]

## Resolution of Pain

Focal tenderness associated with scarred lesions resolves when these implants are resected.[5] Unfortunately, pain relief is much harder to quantitate than pregnancy rates or resolution of focal tenderness. Pain may be due only to the endometriosis, to endometriosis combined with other factors, or to other factors, with endometriosis as a coincidental finding.

## Alternative Therapy

### Medical Suppression

Medical suppression is used in specific clinical circumstances. Danazol and gonadotropin-releasing hormone analogs have produced the most rapid and predictable relief of pain. These are the preferred method of treatment for short-term (6 months or less) use. Oral contraceptives are less expensive and are more generally used for long-term relief of pain.

### Laparotomy Surgery

Laparotomy has been the standard for surgical therapy for endometriosis. Palpation, examination of retroperitoneal spaces, examination of bowel, and delicate handling of deep lesions are enhanced at laparotomy when compared with laparoscopy. Laparoscopic excision of deep bowel lesions is frequently associated with persistence.[19] The indications for laparotomy have been discussed in the text. However, we feel it is most useful in patients with persistent pelvic pain after initial laparoscopic treatment and in those with bulk tumor that is tender and infiltrating a hollow viscus.

## Conclusions

Bipolar coagulators, unipolar knives, thermocoagulators, and lasers have been used to ablate (coagulate, vaporize, or excise) endometriosis. A combination of these modalities is superior to one alone. Careful attention to the nature and presentation of endometriosis can help choose the technique most useful in a specific clinical situation. However, further study is needed to determine the most appropriate technique or the technique that will be the easiest to teach and to apply for a given clinical situation.

## References

1. Diamond MP, Daniell JF, Johns DA, et al. Postoperative adhesion development after operative laparoscopy: evaluation at early second-look procedures. *Fertil Steril.* 1991; 55:700–704.
2. Martin DC, Hubert GD, Vander Zwaag R, et al. Laparoscopic appearance of peritoneal endometriosis. *Fertil Steril.* 1989;51:63–67.
3. Murphy AA, Green WR, Bobbie D, et al. Unsuspected endometriosis documented by scanning electron microscopy in visually normal peritoneum. *Fertil Steril.* 1986;46:522–524.
4. Nisolle M, Paindaveine B, Bourdon A, et al. Histologic study of peritoneal endometriosis in infertile women. *Fertil Steril.* 1990;53:984–988.
5. Martin DC (ed). *Laparoscopic Appearance of Endometriosis.* 2nd ed., vol. I. Memphis: Resurge Press; 1990.
6. Nezhat C, Crowgey SR, Nezhat F. Videolaseroscopy for the treatment of endometriosis associated with infertility. *Fertil Steril.* 1989; 51:237–240.
7. Cornillie FJ, Oosterlynck D, Lauweryns JM, et al. Deeply infiltrating pelvic endometriosis: histology and clinical significance. *Fertil Steril.* 1990;53:978–983.
8. Martin DC. Laparoscopic and vaginal colpotomy for the excision of infiltrating cul-de-sac endometriosis. *J Reprod Med.* 1988;33:806–808.
9. Davis GD, Brooks RA. Excision of pelvic endometriosis with the carbon dioxide laser laparoscope. *Obstet Gynecol.* 1988;72:816–819.
10. Martin DC, Berry JD. Histology of chocolate cysts. *J Gynecol Surg.* 1990;6:43–46.
11. Grunert GM, Franklin RR. Management of

recurrent endometriosis. In: Wilson EA, ed. *Endometriosis*. New York: Alan R Liss; 1987: 173–184.

12. Semm K. Postoperative care after endoscopic abdominal surgery. In: Semm K, Friedrich ER, eds. *Operative Manual for Endoscopic Abdominal Surgery*. Chicago: Year Book Medical Publishers; 1987:228–238.

13. Reich H, McGlynn F. Treatment of ovarian endometriosis using laparoscopic surgical techniques. *J Reprod Med*. 1986;31:577–584.

14. Martin DC. $CO_2$ laser laparoscopy for endometriosis associated with infertility. *J Reprod Med*. 1986;31:1089–1094.

15. Adamson GD, Lu J, Suback LL. Laparoscopic $CO_2$ laser vaporization of endometriosis compared with traditional treatments. *Fertil Steril*. 1988;50:704–710.

16. Olive DL, Martin DC. Treatment of endometriosis-associated infertility with $CO_2$ laser laparoscopy: the use of one- and two-parameter exponential models. *Fertil Steril*. 1987; 48:18–23.

17. Kojima E, Yanagibori A, Yuda K, et al. Nd:YAG laser endoscopy. *J Reprod Med*. 1988;33:907–911.

18. Keye WR, Hansen LW, Astin M, et al. Argon laser therapy of endometriosis: a review of 92 consecutive patients. *Fertil Steril*. 1987;47:208–212.

19. Martin DC, Hubert GD, Levy BS. Depth of infiltration of endometriosis. *J Gynecol Surg*. 1989;5:55–60.

# Laparoscopic Ovarian and Parovarian Surgery

*Michael P. Steinkampf and Ricardo Azziz*

## CHAPTER OUTLINE

## Laparoscopic Oophorectomy and Ovarian Cystectomy

### Indications

Indications for laparoscopic removal of the ovary include pelvic pain from ovarian adhesions not amenable to simple adhesiolysis, chronic inflammation, nonmalignant ovarian neoplasms in which preservation of ovarian function is not desired, or rarely castration for the treatment of breast cancer and other estrogen-sensitive disorders.

In general, ovarian cystectomy is preferable to oophorectomy in women who desire future fertility or when only a single ovary is present. Oophorectomy is preferable in postmenopausal women, in order to remove the entire tumor for pathology, and minimize spillage. Nonmalignant ovarian tumors amenable to laparoscopic treatment include endometriomas, dermoids, and serous and mucinous cyctadenomas.

### Patient Selection and Preoperative Evaluation

Table 12.1 outlines the factors to consider in deciding which patients should undergo an attempt at laparoscopic treatment of their adnexal mass. Table 12.2 outlines the indications for the management of adnexal masses by

TABLE 12.1. Considerations in the selection of patients for laparoscopic management of an adnexal mass.

Age: < or > 50 years
Menopausal status
Family history
Systemic symptoms
Endocrine functionality
Sonographic appearance
Serologic markers

TABLE 12.2. Indications for the management of an adnexal mass by laparotomy.

Size > 10 cm?
Torsion?
Bilaterality, unless endometriosis suspected
Sonography demonstrating either:
  −A complex mass, particularly containing papillations or thick septae
  −A multicystic mass, unless endometriosis suspected
  −A solid mass
  −Ascites
Presence of endocrine or systemic symptoms
CA-125 >35 U/mL in postmenopausal patients

laparotomy. A thorough history and physical examination generally suggest the etiology of the mass. Worsening dysmenorrhea and infertility are characteristic of pelvic endometriosis, whereas a history of sexually transmitted diseases and pelvic pain suggests an inflammatory mass. Laboratory testing should be individualized depending on the patient's clinical presentation. Pelvic sonography, particularly using a transvaginal probe, may be useful in guiding therapy. Masses that are bilateral, predominantly solid, or have significant papillations or excrescences are more likely to be malignant, and these patients should be prepared for radical surgery if ovarian malignancy is detected at laparoscopy. If ascites is detected preoperatively, in association with an ovarian mass(es) and in the absence of prior ovarian stimulation, the patient should proceed directly to a laparotomy, since the likelihood of a cancerous process is great. Patients of reproductive age whose adnexal tumor is predominantly cystic should be observed for at least 6 weeks, since functional ovarian cysts will spontaneously regress over this period. The use of oral contraceptives to hasten resolution of functional ovarian cysts has been recommended, but we have abandoned this treatment after failing to confirm efficacy in a controlled study.[1] Furthermore, preoperative estrogen/progestin treatment may increase the risk of pulmonary embolism.[2]

Major concerns in the laparoscopic treatment of ovarian masses include spilling the cyst contents and its possible consequences, and misdiagnosing an ovarian malignancy.

## Intraoperative Cyst Rupture

A major advantage of laparoscopy, the use of small incisions, necessarily increases the risk of cyst rupture. This has been suggested to increase morbidity in patients with both benign and malignant tumors. Occasionally a mucinous cystadenoma that spontaneously perforates results in extensive intraabdominal production of mucin, possibly by transformation of the peritoneal mesothelium to a mucin-secreting epithelium (pseudomyxoma peritonei). In these patients removal of the cyst and evacuation of the mucin does not prevent intraabdominal reaccumulation. Pseudomyxoma peritonei is almost invariably found at the initial operation, and does not appear to be a complication of cyst rupture at surgery, either by laparotomy or laparoscopy. Although spontaneous or iatrogenic rupture of ovarian teratomas can induce peritoneal granuloma formation and adhesions, these complications have not been reported with intraoperative rupture. Mage and colleagues removed 91 cystic teratomas laparoscopically without complication.[3] Nezhat and associates performed second-look laparoscopy on four patients in whom dermoid cysts had been excised laparoscopically and found no evidence of granuloma formation.[4] Thus, it would appear that the risk of complications from rupture of benign cysts during laparoscopy is small. Obviously, extensive irrigation and aspiration of the pelvis should follow the drainage (either spontaneous or intentional) of cyst contents.

The adverse effects of spill from a malignant cyst at the time of laparoscopic removal is less certain. Ovarian cancer generally spreads by peritoneal dissemination, and it seems reasonable that the dissemination of malignant cells into the abdominal cavity would increase the risk of tumor recurrence. On the other hand, it is likely that the manipulation of tumors during any attempt at removal results in the sloughing of some cancerous cells into the peritoneal cavity. Early studies on the prognostic effect of ovarian tumor rupture at laparotomy were inconclusive. Parker and colleagues noted that rupture of the ovarian tumor capsule had no effect on survival,[5] whereas a retrospective study of data from the Mayo Clinic indicated that survival was decreased in those patients.[6] These studies are difficult to interpret because of small patient numbers and the failure to account for confounding factors that might affect the risk of recurrence. In a multivariate analysis of 519 patients with stage I ovarian cancer, Dembo and coworkers found that histologic tumor grade was the most powerful predictor of recurrence, with dense adherence and large-volume ascites also significant predictors.[7] When confounding factors were accounted for, intraoperative cyst rupture was not found to worsen the patient's prognosis. Similarly, in a recent series of 222 patients with stage I or II ovarian cancer analyzed with multivariate techniques, Young and colleagues were unable to identify intraoperative tumor rupture as a prognostic factor for disease-free survival.[8] Thus, intraoperative rupture of a recognized ovarian cancer does not seem to affect the risk of tumor recurrence.

## Misdiagnosing an Adnexal Malignancy

Laparoscopic management of ovarian masses that are subsequently found to be malignant may delay definitive surgery and possibly worsen prognosis. Tumor implantation after laparoscopic biopsy of malignant ovarian tumors with delay in definitive therapy has been reported.[9] From an anecdotal and unselected survey of gynecologic oncologists, Maiman and coworkers found that a delay of several weeks in the performance of definitive surgery, was noted in many patients with a malignancy who had undergone laparoscopy for a pelvic mass. Prior to the laparoscopy over one-half of these masses had "benign" characteristics (less than 8 cm in diameter, cystic, and unilateral).[10] Despite this anecdotal report, the frequency with which ovarian cancer is encountered during operative laparoscopy of properly selected patients is generally less than 1%. Furthermore, the malignancy is generally recognized at the time of the laparoscopy. Mage and colleagues found that among 481 patients of reproductive age with cystic adnexal masses evaluated by laparoscopy, and predicted to be benign by sonographic criteria (generally completely anechoigenic cysts of < 8 cm), only 5 eventually demonstrated an ovarian malignancy. All five patients were recognized at the time of the endoscopy. Four hundred and twenty patients (87.4%) were able to be treated laparoscopically, while 61 had a laparotomy for a suspected malignancy or extensive adhesions.[3] In an other report by Hauuy and colleagues, of 169 cysts predicted benign and treated laparoscopically none were malignant.[11] Parker and Berek described screening criteria for predicting a benign adnexal mass in postmenopausal women including: ultrasound findings of a cystic adnexal mass < 10 cm with distinct borders and no evidence of irregular solid parts, thick septa, ascites, or matted bowel; and a normal serum CA-125 value (<35 U/mL).[12] A laparoscopic resection was able to be performed in 22 (88%) of these patients, while all 25 demonstrated benign lesions. Thus, with proper patient selection the vast majority of cysts operated upon, whether pre or post menopausally, are benign. Furthermore, a high index of suspicion at the time of the laparoscopy will generally identify those few malignancies that have escaped the selection process.

Table 12.3 denotes the principles for handling an adnexal mass laparoscopically. If a malignancy is encountered at the time of laparoscopy, or pathologically noted in the immediate postoperative period, a prompt staging laparotomy should be performed, after appropriate consultation with a gynecologic oncologist. While the laparoscopic treatment of a

TABLE 12.3. Principles of laparoscopic management adnexal masses.

Properly select patients by history, age, menopausal status, sonographic appearance, and tumor markers

At surgery:

–Examine pelvis and abdomen for mets, excessive bowel adhesions at mass, peritoneal excresences, etc.

–Obtain washings, particularly in postmenopausal patients

–Minimize spillage

–Open cyst and examine lining

–If the cyst appears functional or cannot be removed always obtain a biopsy of cyst wall

–Enucleate or excise, do not drain

–When in doubt, obtain a frozen section

stage I ovarian cancer has been reported,[14] the difficulty in performing a thorough sampling of periaortic and iliac nodes for proper staging precludes the routine use of this approach.

We suggest that a frank and thorough discussion of the potential benefits and complications of laparoscopic ovarian surgery be carried out with the patient before the procedure. We have found that most patients are willing to accept the small risk of inadvertent disruption of a malignancy in return for the obvious benefits that laparoscopic surgery offers.

## Technique: Oophorectomy or Salpingo-oophorectomy

The technique of oophorectomy or salpingo-oophorectomy employs the same principles as for removal by laparotomy: lysis of periovarian adhesions, control of the blood supply, and sharp excision. It is most important to identify the course of the ureter and the iliac vessels before dissection. The left ureter will often be more difficult to locate because of its proximity to the root of the sigmoid mesentery. If necessary, the retroperitoneal space can be opened between the round and infundibulopelvic ligaments to facilitate identification. It is also important to free the ovary and tube fully from surrounding structures before removal in order to minimize the chance of resecting a portion of bowel or ureter, or of leaving a piece of ovarian cortex attached to the pelvic sidewall.

A simple oophorectomy can be accomplished by 1) placing a loop ligature into the abdominal cavity over the ovary; 2) grasping the ovary with a 5- or 10-mm claw forceps, placed through a contralateral suprapubic incision and through the suture loop; 3) drawing the ovary through the loop ligature, toward the midline, and ligating the meso-ovarium; 4) three loop ligatures should be placed, preferably using O-chromic; care must be taken not to draw or kink the ureter into the ligatures, and inspection of its course should be made before excision of the ovary; and 5) after hemostasis the meso-ovarium is incised with scissors, leaving at least a 3-mm pedicle. While the method described makes use of the suture ligature, equally satisfactory results can be obtained with bipolar cauterization (Figs. 12.1, 12.2, and 12.3). After ovarian excision, any remaining bleeding can be cauterized using bipolar forceps.

Alternatively, a complete adnexectomy can be performed: 1) the adnexa and ovary is freed from surrounding adhesions; 2) using bipolar cauterization, the infundibulopelvic laterally and the tubal isthmus and utero-ovarian ligament medially are thoroughly desiccated. It is most important to occlude the vessels completely with the bipolar paddles before cauterization and to desiccate at least a 5-mm wide strip. As indicated above, the ureter and underlying iliac vessels must be clearly identified; 3) the cauterized tissue is incised with scissors. For added protection, particularly if the vessels are prominent, the cut infundibulopelvic ligament can be additionally ligated with one or two loop ligatures; 4) placing gentle traction medially on the adnexa, the intervening peritoneum is progressively cauterized and incised, although this tissue is relatively avascular; and 5) after the adnexa is completely excised, any bleeding points on the pelvic sidewall can be controlled with the bipolar cautery.

Removal of the ovary from the abdominal cavity is often the most difficult part of the oophorectomy. For small ovaries, the entire organ can be removed through a 10-mm trocar placed either in the umbilical or suprapubic area. A morcellator can be also be used, but this may hinder adequate pathologic examina-

FIGURE 12.1. An oophorectomy can be performed by
initially coagulating with bipolar the utero-ovarian ligament, after fully identifying
the course infundibulopelvic
ligament and ureter. Medial
traction on the ovary can be
applied using a 5- or 10-mm
claw forceps.

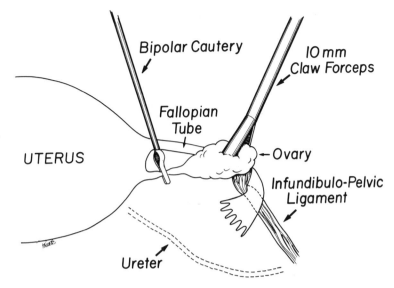

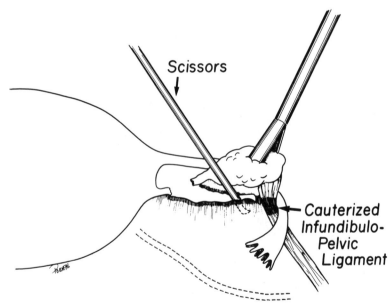

FIGURE 12.2. The vessels entering the ovarian hilum from
the infundibulopelvic ligament
are cauterized. At least a 5-
mm area of cauterization
should be performed. With
continued medial traction on
the ovary, the utero-ovarian
ligament is incised with
hook scissors, and the meso-
ovarium dissected.

tion. Enlargement of either the umbilical or suprapubic incisions can also be employed for removal of larger ovaries. Finally, the ovary may be removed through a colpotomy incision. This method seems to be associated with less postoperative pain than a minilap incision. Any cystic components within the ovary may be aspirated through the vagina before removal. Although the colpotomy incision may be performed vaginally, we prefer to place a sponge stick into the posterior vaginal fornix and incise the vagina laparoscopically, with either a laser or needle cautery. If this approach is taken, it is imperative to confirm that the sigmoid colon is well away from the site of the planned incision, and dissection of the colon from the cul de sac may be performed if indicated.

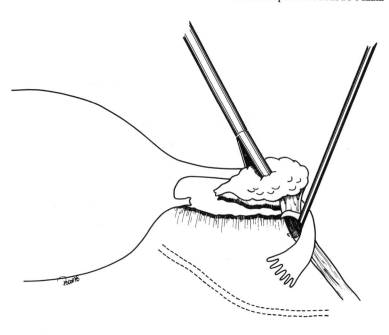

FIGURE 12.3. The cauterized infundibulopelvic ligament is now incised with hook scissors. If the vessels are prominent within the infundibulopelvic ligament, a loop ligature can be applied after cauterization, for added protection against postoperative bleeding. Any remaining bleeding after ovarian excision can be cauterized using bipolar forceps.

## Technique: Ovarian Cystectomy

As for laparotomy, laparoscopic removal of an ovarian cyst should be preceded by careful inspection of the pelvic peritoneum, contralateral ovary, and the abdominal contents. If signs of malignancy such as peritoneal implants, ascites, or capsular excrescences are noted, laparoscopic removal of the cyst should not be attempted. If the cyst appears functional (i.e., a follicular or corpus luteum cyst), simple aspiration or fenestration by removal of the roof of the cyst with scissors may be performed. To minimize the possibility of a missed malignancy, a section of the cyst wall should always be removed for pathological examination after aspiration.

The approach to laparoscopic cystectomy differs somewhat depending on whether the tumor is an endometrioma or whether it is a benign neoplasm. Endometriomas generally are involved in dense adhesions to the pelvic sidewall and/or sigmoid, while other tumors are not. Furthermore, the endometrioma often will drain freely during dissection of the ovary from surrounding structures, and the enucleation site will be dictated by the drainage site. Finally, whereas the ovarian cortex overlying benign neoplasms is generally healthy (although possibly thinned out), that covering an endometrioma is often fibrotic and infiltrated with endometriosis. Usually limited excision of the abnormal ovarian cortex overlying the endometrioma (and often surrounding the drainage site) is required, along with cystectomy. If a tumor other than an endometrioma is suspected, peritoneal washings should be obtained before cystectomy. The washings can be discarded if the cyst, once removed, is felt to be definitively benign.

An ovarian cystectomy can be performed as follows (Fig. 12.4):

1. The ovary is freed from surrounding adhesions and the ureter and pelvic sidewall vessels are clearly identified.
2. An incision is made over the cyst with scissors, through the area where the ovarian cortex is maximally thinned. The incision should be parallel to the long axis of the ovary and as far posterior as possible to minimize the possibility of adhesions to the bowel, uterus, or tube.
3. If needed, the ovary can be rotated with the use of a blunt probe. A grasper placed at the utero-ovarian ligament can also be used, but the ligament generally tears if the cyst is larger than 3 cm.

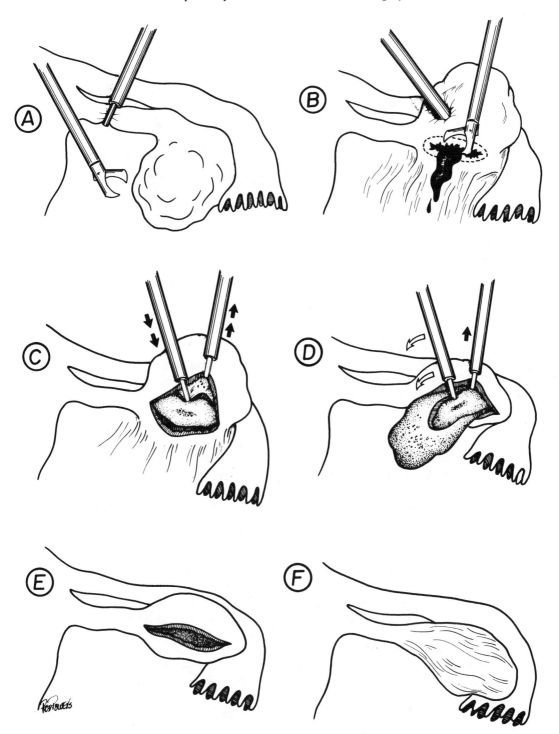

FIGURE 12.4. Laparoscopic ovarian cystectomy. The dissection planes are easiest to attain if the cyst remains distended during the initial phase of enuclea-tion. Nevertheless, this may not always be possible, since many ovarian endometriomas will leak during their initial dissection from the pelvic sidewall.

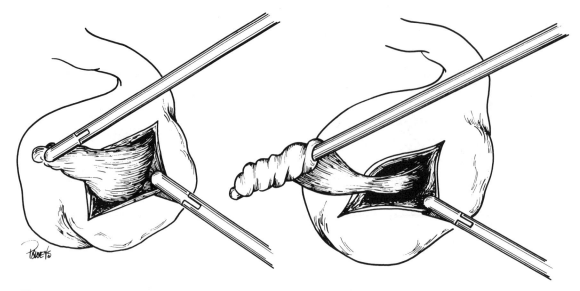

FIGURE 12.5. To facilitate cyst enucleation the cyst wall can be grasped with biopsy forceps and twisted while applying gentle traction, peeling the cyst wall from the underlying ovarian bed.

4. Alternatively, if the ovarian cortex overlying the cyst is exceedingly thin or the cyst is very large, sharp dissection around the base of the cyst with scissors, circumferentially resecting part of the cortex, can be performed.

5. Bluntly, a plane is created between cyst wall and ovarian cortex by spreading the tips of the scissors. For countertraction, the edge of the cortex can be grasped using a biopsy forceps or adhesion grasper.

6. Although some laparoscopic surgeons routinely empty the cyst before removal, we find that an intact cyst facilitates initial dissection. Once an adequate dissection plane is created circumferentially around the cyst, the cyst is aspirated and opened. We try to minimize spillage of cyst contents by first aspirating through a large-bore (18 or 16 gauge) spinal needle placed transabdominally. Placing a suction cannula near the drain site also helps minimize spill. Drainage of dermoids or mucinous cystadenomas generally requires fenestration, followed by extensive irrigation and aspiration.

7. Once opened, inspection of the inner aspect of the cyst wall is performed to detect the presence of excrescences or papillations, suggestive of ovarian malignancy. If solid areas are found within the cyst wall at laparoscopy or after removal, a frozen section is obtained. If malignancy is detected a staging laparotomy is performed.

8. After the cyst is opened and inspected, the edges of the cyst wall (and no longer the ovarian cortex) are grasped. Continued dissection of the cyst wall is performed, using the scissors in blunt fashion.

9. The cyst wall is then peeled from the ovarian bed. Twisting the cyst wall over a biopsy forceps while applying gentle traction may facilitate removal (Fig. 12.5).

10. After cyst enucleation inspection of the cyst bed should be performed and any remaining fragments removed.

11. Hemostasis in the ovary can be obtained with a bipolar cautery. Contrary to what has often been assumed, hilar vessels do not penetrate into the cyst wall and significant bleeding is not often encountered if a proper dissection plane was initially created.

12. The cyst tissue can be removed from the pelvis, as described above for oophorectomy.

13. The ovarian incision may be covered with

Interceed (Johnson and Johnson, Inc.) to minimize adhesion formation. Suturing of the ovary is rarely needed, and only in circumstances where the normal ovarian cortical anatomy has been severely disrupted. More frequently, redundant thinned out ovarian cortex is circumferentially resected.

14. As for any laparoscopic procedure, thorough lavage of the pelvis is performed with lactated Ringer's solution at the end of the surgery.

## Results of Laparoscopic Management of Adnexal Cystic Masses

Many authors have demonstrated the success of laparoscopic ovarian surgery. Reich reported 116 laparoscopic oophorectomies without complication.[14] Perry and Upchurch reported 12 patients undergoing a unilateral and five a bilateral salpingo-oophorectomy.[15] Only one patient required a laparotomy for postoperative bleeding. We have performed more than 40 oophorectomies or adnexectomies without significant complications.

Mage and colleagues reported that of 481 patients undergoing a laparoscopy for a presumed benign cyst, 42 (8.7%) underwent a laparotomy for inability to perform the surgery endoscopically due to dense adhesions and/or excessively large tumors (>10 cm).[3] In 19 of 481 (3.9%) patients a laparotomy was performed after the laparoscopy for the presence or suspicion of a malignancy. Among the 420 patients treated laparoscopically for ovarian cysts, only three (0.7%) suffered significant complications (pelvic infection in two, and acute pain in one). Hauuy and colleagues reported on 165 attempts at laparoscopic treatment of ovarian cysts.[16] The operation was successful in 158 (93%). Failure rate was highest for endometriomas (18.1%) and dermoids (5.7%). We have had to proceed to a laparotomy in three of 30 (10%) patients with endometriomas secondary to the density of periovarian adhesions.

The fertility rate after laparoscopic treatment of endometriomas is unclear. Reich and McGlynn reported a pregnancy rate of 60%

(12/20) among patients treated with laparoscopy only.[17] Kojima and colleagues reported a 37.5% (6/16) pregnancy rate after surgery.[18] Daniell and associates noted that 12 of 32 (38%) patients treated by laparoscopy achieved pregnancy after their initial surgery.[19] In our practice, among 20 infertile patients with laparoscopically treated endometriomas 6 (30%) became pregnant, with one miscarriage. We suspect that the success of laparoscopic ovarian surgery will depend not only on the skill of the surgeon, but more importantly on proper preoperative evaluation and patient selection.

# Laparoscopic Treatment of Anovulation

Polycystic ovary syndrome (PCOS) is a disorder of chronic anovulation and infertility. The ovaries typically are symmetrically enlarged, with a smooth, thickened capsule and multiple ovarian follicular cysts 4 to 8 mm in diameter. Wedge resection of the ovaries has been known to result in temporary normalization of ovarian function, with pregnancy resulting in 60% to 70% of infertile women.[20,21] The mechanism for this effect is unclear, but may involve reduction in ovarian androgen production through a decrease in stromal mass or disruption of parenchymal blood flow. A number of alternatives to wedge resection by laparotomy have been proposed to decrease the morbidity and the associated postoperative adhesion formation.

## Preoperative Evaluation

Patients with PCOS usually have a history of infrequent, irregular menses from puberty; the sudden onset of amenorrhea, especially with progressive virilization, should alert one to the possibility of a hormonally active adrenal or ovarian tumor. When appropriate, other causes of androgen excess should also be ruled out including the hyperandrogenic–insulin resistant–acanthosis nigricans (HAIRAN) syndrome, late-onset adrenal hyperplasia, or

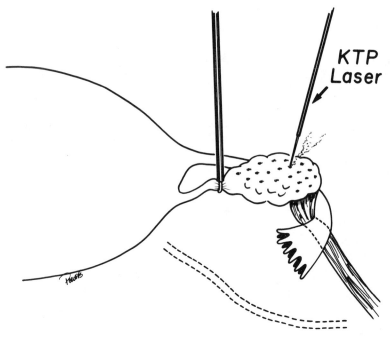

FIGURE 12.6. Laparoscopic cauterization for the treatment of the PCOS. The surface of the ovary is fulgurated at evenly spaced points. If unipolar cautery is used, four to eight points per ovary are required. However, if the laser is used the number of punctures required may be as high as 25 to 40 per ovary.

Cushing's syndrome. A basic infertility evaluation including semen analysis, hysterosalpingography, and ovulatory monitoring with basal body temperature charting, endometrial biopsy, or luteal progesterone assay should also be performed, if applicable. Because of the risk of postoperative adhesions, we feel that only patients who have failed to ovulate with clomiphene citrate should be considered candidates for the laparoscopic treatment of PCOS. Patients should be counseled about the option of gonadotropin treatment before surgery is performed.

## Technique of Laparoscopic Ovarian Cauterization for PCOS

Laparoscopy is performed in the standard manner. After careful inspection of the pelvis, the utero-ovarian ligament is held with an atraumatic grasper and the surface of the ovary is fulgurated at evenly spaced points. If unipolar needle cautery is used, four to eight points per ovary are satisfactory, with cautery maintained until the ovarian capsule and cortex is penetrated. If the laser ($CO_2$ or KTP) is used, the number of punctures required may be higher (Fig. 12.6), with 25 to 40 reportedly used by

some surgeons.[22] After cauterization, the pelvis is irrigated and inspected for bleeding, although this is a rare complication. Although laparoscopic wedge resection is feasible, the results have not been shown to be superior to simple fulguration of the ovary.

## Results of Laparoscopic Cauterization for PCOS

Campo and coworkers performed multiple ovarian biopsies at laparoscopy in 12 patients with PCOS who had not responded to clomiphene; pregnancy subsequently occurred in five patients.[23] Gjonnaess described laparoscopic cauterization of the ovaries, with pregnancy occurring in 24 of 35 patients so treated.[24] More recently, Daniell and Miller noted comparable results with laser fulguration.[22] About half of their patients who were refractory to clomiphene ovulated spontaneously after surgery, and 85% of patients previously dependent on clomiphene for cyclic ovarian function subsequently ovulated without medication. Pregnancy was achieved in 56% of patients. In their hands, the KTP laser was more useful than the $CO_2$ laser because of the decrease in plume formation.

# Laparoscopic Resection of Parovarian Cysts

Parovarian cysts may present as an adnexal mass and are usually detected by pelvic examination and/or sonography, which reveals a simple uniloculated cystic structure in the adnexa. Genadry and colleagues reviewed 132 benign parovarian cysts and observed that 51% of tumors greater than 3 cm in diameter were of mesothelial (peritoneal inclusion) origin, 19% were paramesonephric, and none were of mesonephric (Wolffian) origin.[25] Most of these cysts (79%) were encountered in women between the ages of 20 and 49 years. Mesothelial cysts usually comprise a single layer of epithelium or mesothelium, are encapsulated in a thin fibrous connective tissue layer and can reach >10 cm in size. The mesosalpingeal vasculature surrounds but does not penetrate the connective tissue layer encapsulating the cyst.

## Indications and Patient Selection

Often a parovarian cyst will be diagnosed by pelvic examination, or incidentally during pelvic ultrasonography or diagnostic laparoscopy. At the time of the laparoscopy it is most important to determine whether there are any solid components within the parovarian cyst, or peritoneal implants suggesting malignant transformation. Furthermore, it is important not to confuse a tumorous extension of an ovarian neoplasm into the mesosalpinx with a parovarian cyst. Benign parovarian cysts are rarely bilateral.

If the appearance of the cyst on sonography and laparoscopic inspection of the adnexa suggest that the structure is benign, laparoscopic resection can proceed.

## Technique

Semm prefers to enucleate the cysts without prior drainage,[26] but Herbert and associates describe a technique that involves the initial aspiration of the cyst.[27] The authors prefer not to drain the cyst before enucleation, to facilitate dissection. However, exceedingly large tumors may require partial aspiration before resection. An 18- or 20-gauge spinal needle is placed through the midline of the anterior abdominal wall and the cyst partially aspirated. Following is the authors' preferred method of removing parovarian cysts, using a standard three-puncture operative laparoscopy approach (Fig. 12.7):

1. Once the cyst has been clearly identified the peritoneum overlying the mass, halfway between the tube and the ovary, is picked up with micrograspers and incised with hook or microscissors. The incision is performed parallel to the long axis of the tube. Care should be taken not to enter the cystic cavity at this time. Although the fallopian tube may often be stretched and distorted, the surgeon should avoid any manipulation that may endanger this structure, since the fallopian tube returns to normal once the parovarian cyst is removed.

2. Hook scissors are now introduced through the incision, between the cyst wall and overlying peritoneum, and circumferential dissection begun bluntly, by spreading the tips of the scissors.

3. Once the cyst has been exposed a biopsy forceps (with a central grasping pin) is used to grasp the cyst firmly. At this time it is important not to relax the forceps, in order to avoid leakage of cyst fluid and loss of the dissection planes. Enucleation of the parovarian cyst away from surrounding connective tissue and vasculature is made easiest when it is distended.

4. Alternatively, if the cyst is quite large the biopsy forceps may be relaxed, allowing fluid to drain into the cul de sac and reducing cyst size. If needed the mesosalpingeal incision is extended parallel to the tube.

5. In general, small peritoneal vessels can be transected with the hook scissors with minimal bleeding. Larger vessels should be cauterized before incision.

6. Continuous traction of the cyst toward the midline and progressive circumferential dissection with the closed scissor tips will free the cyst from the surrounding connective tissue and peritoneum.

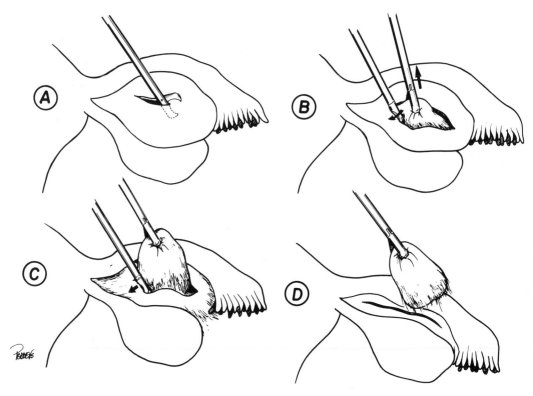

FIGURE 12.7. Laparoscopic resection of a parovarian cyst. Dissection is generally facilitated if the cyst is intact. Bleeding is generally minimal and does not require cauterization. The peritoneum does not have to be sutured closed after resection of the cyst.

7. If there remains a thicker pedicle of coalesced connective tissue attached between the bed and base of the cyst, it is cauterized slightly with bipolar forceps and transected. Bleeding is generally minimal and does not require cauterization. If there is oozing from the parovarian cyst bed, it is preferable to apply pressure with a suprapubic blunt probe for approximately 5 min, followed by extensive irrigation. The placement of catgut loop ligatures at the base of the parovarian cyst is usually unnecessary, and has the potential of creating significant postoperative adhesions. As stated above, no vessels directly penetrate into the ovarian cyst wall, and careful dissection with a blunt-edge scissors should free the cyst in its entirety without the formation of an artificial "pedicle" of coalesced connective tissue.

8. Once the cyst has been enucleated from its mesosalpingeal location it is allowed to drain and removed through a 5- or 10-mm suprapubic sleeve.

9. The peritoneal defect that is left behind does not require suturing. Furthermore, excessive cauterization of the area should be avoided.

## Results

We have removed more than 20 parovarian cysts, ranging from 3 to 7 cm, in the manner described without difficulty. Minimal bleeding is encountered that usually ceases spontaneously or after the application of pressure. Rarely is cauterization required. Cysts >5 cm may require partial aspiration before dissection to reduce the size of the peritoneal incision.

# References

1. Steinkampf MP, Hammond KR, Blackwell RE. Hormonal treatment of functional ovarian cysts: a randomized, prospective study. *Fertil Steril.* 1990;54:775–777.

2. Vessey MP, Doll R, Fairbairn AS, et al. Postoperative thromboembolism and the use of oral contraceptives. *Br Med J.* 1970;3:123–126.

3. Mage G, Canis M, Manhes H, et al. Laparoscopic management of adnexal cystic masses. *J Gynecol Surg.* 1990;6:71–79.

4. Nezhat C, Winer WK, Nezhat F. Laparoscopic removal of dermoid cysts. *Obstet Gynecol.* 1989;73:278–280.

5. Parker RT, Parker CH, Wilbanks GD. Cancer of the ovary. *Am J Obstet Gynecol.* 1970;108:878–888.

6. Webb MJ, Decker DG, Mussey E, et al. Factors influencing survival in stage I ovarian cancer. *Am J Obstet Gynecol.* 1973;116:222–228.

7. Dembo AJ, Davy M, Stenwig AE, et al. Prognostic factors in patients with stage I epithelial ovarian cancer. *Obstet Gynecol.* 1990;75:263–273.

8. Young RC, Walton LA, Ellenberg SS, et al. Adjuvant therapy in stage I and stage II epithelial ovarian cancer: results of two prospective randomized trials. *N Engl J Med.* 1990;322:1021–1027.

9. Hsiu JG, Given FT, Kemp GM. Tumor implantation after diagnostic laparoscopic biopsy of serous ovarian tumors of low malignant potential. *Obstet Gynecol.* 1986;68(Suppl 3):90S–93S.

10. Maiman M, Seltzer V, Boyce J. Laparoscopic excision of ovarian neoplasms subsequently found to be malignant. *Obstet Gynecol.* 1991;77:563–565.

11. Hauuy JP, Madelenat P, Bouquet de la Joliniere, Dubuisson JB. Laparoscopic surgery of ovarian cysts. The indications and the units as found in a series of 169 cysts. *J Gynecol Obstet Biol Reprod.* 1990;19:209–216.

12. Parker WH, Berek JS. Management of selected cystic adnexal masses in postmenopausal women by operative laparoscopy: a pilot study. *Am J Obstet Gynecol.* 1990;163:1574–1577.

13. Reich H, McGlynn F, Wilkie W. Laparoscopic management of stage I ovarian cancer. *J Reprod Med.* 1990;35:601–605.

14. Reich H. Laparoscopic oophorectomy without ligature or morcellation. *Contemp OB/GYN.* 1989;34(3):34–46.

15. Perry CP, Upchurch JC. Pelviscopic adnexectomy. *Am J Obstet Gynecol.* 1990;162:79–81.

16. Hauuy JP, Madelenat P, de La Joliniere JB, et al. Chirurgie per-coelioscopique des kystes ovariens. Incidation et limites a propos d'une serie de 169 kystes. *J Gynecol Obstet Biol Reprod.* 1990;19:209–216.

17. Reich H, McGlynn F. Treatment of ovarian endometriomas using laparoscopic surgical techniques. *J Reprod Med.* 1986;31:577–584.

18. Kojima E, Morita M, Otaka K, et al. YAG laser laparoscopy for ovarian endometriomas. *J Reprod Med.* 1990;35:592–596.

19. Daniell JF, Kurtz BR, Gurley LD. Laser laparoscopic management of large endometriomas. *Fertil Steril.* 1991:55:692–695.

20. Adashi EY, Rock JA, Guzick D, et al. Fertility following bilateral ovarian wedge resection: a critical analysis of 90 consecutive cases of the polycystic ovary syndrome. *Fertil Steril.* 1981;36:320–325.

21. McLaughlin DS. Evaluation of adhesion reformation by early second-look laparoscopy following microlaser ovarian wedge resection. *Fertil Steril.* 1984;42:531–537.

22. Daniell JF, Miller W. Polycystic ovaries treated by laparoscopic laser vaporization. *Fertil Steril.* 1989;51:232–236.

23. Campo S, Garcea N, Caruso A, et al. Effect of celioscopic ovarian resection in patients with polycystic ovaries. *Gynecol Obstet Invest.* 1983;15:213–222.

24. Gjonnaess H. Polycystic ovarian syndrome treated by ovarian electrocautery through the laparoscope. *Fertil Steril.* 1984;41:20–25.

25. Genadry R, Parmley T, Woodruff JD. The origin and clinical behavior of the parovarian tumor. *Am J Obstet Gynecol.* 1977;129:873–880.

26. Semm K. *Operative Manual for Endoscopic Abdominal Surgery.* Chicago: Year Book Medical Publishers; 1987.

27. Herbert CM, Segars JH, Hill GA. A laparoscopic method for the excision of large retroperitoneal parovarian cysts. *Obstet Gynecol.* 1990;75:139–141.

# 13

# Laparoscopic and Hysteroscopic Myomectomy

*Bradley S. Hurst and William D. Schlaff*

CHAPTER OUTLINE

Uterine fibroids are benign smooth muscle tumors that are found in at least 20% of women over age 30 years. The incidence of fibroids increases with age until the time of menopause. Fibroids may be identified in up to 50% of nulliparous women at the age of 50 years.[1] Most women with uterine leiomyomata are asymptomatic. Symptoms that may be attributed to myomas include pelvic pain, pelvic pressure, urinary frequency as a result of direct compression of the bladder, constipation or tenesmus as a result of compression of the colon, abdominal bloating, or abnormal uterine bleeding. Submucous myomas or large intramural myomas may be associated with recurrent pregnancy loss and infertility.

## Indications

Surgery is indicated for patients when significant symptoms are directly attributed to the uterine fibroids. Additionally, surgery is indicated for myomas that are rapidly growing and, therefore, possibly malignant. The traditional surgical procedure of choice for a patient who desires to maintain her reproductive

125

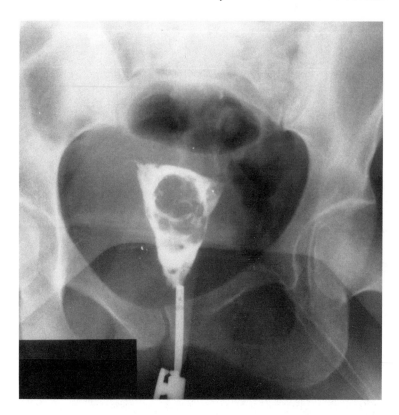

FIGURE 13.1. Hysterosalpingogram with large intrauterine filling defect due to a submucous myoma.

potential is abdominal myomectomy. Hysterectomy, either by abdominal or vaginal route, is the most common surgical procedure for symptomatic patients for whom childbearing is not desired. With the development and improvement of endoscopic equipment and surgical techniques, laparoscopic and hysteroscopic myomectomy is now possible.

## Preoperative Evaluation

The goal of the preoperative evaluation is to determine if surgery is required and, if so, what procedure is optimal. Objective causes should be sought and excluded before surgery for patients with infertility, multiple pregnancy loss, or physical symptoms associated with fibroids. Abnormal uterine bleeding due to cervical factors, ovulatory dysfunction, and endometrial abnormalities such as polyps, hyperplasia, or adenocarcinoma should be excluded before myomectomy. When no other objective findings are identified, the patient must decide if her symptoms are sufficiently severe to warrant surgery.

Radiographic imaging may help to determine whether or not the endoscopic approach is appropriate and advisable. Ultrasonography may provide information about the size, number, and location of fibroids. Magnetic resonance imaging (MRI) is frequently helpful and may give specific information about the location of the myoma(s). MRI may be useful in defining whether the myoma is in a submucous, intramural, subserous, or pedunculated location. Hysterosalpingography is indispensable in the preoperative assessment of the patient suspected of having fibroids. A hysterosalpingogram (HSG) will show the size of any submucous myomas and may give a hint as to the site and extent of the myometrial attachment by evaluation of the filling defect (Fig. 13.1). Furthermore, an HSG will define the relationship of the myoma to the fallopian tube(s) and will provide a preoperative assessment of tubal patency.

# Preoperative Preparation

The ability to perform an endoscopic myomectomy is greatly limited by the size, position, and number of myomas. Although no prospective studies have been conducted, gonadotropin-releasing hormone (GnRH) analogs are frequently used preoperatively. Preoperative suppression with GnRH analogs provides several potential benefits when endoscopic surgery is proposed. First, GnRH analogs may reduce uterine bleeding and allow for a normalization of hemoglobin by the time of surgery in patients who are anemic.[2] Second, GnRH analogs decrease the uterine volume and the size of myomas, which may make them easier to remove.[3] Third, uterine blood flow has been shown to be decreased with GnRH analog treatment. If preoperative ovarian suppression is elected, one should treat for 2 to 4 months before surgery. GnRH analog therapy may be particularly useful in patients who have a submucous myoma where the most difficult step is to bring the resected myoma out through the cervical canal.

The patient should always be prepared for an abdominal myomectomy. Laparotomy may be necessary due to bleeding or technical difficulty with laparoscopic or hysteroscopic myomectomy. The patient should be informed that a hysterectomy may be necessary if attempts at uterine repair are unsuccessful. Although hysterectomy is rarely necessary during abdominal myomectomy, there are no reports that address the incidence of hysterectomy when endoscopic myomectomy is performed.

Autologous blood should be available before surgery whenever possible. If impossible, the patient should be cross-matched for a possible transfusion. Unlike most endoscopic surgery, the patient may well require admission for close postoperative observation for bleeding, fever, infection, or other complications that might arise from myomectomy. If there is no immediate postoperative complication, there is no need to require a prolonged recuperation or to schedule an extended leave from work.

# Laparoscopic Myomectomy

## Patient Selection

Endoscopic myomectomy should be attempted only by those with extensive experience in operative endoscopic procedures. The potential morbidity associated with this procedure includes massive blood loss, infection, and extensive postoperative adhesions. With these cautions in mind, several operative principles should be observed when laparoscopic myomectomy is performed.

Laparoscopic myomectomy is most likely to be successful when fibroids are single and pedunculated. Although laparoscopic myomectomy may be possible when fibroids are either large or quite numerous, one must question whether the endoscopic approach is safest for the patient and is least likely to result in operative complications or postoperative adhesions. If subserous or pedunculated myomas are confirmed either by ultrasound or MRI, it may be possible to remove them laparoscopically. However, deep intramural myomas may result in unacceptable blood loss if approached with the laparoscope, and it continues to be our recommendation to approach these by laparotomy.

Although fever is quite common after myomectomy, infection is much less common. Nevertheless, prophylactic antibiotics are frequently used for laparoscopic myomectomy, although there are no prospective trials evaluating their efficacy.

## Instrumentation

Laparoscopic instruments necessary for myomectomy are similar to those required for other extensive laparoscopic procedures. An operating laparoscope or a straight laparoscope may be used. A second laparoscope, a "teaching head," or a video monitor system is necessary to allow visualization by the assistant. Three or four incisions may be required so appropriate instruments must be available. A laparoscopic needle and syringe is necessary if the myometrium is to be injected with vasopressin (20 U in 20 cc of normal saline). Al-

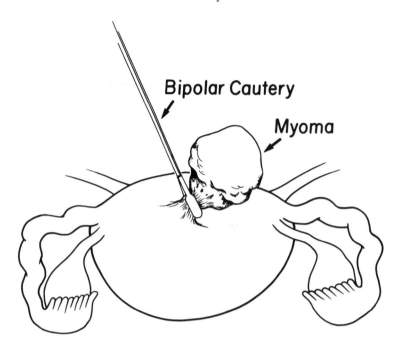

Bipolar Cautery

Myoma

FIGURE 13.2. Technique for removal of a pedunculated myoma. The fibroid is grasped and held to allow a bipolar cautery to be placed at the base of the entire pedicle.

ternately, this can be done transabdominally with a spinal needle under direct laparoscopic visualization. A $CO_2$, KTP, Argon, or Nd:YAG laser may be used to make the serosal incision, but lasers are certainly not necessary. The incision may be made effectively with a monopolar microcautery tip or a laparoscopic knife. A grasper with teeth is essential, and must be large enough to grasp the fibroid and provide adequate traction. Sharp scissors are necessary to dissect the myoma from the pseudocapsule. This can also be accomplished with lasers, particularly the sapphire tip of a Nd:YAG laser. An instrument for morcellation should be available. Bipolar cautery, monopolar cautery, diathermy, or a laser with coagulation capabilities is essential to establish myometrial hemostasis. For a pedunculated myoma, large bipolar paddles may be quite helpful. A rapid irrigating and aspirating system is required. Instruments to perform vaginal or abdominal surgery should be available at the time of myomectomy. If myomas are too large to be removed through the laparoscope, they may be removed through a posterior colpotomy or a minilaparotomy incision.

A Foley catheter is placed to be sure that the pelvis will not be obscured by an enlarging bladder, and a rigid intrauterine instrument is placed to allow good uterine manipulation.

## Technique

Basic operative laparoscopic techniques are used to prepare the patient for surgery. A subumbilical incision is made for the laparoscope, and a midline suprapubic incision is made for suction, irrigation, or operative instruments. The site of operating incisions will depend on the site of the myoma. A retracting instrument will generally be placed through the side opposite the dissecting instrument, which can be placed either in the midline or laterally.

For a patient with a pedunculated myoma, the following steps are recommended. First, the fibroid is grasped and held in a position to allow a bipolar cautery to be placed at the base of the pedunculated fibroid (Fig. 13.2). This bipolar instrument is passed through the incision opposite the retracting instrument. Whenever possible, the bipolar cautery instrument should be placed across the entire pedicle. If this is not possible, the stalk may be coagulated in two or more sections. The bipolar cautery is then activated until coagulation has stopped and there is no current flow. While

FIGURE 13.3. Technique for removal of pedunculated myoma. Monopolar cautery scissors are used to resect stalk.

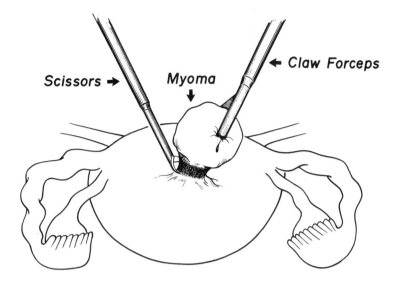

Scissors → Myoma ↓ ← Claw Forceps

continuing to hold the myoma gently with the grasping instrument, the bipolar cautery is replaced with scissors. The stalk is then sharply resected (Fig. 13.3). Monopolar cautery scissors may be used to resect the stalk. If this instrument is used, the current should be applied to the area of the stalk proximal to the bipolar lesion (i.e., between the ground plate and the coagulated site). This will minimize the risk of injury to adjacent tissue. If required, the defect produced by excision of the myoma may then be cauterized with bipolar or monopolar cautery until hemostasis has been accomplished. The fibroid, if less than 1 cm in diameter, can be pulled directly through the 10-mm trocar with the grasping forceps. For a larger myoma, extraction can be accomplished with a morcellator (Fig. 13.4). Nevertheless, this can be quite tedious. Alternatively, the fibroid can be grasped with one instrument and progressively cut into smaller pieces with a monopolar cautery or scissors placed through another channel. In this event, the myoma should be shaved within the anterior cul de sac to reduce the possibility of injury to the bowel. Myomatous fragments can be removed through the 10-mm laparoscope channel. If the myoma cannot be removed in this manner, it may be necessary to remove it through the cul de sac or by minilaparotomy.

If a minilaparotomy is done, however, several preliminary steps must be completed. Lapa-

rotomy will likely result in loss of most or all of the pneumoperitoneum, and will make any further procedures virtually impossible. Hemostasis must be obtained at all operative sites and fluid aspirated from the pelvis if desired. Essentially the procedure must effectively be completed. The fibroid is then grasped with the laparoscopic grasper and held up to the area where the minilap incision will be made. The abdominal incision should be slightly larger than the myoma. Once the incision has been made and the peritoneum has been opened, the grasping instrument is passed through the incision and the myoma directly removed from the abdomen.

Another alternative is removal of the myomas through a colpotomy incision. Again, hemostasis should be established and the pelvis irrigated before colpotomy, since the incision will cause loss of the pneumoperitoneum. The fibroid should be grasped with the laparoscopic grasper so that the fibroid may be directly passed through the colpotomy incision when it is made. The colpotomy is opened under laparoscopic guidance, and the myomas are removed. The incision is closed in the usual manner.

Subserosal fibroids present more of a challenge than pedunculated fibroids. The operative principles followed should be the same as those used at laparotomy. Specifically, the incision should be in the anterior uterus, and as many myomas should be removed through one

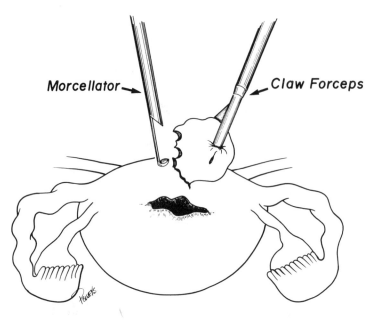

Morcellator → ← Claw Forceps

FIGURE 13.4. Technique for removal of pedunculated myoma. Large claw forceps are used to grasp the myoma. The morcellator is used to decrease the size of the myoma.

FIGURE 13.5. Technique for removal of a subserous myoma. Vasopressin is injected into incision site (*dotted line*). The incision is made down to the myoma.

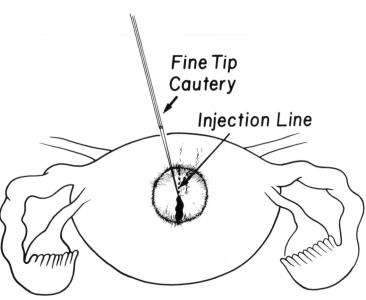

Fine Tip Cautery

Injection Line

incision as possible. Care should be taken to avoid trauma to the surrounding normal tissue.[4] To reduce blood loss, the incision site may be injected with vasopressin. One ampule (20 U) of vasopressin (Pitressin) is diluted in 20 cc of saline and injected directly into the incision site either transabdominally with a spinal needle or via a laparoscopic needle. Blanching of the serosa should be seen. The incision is then made with either a $CO_2$, KTP, Argon, or Nd:YAG laser, monopolar cautery, or a unipolar knife (Fig. 13.5). The choice of instrument is at the discretion of the surgeon, as there are no data that suggest that any one method is superior to the others. The incision is carried down to the myoma. A blunt probe is used to expose the superficial aspect of the myoma from the pseudocapsule (Fig. 13.6). The myoma is then grasped with a claw forceps (Fig. 13.7). Dissecting scissors or thermo-

FIGURE 13.6. Technique for removal of a subserous myoma. A blunt probe is used to expose the superficial aspect of the myoma.

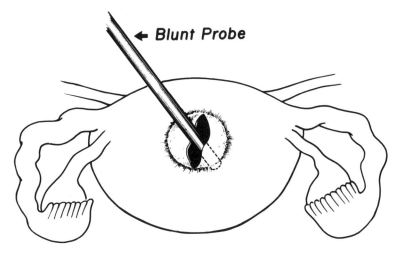

FIGURE 13.7. Technique for the removal of a subserous myoma. The myoma is grasped and countertraction is applied while the myoma is dissected from the pseudocapsule with scissors.

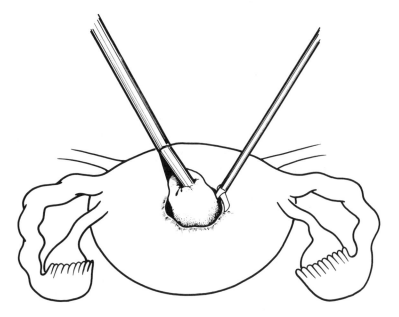

coagulator is inserted through the contralateral lower abdominal incision. Countertraction is applied with the grasping forceps while the myoma is dissected from the pseudocapsule with the scissors or blunt dissection. When the dissection becomes difficult, the grasping forceps and the scissors are reversed and are placed through opposite trocars. This may better enable dissection of the contralateral side. The myoma should never be pulled or twisted from the base, since this may cause disruption of the endometrium. Rather, the base of the myoma should be excised. After the myoma has been removed, it is placed in the posterior cul de sac. Monopolar or laser coagulation of the base may be required to achieve hemostasis (Fig. 13.8).

If additional myomas are found, they should be removed through the same initial uterine incision if possible. The serosa at the incision site is grasped and retracted to provide maximal exposure of the myoma through the myometrium. An incision is made deeper into the myometrium, and the myoma is exposed. Again, the superficial aspect of the myoma is separated from the pseudocapsule by dissec-

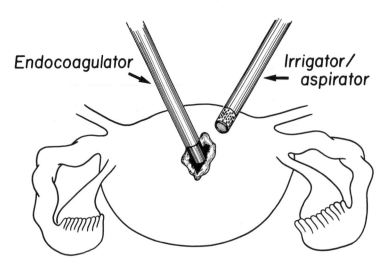

**Endocoagulator**

**Irrigator/ aspirator**

FIGURE 13.8. Technique for the removal of a subserous myoma. The myometrium is coagulated after myomectomy to achieve hemostasis.

tion with a blunt manipulator. The myoma is grasped and sharply cut from the pseudocapsule as previously described. All fibroids collected should be placed in the posterior cul de sac to avoid losing any tissue.

Once the myomectomy has been completed, the myometrium is coagulated until adequate hemostasis is achieved. This may prove to be a long and tedious process. An irrigation/aspiration system is helpful to keep the site clean and to identify small bleeding sites. Hemostasis may be achieved either by bipolar cautery, monopolar cautery, thermocoagulation, Nd:YAG laser, or a defocused $CO_2$ laser. Of these, the defocused $CO_2$ laser is probably the least effective, while all of the other options are acceptable. Both irrigation fluid and blood will dramatically reduce the effectiveness of all these coagulation modalities, so the area should be kept as dry as possible for maximal coagulation.

Depending on the size of the defect, suturing of the myometrium may be unnecessary. Defects involving more than half the depth of the uterine wall generally are sutured using intraabdominal or extracorporeal tying techniques (see Chapter 4). Although there are no available data, it seems appropriate to repair these deep myometrial incisions. The integrity and tensile strength of the uterine wall subsequent to laparoscopic myomectomy has not been studied.

Laparotomy may be necessary in the face of

difficulty or complications, and should never be considered a procedure of last resort. It is foolhardy to continue a procedure laparoscopically if serious morbidity is a distinct possibility. Significant bleeding that cannot be quickly controlled is an indication for immediate laparotomy. Long or deep incisions that cannot be repaired laparoscopically should be handled with a laparotomy using microsurgical techniques in an attempt to limit blood loss and to reduce adhesion formation. If multiple myomas are unexpectedly identified, or if the myomas are too large or too deep in the muscle of the uterus to remove safely, laparotomy should be performed. Laparotomy also should be performed if the endometrium is exposed or disrupted during the procedure to allow for adequate uterine reconstruction. In short, laparotomy should never be perceived as a defeat but, rather, as a prudent step to insure the safety and well-being of the patient.

## Postoperative Care

A patient who has undergone a successful laparoscopic intramural myomectomy may be hospitalized as an inpatient for 24 to 48 hr. Serial hemoglobin levels should be obtained postoperatively. The patient's vital signs should be monitored every 4 hr. There need be no physical restrictions on activity postoperatively if the patient's vital signs are stable. Bleeding may occur from the intraabdominal operative sites, and the patient may become hemodynamically unstable. For a patient with a progressively declining hemoglobin or unstable vital signs, further diagnosis and probable operation are necessary. Laparoscopy may be performed initially to determine whether or not there is bleeding from the incision sites. If the bleeding site(s) is identified, laparoscopic coagulation is acceptable. However, if the site(s) cannot be controlled laparoscopically, or if there are multiple bleeding sites or brisk bleeding, laparotomy should be performed. Fever is quite common after abdominal myomectomy, and this may also occur after a laparoscopic myomectomy. Postoperative fever should be evaluated and managed no differently than after an abdominal procedure. The additional danger, however, comes from an unsuspected bowel injury. A fever that does not respond to aggressive antibiotic therapy should be considered suspicious for a possible unrecognized bowel injury.

Extensive adhesion formation and the risk of bowel obstruction due to adhesions may occur after laparoscopic myomectomy as a result of large defects in the uterus. There are no adjuncts to laparoscopic surgery currently available that have been shown to reduce adhesions after a myomectomy. Interceed barriers have not yet been tested on myomectomy incisions. Hyskon and other adjuvants are of limited use. The Gore-Tex Surgical Membrane (W.L. Gore & Associates, Naperville, IL) appears to be effective at reducing adhesions to the uterus when placed at the time of abdominal myomectomy, but at this point has not been evaluated for laparoscopic myomectomy. The use of early second-look laparoscopy for lysis of adhesions may be warranted after laparoscopic myomectomy.

## Results

Many techniques of laparoscopic myomectomy are described in the literature.[5-7] However, there is scant data to evaluate the outcome and results of the surgery. Furthermore, there are no studies comparing outcome of laparoscopic versus abdominal myomectomy. Therefore, laparoscopic myomectomy should be limited to investigational protocols until key questions relative to the efficacy and safety of the procedure can be determined by appropriate studies. Until such data are available, abdominal myomectomy remains the procedure of choice for large, deep, intramural myomas. The risks associated with resection of pedunculated myomas appears to be lower than those associated with intramural myomectomy and the former may be much more amenable to laparoscopic resection.

## Hysteroscopic Myomectomy

In contrast to the lack of studies available for evaluation of laparoscopic myomectomy, there is a growing body of evidence supporting the use of hysteroscopy for removal of submucous myomas, since the procedure was first described by Neuwirth and Amin in 1976.[8]

### Patient Selection

Hysteroscopic myomectomy should be considered for any patient with a symptomatic submucous myoma. Patients with submucous myomas frequently present with menorrhagia and metrorrhagia. Bleeding may be severe and result in significant anemia. Many experience severe dysmenorrhea. Submucous myomas may be associated with recurrent pregnancy losses and infertility.[9] As with the laparoscopic procedure, before considering hysteroscopic myomectomy a thorough preoperative evaluation is required. The single most important step is identifying the size and attachment of the myoma. An HSG should be performed to determine the size and location of the myoma.[10] In some cases, ultrasound or MRI can also be useful in this regard. Abdominal myomectomy should be considered if there is extensive intramural involvement or if the submucous myoma is attached to a broad portion of the uterine wall.

### Instrumentation and Technique

Hysteroscopic myomectomy becomes more difficult with increasing size of fibroids. Preoperative GnRH analog therapy is useful to reduce the size of fibroids, although no prospective studies have been performed to confirm this. In addition, GnRH analog therapy allows for improvement of hemoglobin concentration when anemia is present.[10] If GnRH analogs are used, therapy should be initiated 2 to 3 months before surgery.

Careful preoperative preparation is critical. If the myoma appears to be large ($\geq 3$ cm) one should consider dilating the cervix preoperatively with laminaria or other hydrophilic adjuncts. As many laminaria as possible should be inserted into the cervix the day before surgery and held in place with a vaginal sponge. These should be removed and replaced the night before surgery to maximize cervical dilatation, thereby insuring the greatest possible chance of successfully removing the myoma transcervically. Prophylactic antibiotics should be considered. Finally, autologous blood should be banked or a cross-match obtained before surgery.

Diagnostic hysteroscopy should be performed before myomectomy is attempted. The size and location of the myoma should be carefully confirmed. If the myoma exceeds the skill of the operator, the procedure should be terminated at this point.

Laparoscopic surveillance is recommended at the time of hysteroscopic myomectomy in the case of large submucous myomas to reduce complications such as uterine perforation. The assistant is able to warn the operator if the dissection is nearing the uterine serosa. Additionally, a perforation is usually immediately evident with laparoscopy.

Once the decision is made to proceed with a hysteroscopic myomectomy, an operating hysteroscope is used. A modified urologic resectoscope with a monopolar cautery loop may be used to shave the myoma (Fig. 13.9).[9] Alternatively, a Nd:YAG laser with a sapphire tip may be used through the operating channel of the hysteroscope.[11] An operating hysteroscope with rigid or semirigid scissors can sometimes be used for pedunculated submucous myomas.

Several distending media are available. Hyskon (32% dextran-70) offers the advantage of high viscosity, which allows for distention

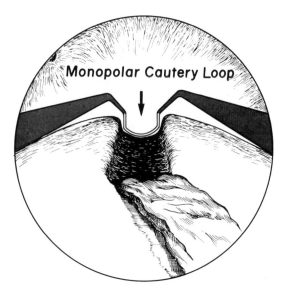

FIGURE 13.9. Technique for hysteroscopic resection of a submucous myoma. Diagnostic hysteroscopy is performed to characterize size and location of the fibroid. Using a modified urologic resectoscope, a monopolar cautery loop is used to shave the myoma to its base.

of the endometrial cavity with less spillage through the cervix, compared to less viscous media. Hyskon is immiscible with blood, and bleeding points may be easily identified. The use of more than 200 to 300 ml of Hyskon is discouraged, since pulmonary edema may result.[12] Visibility is severely compromised in the presence of significant bleeding or clots. In these situations, alternatives to Hyskon include 5% dextrose in water, normal saline, lactated Ringer's solution, 1.5% solution of glycine, or sorbitol. The use of these solutions allows for rapid clearance of blood and myomatous fragments. Total infusion should not exceed more than 2 to 3 liters since significant shifts of electrolytes may occur. Intrauterine vasopressin may be used to reduce uptake of the distention media.[13]

The cervix should be dilated to allow insertion of the hysteroscopic instruments, but not so much that the seal between the cervix and the hysteroscope is lost. For a pedunculated submucous myoma, simple excision with scissors may be possible. The resectoscope may be used as well to coagulate the vascular stalk. The fibroid should be removed with the resectoscope or with graspers and sent for pathologic diagnosis. In uncommon cases, the myoma cannot be removed and is left to degenerate in the uterus.

Even if the myoma is not on a narrow stalk, the initial step is to attempt to coagulate the blood supply to the myoma. The resectoscope is placed beyond the myoma and the flat loop is used to try to control the blood supply. Thereafter, the myoma is progressively shaved in the midline toward the lower uterine segment. To accomplish the shaving, the loop is extended to or past the fibroid and then the cutting current is used as the loop is brought toward the hysteroscope. The current should only be activated when adequate visualization is achieved. The lateral aspects can then be shaved with the loop of the resectoscope. There is no need to remove the intramural aspect of the fibroid. Attempts to do so will result in significantly more uterine bleeding and greatly increase the chance of uterine perforation. Overall, resection into the myometrium is not likely to give better results than simply shaving the myoma to its base.[10]

The Nd:YAG laser, generally with sapphire tip, may also be used to resect the myoma. Deaths from embolization have been reported when carbon dioxide ($CO_2$) has been used to cool the Nd:YAG laser during endometrial ablations. Therefore, fluid should always be used to cool the sapphire tip if the Nd:YAG laser is used. No studies comparing cautery with Nd:YAG laser have been performed. Thus, the surgeon must choose the technique that is more comfortable.

The endometrium may be ablated after myomectomy in patients with a history of heavy uterine bleeding when childbearing is no longer desired.[14] This can be accomplished either by rollerball electrocautery or by Nd:YAG laser. Of these two, the rollerball technique is generally believed to be faster and more efficient. However, no long-term data regarding the safety or advisability of this procedure are available. Again, if visibility is unacceptable or if the patient is at risk of sig-

nificant complications, the procedure should be abandoned and abdominal myomectomy should be performed.

## Results

Results with hysteroscopic myomectomy are generally good when performed by an experienced hysteroscopic surgeon. Most patients with abnormal bleeding have significant improvement. Fifty percent of patients who have a hysteroscopic myomectomy followed by endometrial ablation will have no more uterine bleeding.[15] Long-term studies are not yet available with regard to hysteroscopic myomectomy or endometrial ablation to evaluate the recurrence of abnormally heavy uterine bleeding. Adenomyosis or cryptic endometrial adenocarcinoma are theoretical risks of uterine ablation.

There is minimal data regarding fertility after hysteroscopic resection of myomata. Pregnancy rates of 25% to 33% have been reported,[9,14,16] although there are no prospective studies available to compare hysteroscopic versus abdominal myomectomy with regard to pregnancy. Abdominal myomectomy is generally considered to result in a 50% to 60% pregnancy rate.

## Alternative Techniques

Expectant management should be elected for patients with minimal symptoms unless there is rapid growth of fibroids or if the adnexae cannot be evaluated.[1] Symptoms due to fibroids may improve after a course of GnRH analog therapy, and symptomatic relief may persist even after regrowth of fibroids.[3] For patients with symptomatic fibroids who no longer desire preservation of fertility, hysterectomy is the procedure of choice. Abdominal myomectomy remains the primary procedure for symptomatic patients who desire preservation of fertility. Unfortunately, abdominal myomectomy generally requires longer hospitalization and recovery time. Furthermore, it is probably associated with greater morbidity than endoscopic myomectomy, although this may in part be the result of selection bias.

## Conclusions

Advanced instruments and surgical techniques have made increasingly difficult gynecologic procedures an endoscopic possibility. Laparoscopic and hysteroscopic myomectomy both require highly advanced surgical skills. One must recognize that the availability of equipment and the technical ability to perform these procedures does not allow one to conclude that these procedures are optimal or even appropriate for uterine fibroids or for other indications. Most fibroids that can easily be removed with the laparoscope probably do not require surgical resection at all. The potential complications associated with laparoscopic myomectomy are serious enough that incidental or elective laparoscopic myomectomy is rarely, if ever, indicated. On the other hand, well selected patients may be good candidates for laparoscopic or hysteroscopic myomectomy in the hands of an experienced endoscopist. When an endoscopic myomectomy is performed, technique must be impeccable and hemostasis scrupulously confirmed. The surgeon should have a very low threshold for laparotomy should complications arise.

## References

1. Entman SS. Uterine leiomyoma and adenomyosis. In: Jones HW, III, Wentz AC, Burnett LS, eds. *Novak's Textbook of Gynecology*. 11th ed. Baltimore: Williams and Wilkins; 1988:443–454.
2. Monroe SE, Andreyko J. Treatment of uterine leiomyomas and hirsutism with nafarelin. *J Reprod Med*. 1989;34:1029–1033.
3. Schlaff WD, Zerhouni EA, Huth JAM, et al. A placebo-controlled trial of depot gonadotropin-releasing hormone analog (leuprolide) in the treatment of uterine leiomyomata. *Obstet Gynecol*. 1989;74:856–862.
4. Rock JA, Murphy AA. Anatomic abnormalities. *Clin Obstet Gynecol*. 1986;29:886–911.
5. Murphy AA. Operative laparoscopy. *Fertil Steril*. 1987;47:1–18.
6. Semm K, Mettler L. Technical progress in pelvic surgery via operative laparoscopy. *Am J Obstet Gynecol*. 1980;138:121–127.
7. Gordon AG, Lewis BV, eds. *Gynecological Endoscopy*. Philadelphia: JB Lippincott; 1988:8.9–8.10.
8. Neuwirth RS, Amin HK. Excision of submucous fibroids with hysteroscopic control. *Am J Obstet Gynecol*. 1976;126:95–99.
9. Buttram VC Jr, Reiter RC. Uterine leiomyomata: etiology, symptomatology, and management. *Fertil Steril*. 1981;36:433–445.
10. March CM. Hysteroscopic resection of submucous myomas. *Contemp Obstet Gynecol*. 1990;35:59–66.
11. Donnez J, Schrurs B, Gillerot S, Sandow J, Clercks F. Treatment of uterine fibroids with implants of gonadotropin-releasing hormone agonist: assessment by hysterography. *Fertil Steril*. 1989;51:947–950.
12. Zbella EA, Moise J, Carson SA. Noncardiogenic pulmonary edema secondary to intrauterine instillation of 32% dextran 70. *Fertil Steril*. 1985;43:479–480.
13. Brooks PG, Loffer FD, Serden SP. Resectoscopic removal of symptomatic intrauterine lesions. *J Reprod Med*. 1989;34:435–437.
14. DeCherney A, Polan ML. Hysteroscopic management of intrauterine lesions and intractable uterine bleeding. *Obstet Gynecol*. 1983;61:392–397.
15. Hallez JP, Netter A, Cartier R. Methodical intrauterine resection. *Am J Obstet Gynecol*. 1987;156:1080–1084.
16. Neuwirth RS. Hysteroscopic management of symptomatic submucous fibroids. *Obstet Gynecol*. 1983;62:509–511.

# 14

# Laparoscopic Treatment of Tubo-ovarian and Pelvic Abscess

*HARRY REICH*

CHAPTER OUTLINE

A pelvic abscess is a localized collection of many organisms, inflammatory exudate, and necrotic debris often separated from surrounding tissue by a fibrous pseudocapsule. A tubo-ovarian complex is a tubo-ovarian abscess (TOA) that lacks a classic pseudocapsule and is made up of the agglutination of tube and ovary to adjacent pelvic and abdominal structures after reaction to purulent exudate from the inflamed tube. A true pelvic abscess with a classic pseudocapsule can occur in the ovary and after rupture of a diverticulum. Whatever the terminology, purulent material exists in a collection within the pelvis.

Abscess is the end result of an acute or subacute infection often beginning with an initial stage of peritonitis where aerobic bacteria predominate, followed by the development of an intraabdominal abscess with emergence of anaerobic bacteria as the predominant flora. Abscesses contain many organisms in high concentration, but not in a rapid growth phase, making them less susceptible to antimicrobial agents that require actively growing organisms for efficacy. In addition, the fibrous pseudocapsule, which the host makes in an attempt to control the infection, may inhibit adequate levels of antimicrobial agents from entering the abscess. The anaerobic milieu itself may hinder host defense mechanisms, reducing the ability of neutrophils to phagocytize and kill bacteria. Thus, therapy for abscesses must include some technique to drain the pus, along with appropriate antimicrobial therapy.

Until the early 1970s, clinicians who suspected a pelvic or tubo-ovarian abscess considered extirpative surgery, total abdominal hysterectomy and bilateral salpingo-oophorectomy (TAH/BSO). More recently, unruptured abscesses have been treated with intravenous antibiotics with surgery reserved for poor responders to medical therapy. Although this approach avoids immediate operation, prolonged contact between necrotic and inflamed tissue often causes dense fibrous adhesions that impair reproductive potential. In an effort to avoid this problem, some gynecologists have advocated the use of laparoscopy with early lysis of acute adhesions as an alternative.

The commonly accepted belief that surgical intervention during acute pelvic infection results in greater injury than waiting for the infection to subside was initiated with the report of Simpson.[1] This opinion prevailed until recently, even though the risks associated with surgical intervention had changed drastically since the early part of this century. In reality, it is much easier to operate on acute adhesions. Later these adhesions become dense, fibrotic and vascularized, obliterating the normal anatomic relationships. For example, second-look laparoscopic adhesiolysis soon after infertility surgery is much easier to perform than the original operation.[2]

Electrosurgery, laser surgery, and sharp scissor dissection, all of which are useful for chronic pelvic inflammatory disease, have no place in the treatment of acute inflammatory adhesions. Simply stated, the laparoscopic treatment of acute adhesions, with or without abscess, does not require the high level of technical skill necessary to excise an endometrioma, open a hydrosalpinx, or remove an ectopic pregnancy under laparoscopic control. It is essentially an exercise in careful blunt dissection using a probe or aquadissection with a suction-irrigation device that can be performed by gynecologists experienced in operative laparoscopy using equipment available in most hospitals.

## Why Laparoscopic Treatment Works

Peritoneal defense mechanisms that protect the host from invading bacteria include absorption of the microbes from the peritoneal cavity by the lymphatic system, phagocytosis by macrophages and polymorphonuclear leukocytes, complement effects, and fibrin trapping.[3] Fibrin trapping and sequestration of the bacterial inoculum by the omentum and intestine and the formation of a tubo-ovarian complex act to contain the infection initially, although abscesses eventually may form. Although the deposition of fibrin traps bacteria and decreases the frequency of septicemic death, thick fibrin deposits ultimately represent a barrier to insitu killing by neutrophils, with resultant abscess formation. Once formed, the abscess walls inhibit the effectiveness of antibiotics and the ability of the host to resolve the infection naturally.

Ahrenholz and Simmons[4] studied the role of purified fibrin in the pathogenesis of experimental intraperitoneal infection. Their conclusion was that fibrin delays the onset of systemic sepsis, but the entrapped bacteria cannot be eliminated easily by the normal intraperitoneal bactericidal mechanisms and, as a result, an abscess can form. They also felt that radical peritoneal debridement or anticoagulation may reduce the septic complications of peritonitis. Stated another way, procedures that decrease fibrin deposition and/or facilitate fibrin removal, either enzymatically or surgically, decrease the frequency of intraperitoneal abscess formation; hence, the rational for extensive peritoneal lavage and radical excision of inflammatory exudate in patients with TOA. Success with the laparoscopic and laparotomy treatment of TOA by the author[5] and others[6-8] substantiates the laboratory work of Ahrenholz and Simmons. Laparoscopic drainage of a pelvic abscess, followed by lysis of all peritoneal cavity adhesions and excision of necrotic inflammatory exudate, allows host defenses to control the infection effectively.

## Indications

Women with lower abdominal pain and a palpable or questionable pelvic mass should undergo laparoscopy to determine the true diagnosis, as even "obvious TOAs" may prove to be endometriomas, hemorrhagic corpus luteum cysts, or an abscess surrounding a ruptured appendix. The worldwide average rate of misdiagnosis of pelvic inflammatory disease (PID) is 35% when laparoscopy has been used for confirmation.[9]

The diagnosis of TOA should be suspected in women with a recent or past history of pelvic inflammatory disease who have persistent pain and pelvic tenderness on examination. Fever and leukocytosis may or may not be present.[10] Ultrasound frequently documents a tubo-ovarian complex or what appears to be an abscess. After the presumptive diagnosis of TOA is made, hospitalization should be arranged for laparoscopic diagnosis and treatment soon thereafter.

In patients suspected of having a TOA, intravenous antibiotics should be initiated on admission to the hospital, usually 2 to 24 hr before laparoscopy. Adequate and sustained blood levels of antibiotics are required to combat transperitoneal absorption of aerobic and anaerobic organisms during the operative procedure. This author prefers cefoxitin 2 g intravenously, every 4 hr from admission until discharge, which occurs usually on postoperative day 2 or 3.[11] Newer cephamycins, cefmetazole 2 g every 8 hr, or cefotetan 2 g every 12 hr can also be considered. Oral doxycycline is started on the first postoperative day and continued for 10 days. Although clindamycin and metronidazole both have demonstrated greater ability to enter abscess cavities and reduce bacterial counts therein, cefoxitin is used to simplify therapy to a single intravenous (IV) agent and assess further the efficacy of the laparoscopic surgical procedure; that is, the IV antibiotic alone should not be considered the reason for successful therapy. One pioneer in this area, Dr. Jeanine Henry-Suchet, starts antibiotics during the laparoscopic procedure only after cultures have been taken.[6]

## Instrumentation and Technique

The laparoscopic procedure is always performed under general anesthesia. A high flow $CO_2$ insufflator is valuable to maintain the pneumoperitoneum and compensate for the rapid loss of $CO_2$ during suctioning. A Cohen or Rubin's cannula is then placed in the endocervical canal for uterine manipulation and tubal lavage. A 10-mm laparoscope is inserted through a vertical intraumbilical incision. Lower quadrant puncture sites are made above the pubic hairline and just lateral to the inferior epigastric vessels. The upper abdomen is examined and the patient is placed in a 20° Trendelenburg's position before focusing attention on the pelvis. A Foley catheter is inserted. Through the right-sided ancillary puncture site, either a blunt probe or a grasping forceps is inserted and used for traction and retraction. Through the left-sided suprapubic sleeve, a suction-irrigation cannula (Aquapurator, WISAP Co.) or a suction probe attached to a 50-cc syringe is inserted and used to mobilize omentum, small bowel, rectosigmoid, and tubo-ovarian adhesions until the abscess cavity is entered. Purulent fluid is aspirated while the operating table is returned to a 10° Trendelenburg's position. Cultures should be taken from the aspirated fluid, from the inflammatory exudate excised with biopsy forceps, and from exudate near the tubal ostium. A bronchoscope cytology brush may be useful to obtain these last cultures.

After the abscess cavity is aspirated, the dissection is continued, separating the bowel and omentum completely from the reproductive organs and lysing tubo-ovarian adhesions. Aquadissection is performed by placing the tip of the suction-irrigation cannula against the adhesive interface between bowel-adnexa, tube-ovary, or adnexa-pelvic sidewall, then using both the cannula tip and the pressurized physiologic solution to develop a dissection plane (Fig. 14.1). The dissection can then be extended either bluntly or with continued fluid pressure. A 3-mm or 5-mm grasping forceps places the tissue to be dissected on tension so that the surgeon can identify the distorted tissue plane accurately before aquadissection. When the dissection is completed, the abscess cavity (necrotic inflammatory exudate) is excised in pieces using a 5-mm biopsy forceps.

It is important to remember that after ovulation, purulent material from acute salpingitis may gain entrance to the inner ovary by inoculation of the corpus luteum, which may then become part of the abscess wall. Thus, after draining the abscess cavity and mobilizing the

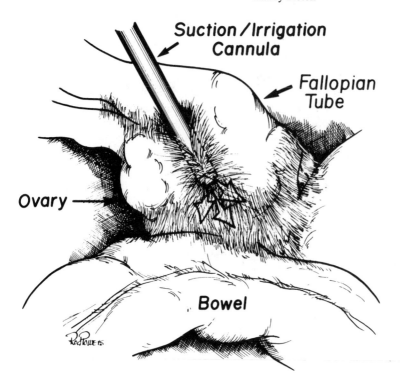

Suction/Irrigation Cannula

Fallopian Tube

Ovary

Bowel

FIGURE 14.1. The aspiration–irrigation cannula, continuously irrigating with a physiologic solution (Ringer's lactate or normal saline), and a blunt probe are used to separate acutely adherent organs.

entire ovary, a gaping hole of varying size may be noted in the ovary that heretofore had been intimately involved in the abscess cavity. This area should be well irrigated; it will heal spontaneously and significant bleeding is rarely encountered.

Next, the grasping forceps are inserted into the fimbrial ostia and spread in order to free the agglutinated fimbriae. Irrigation of the tube through the fimbriated end should be performed to remove infected debris and diminish chances of recurrence. The fimbrial endosalpinx is visualized at this time and its quality assessed for future prognosis.

Tubal lavage with indigo carmine dye through the Cohen cannula in the uterus should be attempted. With early acute abscesses, the tubes are rarely patent because of interstitial edema. In contrast, when the abscess process has been present for longer than 1 week and/or the patient was previously treated with antibiotics, lavage frequently documents tubal patency. Rarely, necrotic material can be pushed from the tube during the lavage procedure.

The peritoneal cavity is extensively irrigated with Ringer's lactate solution until the effluent is clear. The total volume of irrigant often exceeds 20 L. As part of this procedure, 2 L of Ringer's lactate solution are flushed through the aquadissector into the upper abdomen, one on each side of the falciform ligament, to dilute any purulent material that may have gained access to these areas during the 20° Trendelenburg's positioning. Reverse Trendelenburg's position is then used for the "underwater" exam. The laparoscope and the aquadissector are manipulated into the deep cul de sac beneath floating bowel and omentum, and this area is alternately irrigated and suctioned until the effluent is clear. An "underwater" examination is then performed to observe the completely separated tubes and ovaries and to document absolute hemostasis. At the close of each procedure, at least 2 L of Ringer's lactate is left in the peritoneal cavity to prevent fibrin adherences from forming between surfaces during the early healing phase and to dilute any bacteria present.

The umbilical incision is closed with 4-0 Vicryl. The lower quadrant 5-mm and 3-mm incisions are loosely approximated with a vascular clamp and covered with collodion to allow drainage of excess Ringer's lactate solution should increased intraabdominal pressure be present. No drains, antibiotic solutions, or heparin are used. A second-look laparoscopy is encouraged.

Without question, the more acute the abscess, the easier the dissection. Patient and physician delay often makes the laparoscopic procedure more difficult than it need be. However, even chronic abscesses can be treated successfully by careful blunt aquadissection.

## Postoperative Care

Postoperatively, the patient is usually ambulatory and on a "diet as tolerated" after recovery from anesthesia. Temperature elevation rarely persists past the first postoperative day. The patient is usually discharged in 2 to 3 days if she remains afebrile, and examined 1 week after discharge. All restrictions are removed at that time.

## Alternative Techniques

Currently, unruptured abscesses are treated with IV antibiotics. Surgery is reserved for poor responders to medical therapy. This approach often avoids immediate operation but commonly has reproductive consequences. Surgery during the acute phase commonly results in hysterectomy and bilateral salpingo-oophorectomy or, at best, a unilateral salpingo-oophorectomy. Most reports on operative technique for treatment of TOA by laparotomy emphasize that the tissues are edematous, congested, friable, and tear easily. Moreover, they note that capillary and venous oozing can be profuse. Hemostasis is often judged less than ideal in such cases and blood loss requiring transfusion is common. These reports also suggest that meticulous dissection is virtually impossible and caution that the bowel is particularly vulnerable to injury when it is being separated from the pelvic viscera.

In contrast, laparoscopic adhesiolysis using the aquadissection is rarely bloody. Capillary oozing does occur, but it ceases spontaneously as the procedure progresses. In my experience,

blood loss is rarely greater than 100 cc, and blood transfusion has not been reported after laparoscopic treatment of a pelvic abscess.

Complications of treatment of pelvic abscess by laparotomy include superficial and/or deep wound infection, wound dehiscence, bowel injury including delayed perforation secondary to unrecognized injury, bowel obstruction, persistent undrained collections of pus, thrombophlebitis, pulmonary embolism, septic shock, and subdiaphragmatic abscesses. In contrast, neither wound disruption nor dehiscence are possible using a laparoscopic approach, and the other possible complications have not been reported.

## Results

The author has treated 40 pelvic abscesses using laparoscopic surgical techniques from 1976 to 1989.[12] One patient required a TAH/BSO in 1977 for recurrence 1 month postoperatively. All others demonstrated long-term resolution of their TOA. Eight second-look laparoscopies documented minimal filmy adhesions. Similar results were described by others.[6-8]

## Conclusions

The goal in the management of acute tubo-ovarian abscess is prevention of the chronic sequelae of infection, including pelvic adhesions, tubal occlusion, infertility, and pelvic pain, which often lead to further surgical intervention. Laparoscopic treatment in addition to antibiotic therapy is effective and economical. It offers the gynecologist 100% accuracy in diagnosis while simultaneously accomplishing definitive treatment with a low complication rate.[5,6] Preventing infertility may be possible as an estimated 20% of infertility in the United States results from the sequelae of PID.

Laparoscopy allows for conservation of the tube and ovary with subsequent fertility potential. Additionally, laparoscopy has a high degree of patient acceptance due to minimal incision size, short hospital stay, and early return to full activity. The combination of laparoscopic treatment and effective IV antibiotics is a reasonable approach to the spectrum of PID from acute salpingitis to ruptured tubo-ovarian abscess.

Currently, many physicians are reluctant to advocate the routine use of laparoscopy for the diagnosis and treatment of acute pelvic adhesions and pelvic abscess. Whether the combination of laparoscopic surgery and antibiotics ultimately proves superior to antibiotics alone in the prevention of chronic pelvic adhesions must be resolved through multiinstitutional controlled studies, using second-look laparoscopy. However, early experience with laparoscopic treatment of pelvic abscess combined with IV antibiotic therapy is promising and suggests that this technique may achieve better results than early surgery or medical treatment alone.

## References

1. Simpson FF. The choice of time for operation for pelvic inflammation of tubal origin. *Surg Gynecol Obstet.* 1909;9:45–49.
2. Jansen R. Surgery pregnancy time intervals after salpingolysis, unilateral salpingostomy, and bilateral salpingostomy. *Fertil Steril.* 1980;34:222–228.
3. Skau T, Nystrom P, Ohman L, Stendahl O. The kinetics of peritoneal clearance of *Escherichia coli* and *Bacteroides fragilis* and participating defense mechanisms. *Arch Surg.* 1986;121:1033–1040.
4. Ahrenholz DH, Simmons RL. Fibrin in peritonitis. I. Beneficial and adverse effects of fibrin in experimental *E. coli* peritonitis. *Surgery.* 1980;88:41–46.
5. Reich H, McGlynn F. Laparoscopic treatment of tuboovarian and pelvic abscess. *J Reprod Med.* 1987;32:747–751.
6. Henry-Suchet J, Soler A, Loffredo V. Laparoscopic treatment of tuboovarian abscesses. *J Reprod Med.* 1984;29:579–584.
7. Hudspeth AS. Radical surgical debridement in the treatment of advanced generalized bacterial peritonitis. *Arch Surg.* 1975;110:1233–1237.
8. Rivlin M, Hunt J. Surgical management of diffuse peritonitis complicating obstetric/gynecologic infections. *Obstet Gynecol.* 1986;67:652–657.
9. Jacobson L. Differential diagnosis of acute pelvic inflammatory disease. *Am J Obstet Gynecol.* 1980;138:1006–1012.
10. Franklin E, Hevron J, Thompson J. Management of the pelvic abscess. *Clin Obstet Gynecol.* 1973;16:66–72.
11. Sweet R, Ledger W. Cefoxitin: single-agent treatment of mixed aerobic–anaerobic pelvic infections. *Obstet Gynecol.* 1979;54:193–198.
12. Reich H. Endoscopic management of tuboovarian abscess and pelvic inflammatory disease. In: Sanfilippo J, Levine R, eds. *Operative Gynecologic Endoscopy.* New York: Springer-Verlag; 1988:69–76.

# 15

# Laparoscopic Uterine Nerve Ablation, Presacral Neurectomy, and Appendectomy

*C. Paul Perry and Ricardo Azziz*

A number of less frequently used laparoscopic procedures will be discussed. These techniques may be useful in the treatment of certain forms of pelvic pain. Nevertheless, experience with these procedures is still limited, patients should be selected carefully, and the surgery performed only by experienced laparoscopists.

## Laparoscopic Uterosacral Nerve Ablation

In 1955 Doyle reported the vaginal interruption of the uterosacral ligaments for the relief of dysmenorrhea, since the majority of uterine sensory fibers traverse these ligaments. Various surgeons now interrupt these nerves laparoscopically.[1,2]

### Indications and Patient Selection

Patients undergoing laparoscopic surgery and who complain of significant central dysmenorrhea may be considered candidates for laparoscopic uterosacral nerve ablation (LUNA). No significant benefit will result from LUNA if the origin of the pain is extrauterine, including pelvic peritoneal surfaces, distal tubes, or ovaries. Patients with severe dysmenorrhea and minimal extrauterine pathology are the best candidates for this procedure.

If at the time of laparoscopy, distortion of

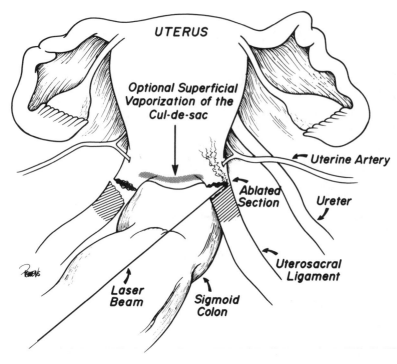

FIGURE 15.1. LUNA: The uterus should be displaced toward the anterior abdominal wall by an intrauterine manipulator. The uterosacral ligament is identified and followed to its insertion on the uterus. Laser energy is applied to the medial aspect of the ligament at its junction with the uterus until totally or partially ablated. Usually a 1.5 to 2 cm long by 1.0 cm deep area of vaporization through the ligament is required. A superficial "U"-shaped area of vaporization, connecting the two interrupted uterosacral ligament segments, may also be performed along the posterior aspect of the utero cul de sac junction, which transects interconnecting fibers otherwise missed.

the pelvic anatomy due to scarring or endometriosis impedes clear identification of the ligament, LUNA should not be attempted.

## Technique

LUNA is relatively easy to perform. KTP, Argon, or contact tip Nd:YAG fiber lasers may be used through the operative channel of the laparoscope or suprapubically. The smoke production and lack of coagulation with the $CO_2$ laser make this instrument less than ideal for this purpose.

The uterus should be displaced toward the anterior abdominal wall by an intrauterine manipulator. The uterosacral ligament is identified and followed to its insertion on the uterus. Laser energy is applied to the medial aspect of the ligament at its junction with the uterus until totally or partially ablated (Fig. 15.1). Total transection can be facilitated by grasping the unroofed uterosacral ligament with atraumatic forceps and stretching toward the midline. Usually a 1.5 to 2 cm long by 1.0 cm deep area of vaporization through the ligament is required. There are some small vessels deep

in the ligament that may require coagulation. A superficial "U"-shaped area of vaporization, connecting the two interrupted uterosacral ligament segments, may also be performed along the posterior aspect of the utero–cul de sac junction. This transects interconnecting fibers otherwise missed. Care must be used to avoid bowel injury during this step.

Incisions too far lateral to the ligament should be avoided since this may result in significant bleeding or ureteral injury. Any bleeding occurring after LUNA should be managed by bipolar, not unipolar, electrocoagulation to decrease the possibility of ureteral injury. If coagulation becomes necessary, the ureter should be identified and atraumatically deviated laterally beforehand with a blunt probe.

Occasionally, total uterosacral ligament excision may be preferable if endometriosis is deeply invasive in this area. This can be accomplished by first making a peritoneal relaxing incision just lateral and parallel to the ligament, and medial to the ureter. The ureter must be clearly visible throughout its pelvic course before performing this maneuver. The uterosacral ligament may then be bluntly isolated, its origin and insertion coagulated with bipolar electrocoagulation, and the entire ligament safely excised. No data are yet available comparing pain relief with this technique and the standard LUNA procedure.

## Results

The success of LUNA for relief of primary dysmenorrhea has ranged from 49% to 70% after 1-year follow-up.[1,2] Relief of secondary dysmenorrhea due to endometriosis by the LUNA procedure was reported to be 71%.[1] Unfortunately, no long-term follow-up studies are available, but it appears that the effectiveness of LUNA may decrease over time.[2] We have performed this procedure in more than 200 patients with endometriosis. About one half of our patients received some initial benefit, some gradually returning to their preoperative pain levels.

Early in our experience with LUNA, two patients required laparotomy for control of bleeding. Acquisition of bipolar electrocoagulation skills will decrease the need for open hemostasis. Further long-term studies are required to determine fully the efficacy and complication rate of this procedure.

# Laparoscopic Presacral Neurectomy

Since its introduction in 1898 by Jaboulay, presacral neurectomy for pelvic pain and dysmenorrhea has enjoyed periods of fluctuating enthusiasm. Cotte was the first surgeon to perform the procedure in the United States and reported some 1500 cases in 1938, with a 98% success rate. Presacral neurectomy was performed frequently throughout the 1940s and 1950s for both primary and secondary dysmenorrhea. Black compiled almost 10,000 cases from the literature, physician questionnaires, and personal experience, and reported an overall success rate ranging from 75% to 80%.[3] The next 20 years were marked by the development of superior medical therapies for dysmenorrhea. Oral contraceptives, nonsteroidal antiinflammatory agents, and gonadotropin-

releasing hormone agonist succeeded in pain control for most patients. However, even today some patients will fail to respond to or do not tolerate conservative therapy.

Recent advances in operative laparoscopy offer the potential for relief of central dysmenorrhea by presacral neurectomy, without the need to resort to laparotomy. Laparoscopic presacral neurectomy (LPSN) may prove to be the treatment of choice in certain carefully selected patients. However, it must not be overused for the fewer we do, the better results we obtain.[1] It should be undertaken only after proper training.

## Indications and Patient Selection

Patients with central, not lateral, primary or secondary dysmenorrhea are considered best candidates. They should have failed other conservative treatments, including LUNA if appropriate. Patients with endometriosis (other than minimal) might best be treated with laparoscopic resection of endometriosis and LPSN, since extrauterine pain responds poorly to LUNA. Low back pain, lateral pelvic pain, and dyspareunia may or may not respond to LPSN.

Patients should be fully informed regarding the potential risks and need for laparotomy. Vascular and ureteral injury along with possible incomplete pain relief or pain recurrence should be discussed.

## Technique

LPSN, unlike LUNA, requires a significant degree of surgical skill. It should be undertaken only by those surgeons familiar with the retroperitoneal anatomy. The presacral nerve is actually the superior hypogastric plexus, which is 1 of about 23 sympathetic collateral plexuses supplying efferent stimulation to the viscera. The superior portion is retroperitoneal and runs from the bifurcation of the aorta to the junction of the vertebral bodies of $L_5$–$S_1$. There it forms the middle hypogastric plexus, which divides at the level of the first sacral vertebral body into the right and left inferior hypogastric plexus. Somatic afferent fibers travel along with these sympathetic nerves transmitting pain sensation to the spinal cord from the various target organs and peritoneal surfaces.

The vast majority of sensory fibers from the uterus and cervix traverse this plexus. Other afferent nerve fibers follow vascular supplies and cannot be interrupted by presacral neurectomy. Sacral parasympathetic fibers referring pain to the low back will usually not be affected. Due to its embryological derivation, the distal third of the fallopian tubes and the ovaries receive their nerve supply from the aortic collateral plexus on the right and the renal collateral plexus on the left. Therefore, presacral neurectomy should not be consistently effective for lateral pelvic pain.[4]

Expert, meticulous dissection is required during LPSN. The boundaries for resection are exactly the same as those at laparotomy: Superiorly, the bifurcation of the aorta; on the right, the right internal iliac artery and right ureter; on the left, the inferior mesenteric and superior hemorrhoidal arteries; and inferiorly, just below the division of the right and left inferior hypogastric plexus and deep, the periosteum of the vertebral bodies (Fig. 15.2).

This retroperitoneal area may be approached from above through the umbilical incision or from below with the suprapubic placement of the laparoscope as described by Perez.[5] Dissection is carried out via a four-puncture technique using atraumatic graspers and a blunt irrigation probe. To assure hemostasis, bipolar coagulation should always be available. A Corson microelectrosurgical needle (Karl Storz, Culver City, CA) or a Nd:YAG laser fiber, with a GRP-4 contact sapphire tip (Surgical Laser Technologies, Malvern, PA), may be used through the operating channel of the laparoscope or one of the three suprapubic incisions. These instruments greatly facilitate isolation of the plexus by hemostatically interrupting fine vessels and nerve fibers that anastomose with the plexus from all directions. The author prefers the umbilical approach with the Nd:YAG fiber placed through the instrument channel of an operating laparoscope. The fiber should be

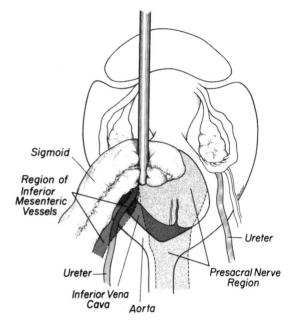

FIGURE 15.2. The anatomic landmarks for a LPSN are depicted.

oriented so it enters the field of vision at 12 o'clock to minimize interference with visibility.

The patient is placed in exenteration stirrups with 30° Trendelenburg and a left lateral tilt, to displace the bowel from the sacral promontory. If required, laparoscopic management of endometriosis is performed first. Next, all structures defining the anatomical extent of dissection are identified. The peritoneum overlying the sacral promontory is then grasped and elevated before incision. A superficial transverse peritoneal incision is made between the inferior mesenteric artery on the left and the right internal iliac artery, about 1 cm cephalad to the right ureteral crossing (Fig. 15.2). The peritoneal edges retract after being cut and require little manipulation to maintain exposure. Blunt dissection, electrosurgery, or laser energy are used to separate the fine nerves and vessels between the undersurface of the peritoneum and the loose connective tissue layer of the presacral space.

The presacral nerve is isolated by developing the avascular space between the nerve and right internal iliac artery down to the periosteum. The plexus usually runs to the left of the midline. Therefore, the next area of dissection should be carried out far enough on the left to assure complete neural resection, but without disturbing the inferior mesenteric artery, the root of the sigmoid mesentery, or the left ureter. This space between the inferior mesenteric artery and the presacral nerve should be dissected bluntly down to the periosteum as well. Care should be taken not to injure the left common iliac vein, which is frequently found in the deep connective tissue of this area. When both the right and left borders of the superior hypogastric portion of the presacral nerve have been developed, the nerve is grasped and elevated off the sacral periosteum. The middle sacral artery and vein are closely adherent to the periosteum and can usually be avoided by careful elevation of the nerve before coagulation. The cephalad portion of the nerve is then coagulated and transected. Gentle traction is applied to the remaining nerve trunk while isolating the middle plexus and right and left inferior hypogastric branches. This dissection should proceed no more than 3 to 4 cm caudal from where the nerve has been transected, so as not to invite troublesome bleeding from the sacral venous plexus. The inferior nerve trunks are then isolated, elevate, and coagulated. Transection is accomplished proximal to the coagulated neural and fatty tissue. The resected tissue should measure about 3 cm in length and can be easily drawn out of the abdomen via one of the suprapubic sites.

## Results

The success rate of LPSN seems to be comparable to the open procedure. Perez has reported only two failures out of the first 25 patients. Follow-up ranges from 6 to 27 months. Only one complication occurred in his series with laparotomy performed for hemostasis.[5] We have performed more than 50 procedures at our institution. Most patients had endometriosis and had not responded to other conservative measures. At this writing we have four failures, all of whom describe persistent lateral or back pain. We have experienced no

complications. The most common reasons for failure are expected to be poor patient selection and incomplete removal of the ganglion. Incomplete removal of the plexus may be due to anatomical variance or lack of presacral neurectomy experience. A 10-year follow-up will be necessary before LPSN can be properly compared with traditional presacral neurectomy.

## Laparoscopic Appendectomy

When the diagnosis of appendiceal pathology is established on laparoscopy, a potential for laparoscopic appendectomy exists. The advantages of laparoscopic appendectomy include a shorter recovery time, improved cosmesis, and the possibility of combining a diagnostic and therapeutic procedure. The disadvantages are that the patient may still need to remain in the hospital for 2 or 3 days until bowel function recovers.

The diagnosis of appendicitis by laparoscopy appears to be quite effective.[6] Spirtos and colleagues[6] visualized 93% of 86 appendices. In six patients, the appendix was not able to be visualized secondary to adhesions, four of which were acutely purulent or ruptured appendicitis. Of the remaining 80 patients, 56 were thought to have appendicitis by laparoscopic exam, which was confirmed histologically in 47 (84%). This 16% false-positive rate is no higher than that observed with appendectomy via laparotomy for suspected appendicitis. Fortunately, the number of cases of appendicitis missed by laparoscopy is relatively low, ranging from 0% to 2% in most reports. In the study by Spirtos et al.,[6] laparotomy was avoided in 20 patients suspected initially of having appendicitis.

### Indications and Patient Selection

The indications for a laparoscopy appendectomy include endometriosis of the appendix, adherence of the appendix to the adnexa via inflammatory or postsurgical adhesions, chronic right midquadrant pain without evidence of pelvic pathology, and chronic/subacute appen-

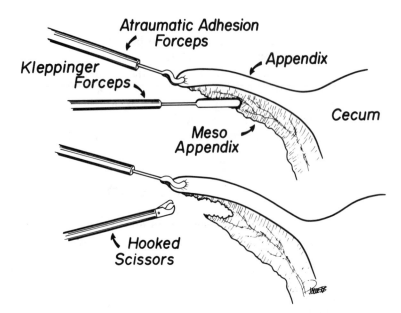

FIGURE 15.3. With an atraumatic grasping forceps (Storz No. 26177AG) placed through the right lower quadrant suprapubic incision, the appendical tip is grasped and placed on traction. Using a bipolar forceps placed through the midline suprapubic incision, the mesoappendix is cauterized to a point 0.5 cm below the junction of the appendix and cecum (top). Care should be used to keep the bipolar forceps 0.5 cm away from the cecum proper. Using hook scissors, the mesoappendix is progressively incised as it is cauterized (bottom).

dicitis. Contraindications include perforated or acutely purulent appendicitis, inability to visualize the appendix fully, or an unconsented, uninformed patient. A retrocecal appendix is not necessarily a contraindication to laparoscopic removal if full visualization of the organ and the mesoappendix is possible with manipulation.

## Technique

The patient's legs should be placed frog-legged and low, not in the usual lithotomy position. The left arm should be tucked parallel to the patient (for right-handed surgeons). Second puncture sites should be oriented toward the right lower quadrant of the pelvis. A puncture site placed halfway between the umbilicus and pubis may be more useful than a suprapubic incision in the left lower quadrant.

With an atraumatic grasping forceps (Storz Co., No. 26177AG) placed through the right lower quadrant suprapubic incision, the appendiceal tip is grasped and placed on traction. Using a bipolar forceps placed through the midline suprapubic incision, the mesoappendix is serially cauterized and cut with hook scissors, to a point 0.5 cm below the junction of the appendix and cecum (Fig. 15.3). Care should be taken to keep the bipolar forceps

0.5 cm away from the cecum proper. Alternatively, the appendix must be trimmed as much as possible of surrounding fatty tissue, in order to facilitate extraction. Using the atraumatic grasper, the appendiceal base is grasped and milked to push fecal matter into the cecum. A loop suture is placed through the midline puncture, with the use of an Endoloop applicator, if needed. At least one of the loop ties should be of synthetic reasorbable material (0-Vicryl or Dexon), and the rest may be of chromic catgut. The appendiceal tip is regrasped by placing the grasper through the loop. The appendix is then pulled through the loop (Fig. 15.4). A micrograsping forceps (WISAP No. 7678) is used to direct the loop suture toward the base of the appendix. Use a knot guide (WOLF No. 838355 or WISAP No. 7669), placed through the midline suprapubic incision, to secure a knot at the appendiceal base while placing traction on the appendix. Three loop ties should be placed consecutively at the appendiceal base. After using the atraumatic grasping forceps to milk the appendiceal base toward the tip, a fourth loop tie is placed approximately 1 cm distal to the appendiceal base (Fig. 15.5).

The 5-mm midline suprapubic cannula is then removed and replaced with a 10-mm sleeve. The base of the appendix just distal to

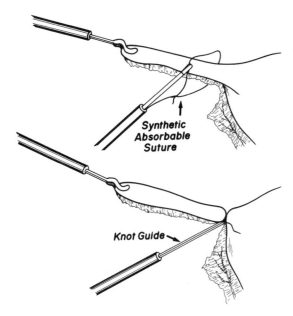

FIGURE 15.4. Using the atraumatic grasper, the appendiceal base is grasped and milked to push fecal matter into the cecum. A loop ligature (0-Vicryl, Dexon, or chromic) is placed through the midline puncture. The appendiceal tip is regrasped and pulled through the loop, using a micrograsping forceps (WISAP No. 7678) to direct the ligature toward the base of the appendix. Three loop ligatures are placed.

the fourth loop tie is fixed with the atraumatic grasper. The appendix is cut free with hook scissors, between the loop ties, and the cut appendiceal stump passed to a claw forceps (WISAP No. 7655KG or WOLF No. 8385) and placed through the 10-mm suprapubic incision. Using the claw forceps the appendix is removed. The scissors, grasper, and claw forceps are then removed from the operating field, along with the appendix. The exposed mucosa of the appendiceal stump is lightly cauterized with bipolar or painted with iodine. Some operators recommend placing a purse-string suture around the appendiceal stump but this is probably unnecessary, whether by laparotomy or laparoscopy. If there is a great concern regarding contamination of the peritoneal cavity, an appendix extractor (WISAP No. 7676) can be used.

Postoperatively, patients remain in the hospital until tolerating regular diet, which may take 2 or 3 days. More recently we have been discharging these patients on the day of surgery, on a clear liquid diet, without problems.

FIGURE 15.5. Using the atraumatic grasping forceps the appendix is milked toward the tip, and a fourth loop is applied approximately 1 cm distal from the tied appendiceal base. The appendix is then cut with hook scissors. The severed appendiceal end is passed to a claw forceps (WISAP No. 7655KG or WOLF No. 8385) placed through a 10-mm suprapubic incision, and the appendix removed. The scissors, grasper, and claw forceps are then removed from the operating field. The exposed mucosa of the appendiceal stump are lightly bipolared or painted with iodine.

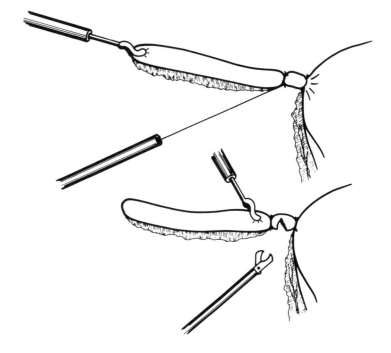

## Results

Using a technique similar to that described above, Gotz and colleagues were able to perform a total of 388 appendectomies.[7] In only 3% of patients was it necessary to abandon the laparoscopic approach for laparotomy. Only 12% of the appendices were proven to be histologically normal. Acute inflammation was noted in 74%, including five perforations, 11% demonstrated subacute and 3% chronic appendicitis.

## References

1. Feste JR. Laser laparoscopy, a new modality. *J Reprod Med.* 1985;30:413–417.
2. Lichten EM, Bombard J. Surgical treatment of primary dysmenorrhea with laparoscopic uterine nerve ablation. *J Reprod Med.* 1987;32:37–41.
3. Black WT. Use of presacral sympathectomy in the treatment of dysmenorrhea. *Am J Obstet Gynecol.* 1964;89:16–22.
4. Curtis AH, Anson BJ, Ashley FL, et al. The anatomy of the pelvic autonomic nerves in relation to gynecology. *Surg Gynecol Obstet.* 1942;75: 743–750.
5. Perez JJ. Laparoscopic presacral neurectomy results of the first 25 cases. *J Reprod Med.* 1990;35:625–630.
6. Spirtos NM, Eisenkop SM, Spirtos TW, et al. Laparoscopy—a diagnostic aid in cases of suspected appendicitis. *Am J Obstet Gynecol.* 1987;156:90–94.
7. Gotz F, Pier A, Bacher C. Modified laparoscopic appendectomy in surgery: a report on 388 operations. *Surg Endosc.* 1990;4:6–9.

# 16

# Techniques and Instrumentation of Operative Hysteroscopy

*Howard A. Zacur and Denise Murray*

## CHAPTER OUTLINE

Hysteroscopy is a term derived from the Greek words to view (*skopeo*) and uterus (*hystera*). As a procedure it was first performed successfully in a human patient in 1869 by Pantaleoni, who used a tube with an external light source to detect "vegetations within the uterine cavity."[1] No attempt was made by Pantaleoni at this time to distend the uterine cavity during this procedure. During the past 100 years developments in optics, fiberoptics, instruments, and distending media have resulted in equipment and techniques that now allow us to diagnose and treat intrauterine disorders using hysteroscopy. This chapter reviews these instruments and their accessories, as well as the distending media, lighting, indications, contraindications, and preoperative preparation for this procedure.

# Instruments

## Hysteroscope

In general, hysteroscopes may be classified as rigid or flexible, designed for diagnostic or operative use, and possessing fixed or variable focusing. Key specifications of the hysteroscope are its scope diameter, lens offset, sheath diameter, and ability to be used with a variety of distending media.

### Rigid Hysteroscopes

Rigid hysteroscopes are currently the most commonly used, and are usually preferred for operative procedures because they contain one or more channels within the sheath through which to pass instruments. The hysteroscope is composed of an endoscope, which is usually enclosed in a metal tube or "sheath," through which distending media or instruments may pass. Sheath diameters may be as small as 3.3 mm (10 Fr) for diagnostic use or as large as 8 mm (24 Fr) for operative use.

#### Optics of Rigid Hysteroscopes

The lens system employed in rigid endoscopes may be divided into three types: classical, Hopkins, and graded index-lens system (GRIN)[2] (see Fig. 3.3). In the classical system the width of the lenses is far less than the length of the telescope and the distance between the lenses is relatively large. Using the Hopkins rod system, the lenses are large in diameter and the separation between the lenses is small. In fact, most of the telescope is occupied by lenses. In the GRIN system the entire telescope is occupied by a slender rod of glass (see Chapter 3).

The picture through the hysteroscope will be affected by the degree of field of view allowed by the outer lens of the hysteroscope, as well as by the angle of this lens to the central axis of the telescope. Most hysteroscopes possess an outer lens that will provide a 60° to 90° field of view depending on the distending medium. This view will be wider in gaseous than aqueous media due to a more optimal refractive index. The outer lens of the hysteroscope may be centered along the axis of the endoscope so that a 360° rotation of the telescope will not result in a change in view. This is called

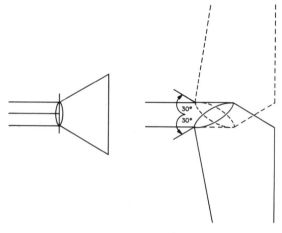

FIGURE 16.1. **Left:** A 60° field of view lens centered at 0° to axis of scope (i.e., 0° viewing angle). **Right:** A 60° field of view when viewing angle is 30° (*solid line*). When the endoscope is rotated 180° (*dashed line*) the potential field of view is much greater than the 0° telescope (reproduced with permission of Prescott, R. Optical Principles of Endoscopy *J Medical Primatology.* 1976; 5:134 and S. Karger, AG, Publishers, Basel).

a 0° scope (Fig. 16.1). Alternatively, the lens may be offset (fore-oblique) by 25° to 30° to the axis of the telescope. When the telescope is rotated 360°, an expanded field of view is seen (Fig. 16.1).

Last, the lens system may focus only when the telescope is in contact with the object to be viewed (e.g., contact hysteroscope) or may provide a magnified or reduced image of the object to be viewed depending on whether the endoscope is brought closer to or taken farther away from the object to be viewed. Under these conditions the hysteroscope view is described as "panoramic."

#### Operative Hysteroscopes

Generally, two operative hysteroscopic set-ups are available. One relies on operative sheaths through which the diagnostic hysteroscope (generally 4 mm in diameter) is placed. The other consists of a hysteroscope constructed with an offset eyepiece and a straight operating channel. When using the first type of hysteroscopic set-up there are two types of operative sheaths. The first has a single channel designed for the insertion of flexible 7 Fr instruments (Figs. 16.2 and 16.3). The disadvantage of this

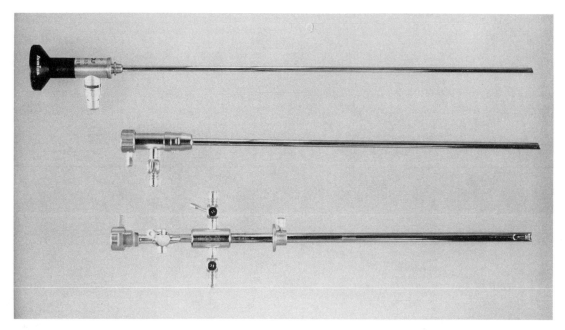

FIGURE 16.2. **From top to bottom:** 25° hysteroscope, 4 mm in diameter, 7-mm diagnostic sheath, and 7-mm operative sheath for the placement of flexible 7 Fr. instruments (Richard Wolf Medical Instruments Corp., Rosemont, IL).

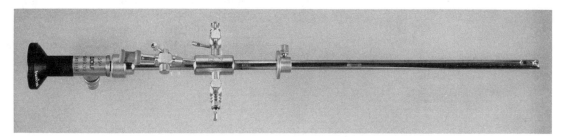

FIGURE 16.3. Hysteroscope within operative sheath for flexible instruments.

set-up is the relatively small size of the instrument jaws and the loss of cutting power because the shaft of the scissors must be flexible. The other type of operative sheath consists of a fixed rigid instrument tip (i.e., scissors, biopsy forceps, or foreign body forceps) attached to the dorsal aspect of the distal end of the sleeve, such that the instrument tip is in full endoscopic view. The disadvantage of this instrumentation is that the sheath must be changed to vary the tips used, which requires that the entire hysteroscope be removed. Furthermore, since the tip is fixed to the sheath, which in turn is fixed to the hysteroscope, the entire endoscopic unit must be moved when the instrument tip needs

to be advanced, reducing the viewing field.

The operating right-angle hysteroscope has a single operative channel through which 3-mm instruments can be placed (Fig. 16.4). Because the lenses have a 10° angle of view, it may be somewhat more difficult to visualize the tubal ostia. However, the instruments are significantly larger and stronger than the flexible ones used above (Fig. 16.5).

### Contact Hysteroscopes

Contact hysteroscopes rely on GRIN lens construction for optics and do not require either a

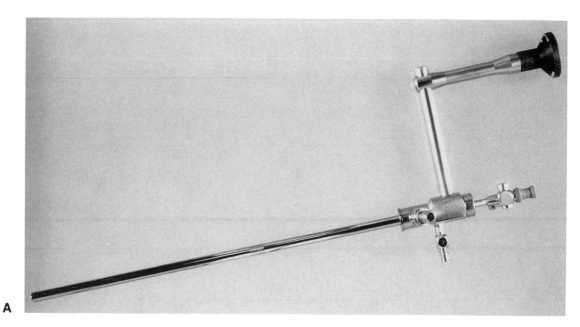

A

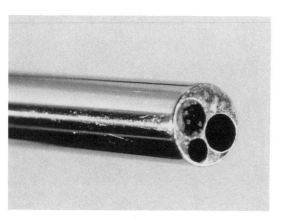

B

FIGURE 16.4. **A:** Operative hysteroscope (0° viewing angle, 7-mm diameter) with straight operating channel for the placement of 3-mm rigid instruments and displaced eye piece. **B:** Tip of rigid operative hysteroscope with operative instrumentation (**larger**) and insufflation (**smaller**) ports (Richard Wolf Medical Instruments Corp., Rosement, IL).

distending medium or fiberoptic light for illumination and visualization. These endoscopes require a light-collecting chamber located near the eyepiece that will transmit light down the endoscope glass guide toward the object of interest. In order to be viewed the endoscope must either be touching or almost touching the surface of interest. Light is transmitted down the glass guide of the endoscope toward the surface that will reflect the light back toward the eyepiece of the endoscope. Because of the rigid glass guide there is no distortion from transmitted images, and these may be magnified 1.6 times without the need for special lenses. Greater magnification to 100× is possi-

ble depending on the eyepiece used. Major advantages to the contact hysteroscope include no need for a special light source, excellent visualization even in the presence of bleeding, and no need for use of a distending medium. Major disadvantages to the contact hysteroscope include lack of a panoramic view, which increases the chance that a lesion may be missed, and the inability to operate through the scope (e.g., take a directed biopsy).

## Microhysteroscopes

Microhysteroscopes as described by Hamou[3] are instruments that can provide a panoramic

FIGURE 16.5. Close-up of jaws of 3-mm rigid scissors **(top)** and biopsy forceps **(middle),** and 7 Fr (2.1 mm) flexible scissors **(bottom).** Note the much larger jaws of the 3-mm scissors (Richard Wolf Medical Instruments Corp., Rosemont, IL).

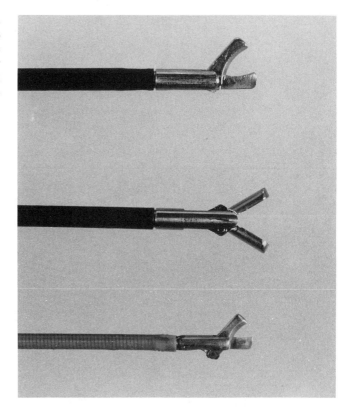

view of the uterine cavity that has been distended, but they can also provide contact and magnified views up to 150× as well. This instrument thus combines the advantages of the panoramic and contact hysteroscope. It is able to accomplish this task using a variable-focusing lens.

### Flexible Hysteroscopes

Development of a steerable and flexible hysteroscope was initially described by Brueschke and Wilbanks in 1974.[4] This instrument had an outer tip diameter of 8.5 mm and contained an operating channel and light source. Previously, flexible endoscopic equipment had been used for the diagnosis of gastrointestinal disorders. Extremely small diameter flexible hysteroscopes have recently been introduced with outer tip diameters of only 3.6 mm, making these instruments potentially ideal for office diagnostic procedures. These scopes may be used for diagnostic or operative indications, and do not require an outer "sheath" (Fig. 16.6).

Drawbacks to the use of flexible hysteroscopes include the fact that only a gaseous distending medium is recommended and resolution is reduced because fiberoptics are employed for visualization, as well as lighting, and the ground substance (adhesive) between the glass fibers results in reduced resolution.

## The Distending Media

Hysteroscopic visualization of the uterine cavity without a contact hysteroscope will require a means of expanding the uterine cavity for panoramic viewing with rigid or flexible hysteroscopes. Lack of suitable distending medium delayed the early development of the hysteroscope. One explanation for the failure to use distending media earlier were the beliefs by investigators at the time that the medium could either contaminate the uterine environment with vaginal pathogens or that the uterus as a muscular organ would not be distendable by the medium.

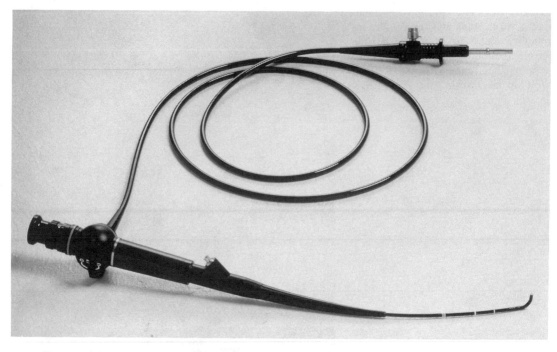

FIGURE 16.6. Flexible operating hysteroscope (Courtesy of Olympus Corp., Lake Success, NY).

It was not until 1925 when Rubin used $CO_2$ gas to distend the uterine cavity for viewing by the hysteroscope that the successful use of a distending medium was reported.[5] In his early studies Rubin found that the procedure produced the best results when performed during the early follicular phase of the menstrual cycle. Traumatic bleeding during the procedure was further minimized by coating the hysteroscope sheath with epinephrine. Despite Rubin's early success with this method, bleeding still obscured vision, preventing others from easily using this procedure until the technique was improved in the 1960s. In 1949 Norment used an air-filled transparent balloon attached to the tip of the hysteroscope to distend the cavity.[6] Visibility was limited, however. Silander, in 1963, modified this approach by using saline instead of air to fill the balloon. Improved visibility was reported, but the field of view was limited and abnormal structures such as small polyps were not recognized due to compression by the balloon.[7]

Distending media for hysteroscopy may be divided into three general classes: 1) liquid nonviscous, 2) liquid viscous, and 3) gaseous.

## Liquid Nonviscous Media

Liquid medium (water or saline) for uterine distention was initially tried by Heineberg in 1914, who used a water irrigation system to clean the hysteroscope of blood and mucus and distend the uterine cavity.[8] Mikulicz-Radecki and Freund[9] and later Gauss[10] used water irrigation systems to rinse the hysteroscope lens but bleeding still obscured their views.

To allay fears that fluids passing into the uterine cavity could be passed in turn into the abdominal pelvic cavity, Schroeder in 1934 measured intrauterine pressures to determine the conditions under which fluid would pass from the uterus into the abdomen.[11] He found that intrauterine pressures exceeding 55 mm Hg allowed liquid to pass into the fallopian tubes. He also noted that suspending a reservoir containing the fluid for uterine distention 650 mm above the patient resulted in an intrauterine pressure of 25 to 30 mm Hg, and placement at 950 mm above the patient resulted in an intrauterine pressure of 35 mm Hg. Under these conditions fluid would remain within the uterine cavity.

Although water or saline were the first non-viscous liquid media used as a distending media for hysteroscopy, other fluids were and are being tried. In 1970 use of a 5% dextrose solution was used by Norment and Sikes[12] and then Quinones and colleagues.[13] Large volumes of fluid were required and visualization was difficult in the presence of bleeding. More recently, use of Ringer's lactate, 1.5% glycine or 4.4% sorbitol solutions have been mentioned as alternative media for uterine distention. These solutions are frequently used as irrigants for urological procedures (e.g., transurethral prostatectomy).

Advantages of the liquid nonviscous distending media include their availability, low cost, and ease of use. Unfortunately, crystalloid solutions are miscible with blood and extensive flushing is required to provide a clear field of view. When use of electrosurgical instruments is anticipated, normal saline should *not* be used because of its conductive nature.

## Liquid Viscous Media

In 1968 Menken used a viscous material, polyvinylpyrrolidone, to distend the uterine cavity.[14] Although it was inert and nonconductive, it was yellowish in color and not biogradable, attributes that limited its usefulness. In 1970, Edstrom and Fernstrom described the use of 32% dextran-70 in 10% dextrose in water as a distending medium for hysteroscopy.[15] This solution was quite viscous, but it was clear and allowed the hysteroscope to be used for diagnostic as well as therapeutic use.

Dextran is a polysaccharide first isolated from beet sugar, where it is formed by the action of the bacteria *Leuconostoc mesenteroides*. Hundreds of glucose molecules make up the polysaccharide molecule and these molecules are bound together through 1:6 and 1:4 glucosidic linkages. Two forms of dextran exist, one with a molecular weight of 70,000 kd and the other with a molecular weight of 40,000 kd. Hyskon, which is currently available and approved for hysteroscopic use, is a 32% solution of the 70,000 molecular weight form. This fluid is clear, sterile, electrolyte-free, nonconductive, and not easily miscible

with blood. Instruments must be thoroughly cleaned to prevent crystallization of this viscous material, which will occlude channels and valves.

## Gaseous Media

Renewed interest in use of $CO_2$ for hysteroscopy occurred after the work of Lindemann in 1971, who designed special equipment for its administration.[16] The problem of gas leakage from the cervix was solved by using a metal bell doughnut that fit snugly to the cervix by means of suction induced by a small vacuum pump. The hysteroscope could then be passed through a rubber O-ring placed in the center of the bell (Fig. 16.7). A distinctive risk of using gaseous agents as distending media is gas embolism. This risk was almost completely eliminated by the development of an insufflating apparatus designed to limit gas flow to no more than 100 ml of $CO_2$ per minute while keeping the intrauterine pressure at values less than 200 mm Hg. These limits were identified by Lindemann from earlier animal and human studies when the electrocardiogram, $PaCO_2$, and blood pH were monitored.[17]

Use of other gaseous agents to perform hysteroscopy is limited due to the risk of embolism. For example, use of nitrous oxide ($N_2O$) as a distending medium was reported by Hulf and colleagues in 1979.[18] In this study $N_2O$ was compared to $CO_2$ and a rise in $PaCO_2$ was seen only when $N_2O$ was used. This rise was believed to result from the "dead space" induced by $N_2O$ molecules due to their inability to solubilize in blood. Thus, gas media that do not solubilize well in blood increase the risk for embolism. Fortunately, $CO_2$ solubilizes well in blood.

Administration of $CO_2$ during hysteroscopy should be provided only by insufflators designed specifically for this purpose. For example, use of laparoscopy insufflators result in $CO_2$ flow rates 10 to 20 times greater (1–2 liters per min) than hysteroscopic insufflators (0.1 liters per min). Increased flow rates also increases the risk of gas embolism as the increased gas volume will be more difficult to solubilize.

Bleeding and bubbling still limit the effec-

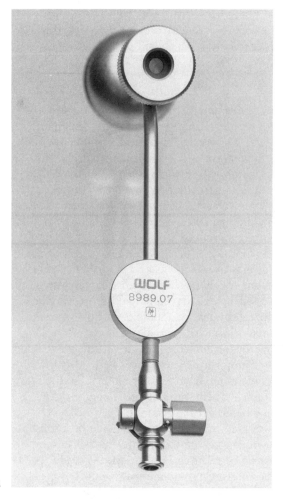

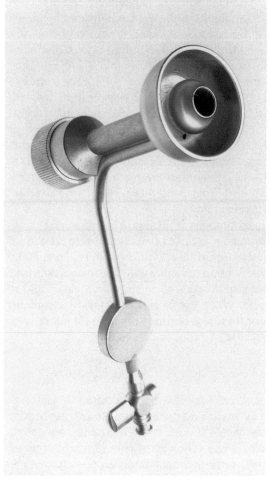

A

B

FIGURE 16.7. 7-mm operative portio adapter. **A:** Portion which faces the hysteroscope. **B:** The side of the portio adapter that faces the cervix is dis-played (Richard Wolf Medical Instruments Corp., Rosemont, IL).

tiveness of $CO_2$ as a distending medium by re-ducing visualization. However, $CO_2$ is easy to use and it is clean. It also has a refractive index of 1.0 allowing it to present a nonmagnified and wider field of view to the operator than either Hyskon (with a refractive index of 1.39) or saline (refractive index 1.37). Other advantages include its availability, rapid absorption, and relative safety.

## Administration of Liquid Distending Media

Early methods of administering low viscosity solutions such as water or saline into the uter-ine cavity relied primarily on raising a fluid-filled reservoir to a predetermined height above the patient, in order to create a specific intrauterine pressure. This technique remains in effect today but has been modified by use of a blood pressure cuff. In brief, uterine-distending solutions made available in soft plastic bags (e.g., 5% dextrose in water solu-tion) are elevated above the patient and en-wrapped by a blood pressure cuff inflated to produce 150 mm Hg pressure. This technique will allow flow of distending medium at rates suitable for performing hysteroscopy. More recently, fluid pumps designed especially for hysteroscopic use have become commercially

FIGURE 16.8. Continuous flow hysteroscopy system.

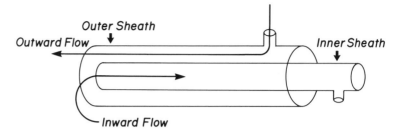

available (e.g., Continuous Flow Resectosurge Pump, ACMI, Stamford, CT).

Previously, methods used to administer high viscosity solutions (e.g., dextran-70) relied on manual injection through a 50-cc syringe connected by intravenous tubing to the hysteroscope. This technique has led to great variations in intrauterine pressures and the volumes of dextran used, and most often has resulted in greater amounts of media being used than were necessary. Use of a Harvard infusion pump to compress the syringe plunger was tried by Lavy et al. to provide additional control over the administration of the dextran.[19] This apparatus was then modified to allow the pump motor to disengage when pressures greater than 150 to 175 cm $H_2O$ were reached (approximately 110–130 mm Hg) and most recently has been further modified and made available commercially (e.g., DeCherney Pump, Cabot Medical Corp., Longhorne, PA). Instead of a motor drive to create pressure, these new infusion pumps use $CO_2$ to force dextran into the uterine cavity at preset flow and pressure rates. Use of reduced volumes of dextran to perform diagnostic and operative hysteroscopy has been the result of this technological advance.

## Maintenance Versus Continuous Flow of Distending Media

Mention should be made of the difference between operative hysteroscopy procedures that rely on a continuous flow of distending media versus those that do not. In brief, when a viscous medium such as dextran is used the fluid may be introduced slowly into the uterine cavity through the hysteroscope. Once the cavity has been distended, only small amounts of additional viscous media need be added to maintain uterine distention. This is not viewed as a continuous flow system since excess fluid usually passes from the uterine cavity around the hysteroscope sheath and emerges from the cervical os. Only small volumes of dextran are usually required to complete most procedures. The major advantage to this system is that the outer diameter of the operating hysteroscope may be kept relatively small.

In contrast, when less viscous media are used, constant flushing of the cavity is required to maintain a clear operating field and a continuous-flow endoscopic sheath is required. These instruments contain an outer sheath through which media flow from the uterine cavity as well as an inner sheath that transmits the fluid into the uterine cavity (Fig. 16.8). The major disadvantage of this system is the size of the outer sheath that must be used.

## Lighting

Development of fiberoptic lighting systems revolutionized endoscopic procedures by providing high intensity light from halogen or Xenon lamps at power outputs of 100 to 300 W. Heat from these lamps was removed by filtering out the infrared spectrum. This allowed sufficient "cold light" to be transmitted along light-emitting fibers so that endoscopic diagnostic and therapeutic procedures could be performed. Light cords may transmit light through fibers or liquid. Fiber-filled cords are less expensive but may transmit less light than liquid-filled cords. Modern-day light generators also can provide brief flashes of brilliant light for still photography (see Chapter 3).

## Accessory Instruments

In addition to the hysteroscopes, other instruments are available for performing intrauterine surgery. These instruments may be passed through the operating channel of the hysteroscope or passed in parallel to the endoscope to aid in diagnosis or therapy. These accessory instruments include biopsy forceps, grasping forceps, scissors, wire cautery loop, roller ball cautery, laser, and fine wire and balloon uterotubal cannulae.

Biopsy forceps may be rigid or flexible and pass within the operating channel of the hysteroscope or alongside it. Tissue samples from the uterine cavity may be taken with these forceps under direct vision. Similarly flexible or rigid scissors may be positioned in the uterine cavity and used to lyse adhesions or septa. Wire cautery loops passed through appropriately insulated hysteroscopes may also be used to lyse adhesions or septa or resect submucous fibroids. The wire loop as described by DeCherney and Polan[20] or roller ball as reported by Townsend et al.[21] may also be employed to electrocauterize the uterine endometrium and ablate it. Such procedures are currently being used to treat some patients with menorrhagia (see Chapter 18). A Nd:YAG laser using a 0.6-mm quartz optical fiber may also be passed through the operating channel of the hysteroscope. Once within the uterine cavity, 40 to 60 W of power may be applied to destroy the uterine endometrium, as reported by Goldrath et al. in 1981.[22] A radiofrequency thermal probe has also been described by Phipps et al., which may be passed through the operating channel of the hysteroscope and into the uterine cavity to accomplish the same task.[23] It must be energized at 27.12 MHz with an incident power level of 550 W to ablate the endometrium thermally.

Last, tubal cannulation devices have been described that may pass through the operating channel of the hysteroscope and into the interstitial portion of the fallopian tube to alleviate obstruction. These cannulae may be used either as a small guidewire probe alone, as reported by Daniell and Miller,[24] or as a guidewire surrounded by a balloon that may be inflated once passed into the interstitial portion of the fallopian tube, as reported by Confino et al.[25] (see Chapter 20).

## Video Imaging

Invention of miniaturized cameras that rely on charge coupled device (CCD) chips have resulted in extremely small ($1 \times 1 \times 1.5$ in) and lightweight (1.6 oz) cameras that are sterilizable, making them ideal for endoscopic use. Using currently available light sources, these cameras may be connected to the hysteroscope and to a video monitor to allow both surgeons and assistants to visualize endoscopic procedures. This may be extremely important for some operative hysteroscopic procedures where technical assistance is required and the assistant must be aware of what the primary surgeon is attempting to accomplish. Using this equipment, the operative procedure may be recorded on video tape and replayed later for the patient or other physicians (see Chapter 6).

## Indications and Contraindications to Hysteroscopy

The indications can be classified under a few general headings as seen in Table 16.1. In essence, hysteroscopy is indicated when any form of intrauterine pathology is suspected, and diagnosis and therapy required. An extensive discussion of indications, contraindications, preparation, and technical procedure for hysteroscopy may be found in Neuwirth's monograph on hysteroscopy.[26]

Contraindications are few and are usually relative. Hysteroscopy is not recommended for patients with acute or chronic uterotubal infection, nor is it usually advised in patients who are actively bleeding or menstruating. However, hysteroscopy to remove an IUD causing infection or a polyp causing bleeding *are* indications for the procedure. Certainly, unintentional instrumentation of the gravid uterus with a hysteroscope is not desirable, although the hysteroscope under planned conditions may serve as a fetoscope.

TABLE 16.1 Indications for Hysteroscopy.

Abnormal Uterine bleeding
  Diagnosis:
    Premenopausal patient
    Postmenopausal patient
  Therapy
    Biopsy and/or directed curettage
    Polyp removal
    Excision of submucous fibroid
    Ablation
Foreign bodies
  Diagnosis:
    Identification
    Localization
  Therapy:
    Removal of IUD
    Removal of suction catheter tip
    Removal of ossified products of conception
    Removal of laminaria
Infertility/recurrent abortions
  Diagnosis:
    Uterine synechiae
    Uterine malformation
    Interstitial tubal occlusion
  Therapy:
    Lysis of synechiae
    Resection of uterine septum
    Removal of interstitial tubal block
    Potential for intratubal insemination
Prenatal diagnosis
  Fetoscopy
  Directed chorionic villus sampling
Contraceptive therapy
  Blockage of utero-tubo ostium with plugs
  Destruction of utero-tubo ostium

## Preoperative Preparation for Hysteroscopic Surgery

Hysteroscopy is usually performed during the early follicular phase of the menstrual cycle to enhance visibility, since the endometrium is thin and less vascular at this time. This may be the only preparation required when hysteroscopy is performed primarily as a diagnostic procedure.

When hysteroscopic surgery is planned, specialized preoperative and postoperative care may be required. For example, removal of large intrauterine polyps or resection of submucous fibroids may be facilitated by preoperative hormonal therapy with Danocrine (400–800 mg/day) or a gonadotropin-releasing hormone analog (GnRH analog) for 1 to 3 months before the procedure. Although not currently approved by the FDA for these indications, use of these medications will usually result in decreased size and vascularity of the uterine polyp or fibroid to be removed. Figure 16.9 shows the preoperative and postoperative hysterosalpingograms of a patient with a large submucous fibroid treated with a GnRH analog before hysteroscopic removal. Use of Danocrine or GnRH analog therapy has also been recommended before proceeding with endometrial ablation since these medications will diminish the thickness of the endometrium, ensuring a greater likelihood that the lining will be completely destroyed.

For certain operative hysteroscopic procedures concomitant laparoscopy or its availability is recommended. This may be of advantage in some cases where lysis of uterine synechiae, excision of uterine septum, removal of fibroids, ablation of the endometrium, or removal of a uterotubal occlusion is required. Laparoscopic visualization under these conditions could potentially prevent or minimize the complication of perforation, as well as monitor successful cannulation of a previously proximally obstructed fallopian tube. In some cases of severe uterine adhesions, laparoscopy may also be used to allow transfundal injection of methylene blue into the scarred uterine cavity to assist the hysteroscopist in identifying the limits of the uterine cavity.

Specialized postoperative therapy may also be required in certain circumstances. Correction of severe uterine synechiae may necessitate temporary intrauterine insertion of an inert foreign body to prevent uterine wall readherence (e.g., IUD or Foley catheter) while also providing exogenous estrogen therapy (e.g., conjugated estrogens given in daily doses of 0.625 mg or 1.25 mg for 25–30 days). Postoperative estrogen therapy without insertion of a foreign body may also be needed after lysis of a uterine septum as recent studies have shown that estrogen given under these conditions stimulates more rapid reepithelization by the endometrium. Preoperative and postoperative broad spectrum antibiotic coverage may also be desirable depending on the circumstances of the individual case.

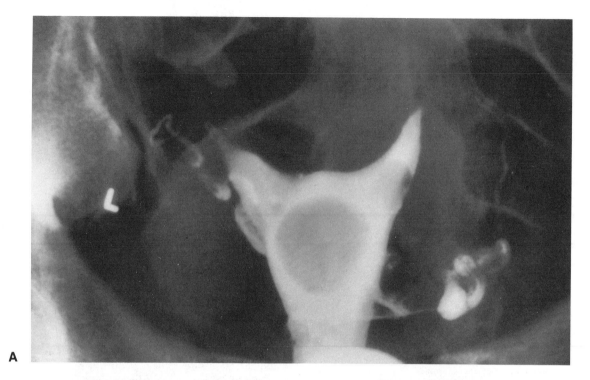

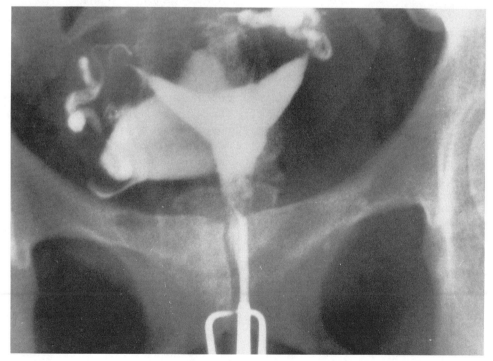

FIGURE 16.9. **A:** Preoperative hysterosalpingogram of a large intrauterine myoma. **B:** Postoperative hysterosalpingogram after pretreatment with GnRH analog and hysteroscopic resection.

Antibiotic use may be employed when previously unsuspected or diagnosed intrauterine infection is discovered, or the procedure is long and operative contamination is suspected.

Removal of large submucous fibroids may result in excessive uterine bleeding. Blood loss in this situation may be controlled by placing a large Foley catheter balloon within the uterine cavity and keeping the balloon expanded for up to 24 hr.

Last, special preoperative therapy may be required in order to lyse severe uterine synechiae through a severely stenotic cervix. In this circumstance cervical dilatation with laminaria and use of intraoperative ultrasonography to guide the hysteroscope may be of help.

# Hysteroscopic Technique

The procedures employed during diagnostic and operative hysteroscopy are relatively straightforward.

## Diagnostic Hysteroscopy

For diagnostic procedures the endocervical canal and uterine cavity must be carefully inspected and both tubal ostia observed. During diagnostic hysteroscopy the endoscope is gently advanced through the endocervical canal and into the uterine cavity under direct vision. When small outer diameter endoscopes are used cervical dilatation may not be needed, although use of large-diameter operating hysteroscopes generally require dilatation. Diagnostic procedures may usually be performed in the outpatient operating room or in the appropriately equipped office. When very small outer diameter endoscopes are used sedation or anesthesia may not be required. For larger diameter telescopes requiring cervical dilatation, a paracervical block with intravenous (IV) sedation or even general anesthesia may prove necessary.

## Biopsy, Polypectomy, Fibroid Removal, and Endometrial Ablation

Directed, biopsy of tissues within the endometrial cavity may be accomplished by passing a biopsy forcep through or alongside the hystero-scope. All types of distending media may be used for this procedure. After the biopsy, blood may accumulate making visualization difficult when $CO_2$ or liquid nonviscous media are used.

Removal of a polyp or a submucous fibroid may be accomplished with the aid of wire loop cautery. As described by Neuwirth, large, broad-based myomas may be shaved to their bases using successive passes of the wire loop.[27,28] If the polyp or fibroid is attached to the uterine side wall by a small pedicle, it may be directly transected. Procedures using the operating hysteroscope with wire loop cautery usually requires liquid viscous nonconductive media. Several, but not all, surgical groups prefer the use of dextran-70 (Hyskon) for these cases. Less viscous media (5% dextrose) is used by other teams but large volumes are frequently required. Lasers passed through the hysteroscope may be used to remove polyps or fibroids, but this remains a relatively new technique. $CO_2$ is required as distending media for these cases as the laser caramelizes the viscous dextran medium.

Ablation of the endometrium has been advocated as an alternative to hysterectomy for corrective treatment of menorrhagia in some patients. Use of the Nd:YAG laser for this purpose has been advocated by Goldrath and colleagues[22] as well as Lomano.[29] In brief, the Nd:YAG laser fiber may either be dragged or brought in close contact with the endometrium (blanching technique) to destroy it. The entire uterine cavity is systematically treated beginning at the cornua. Results may vary depending on whether preoperative medical treatment was used (Danocrine or GnRH analog) and on the wattage of the laser selected.

Electrocautery and thermal destruction of the uterine endometrium have also been recommended as methods of endometrial ablation. Using either the wire loop cautery, roller ball cautery, or thermal probe the entire uterine cavity may be systematically electrocauterized beginning at the ostia and proceeding toward the fundus, then along the anterior, posterior, and lateral uterine walls toward the internal os. Efficacy of therapy is also dependent on preoperative medical treatment designed to reduce the thickness of the endometrium as well as regulation of the wattage used to produce either cautery or heat. Dextran-70 media is usually employed for electrocautery and thermal endometrial destruction whereas $CO_2$ is used for laser procedures as previously mentioned.

## Removal of Foreign Bodies

Foreign bodies found within the uterine cavity include IUDs, suction catheter tips, and laminaria, as well as retained and ossified products of conception. Removal of these foreign bodies may be straightforward or complex. In the simple case the foreign body is located and identified, then grasped with forceps and removed. For complicated cases it may be necessary to excise an embedded object and simultaneous laparoscopy may be of benefit. Either $CO_2$ or liquid media may be employed for these procedures.

## Lysis of Uterine Synechiae or Septa

Scissors or wire loop cautery have usually been used to lyse intrauterine synechiae or to divide uterine septa. Use of the laser is also theoretically possible for this purpose. All of the previously described distending media may be used during this operation, although high molecular weight dextran is usually employed for improved visibility. For filmy synechiae, excision of as much of the adhesion as possible is recommended. In severe cases, wherein the uterine cavity is almost obliterated by very dense adhesions, midsegment transection is usually all that is possible. Placement of an inert foreign body such as an IUD or Foley catheter balloon after lysis may be necessary in treating some cases of severe uterine synechiae to prevent readherence. This is not generally required after transection of a uterine septum, however. Postoperative exogenous estrogen therapy may be of benefit after either lysis of adhesions or uterine septum transection.

## Removal of Interstitial Tubal Obstruction

Alleviation of proximal tubal obstruction is performed by passing a uterotubal cannula through the hysteroscope and into the tubal ostium. This procedure is best performed during the follicular phase of the menstrual cycle to improve visualization. Either $CO_2$ or dextran-70 may be used as distending media. Under direct vision a guidewire alone or guidewire surrounded by a balloon is passed into the tubal ostium and then gently advanced. The procedure is also viewed laparoscopically to detect when the guidewire has passed the obstruction and entered the isthmus of the fallopian tube. Documentation of distal tubal dye spill verifying restoration of tubal patency can also be accomplished at this time. This hysteroscopic technique is relatively new and it is yet unclear how long the alleviation of tubal obstruction will remain.

## References

1. Pantaleoni DC. An endoscopic examination of the cavity of the womb. *Med Press Circ* (Lond.). 1869;8:26–27.
2. Prescott R. Optical principles of endoscopy. *J Med Primatol*. 1976;5:133–147.
3. Hamou J. Microhysteroscopy: a new procedure and its original applications in gynecology. *J Reprod Med*. 1981;26:375–382.
4. Brueschke EE, Wilbanks GD. A steerable fiberoptic hysteroscope. *Obstet Gynecol*. 1974;44:273–278.
5. Rubin IC. Uterine endoscopy, endometroscopy with the aid of uterine insufflation. *Am J Obstet Gynecol*. 1925;10:313–327.
6. Norment WB. Improved instruments for the diagnosis of pelvic lesions by the hysterogram and water hysteroscope. *N C Med J*. 1949;10:646–649.
7. Silander T. Hysteroscopy through a transparent rubber balloon in patients with carcinoma of the uterine endometrium. *Acta Obstet Gynecol Scand*. 1963;42:284–299.
8. Heineberg A. Uterine endoscopy: an aid to precision in the diagnosis of intra-uterine disease. *Surg Gynecol Obstet*. 1914;18:513–515.
9. Mikulicz-Radecki F, Freund A. Ein neues hysteroskope und praktische anwendung in der gynakologie. *Z Gerburtschilfe Gynakol*. 1927;92:13–25.
10. Gauss CJ. Hysteroskopie. *Arch Gynaekol*. 1928;133:18–27.
11. Schroeder C. Uber den ausbau und die leis-

tungen der hysteroskopie. *Arch Gynaekol.* 1934;156:407–419.

12. Norment WB, Sikes H. Fiber-optic hysteroscopy: an improved method for viewing the interior of the uterus. *N C Med J.* 1970;31:251–254.

13. Quinones GR, Alvarado DA, Aznar RR. Tubal electrocoagulation under hysteroscopie control. In Hysteroscopie Sterilization, Miami, 1974, Symposia Specialists.

14. Menken FC. Endoscopic observations of endocrine processes and hormonal changes. In: *Simposio Esteriodes Sexuales.* Bogata; 1968:24–26.

15. Edstrom K, Fernstrom I. The diagnostic possibilities of a modified hysteroscopic technique. *Acta Obstet Gynecol Scand.* 1970;49:327–330.

16. Lindemann HJ. $CO_2$—hysteroscopy today. *Endoscopy.* 1979;2:94–100.

17. Lindemann JH, Mohr J. $CO_2$ hysteroscopy: diagnosis and treatment. *Am J Obstet Gynecol.* 1976;124:129–133.

18. Hulf JA, Corall IM, Knights KM, et al. Blood carbon dioxide tension changes during hysteroscopy. *Fertil Steril.* 1979;32:193–196.

19. Lavy G, Diamond MP, Shapiro B, et al. A new device to facilitate intrauterine instillation of dextran 70 for hysteroscopy. *Obstet Gynecol.* 1987;70:955–957.

20. DeCherney A, Polan ML. Hysteroscopic management of intrauterine lesions and intractable uterine bleeding. *Obstet Gynecol.* 1983;61:392–397.

21. Townsend DE, Richart RM, Paskowitz RA, et al. "Rollerball" coagulation of the endometrium. *Obstet Gynecol.* 1990;76:310–313.

22. Goldrath MH, Fuller TA, Segal S. Laser photovaporization of endometrium for the treatment of menorrhagia. *Am J Obstet Gynecol.* 1981;140:14–19.

23. Phipps JH, Lewis BV, Prior MV, et al. Experimental and clinical studies with radiofrequency induced therapy endometrial ablation for functional menorrhagia. *Obstet Gynecol.* 1990;76:876–881.

24. Daniell JF, Miller W. Hysteroscopic correction of cornual occlusion with resultant term pregnancy. *Fertil Steril.* 1987;48:490–492.

25. Confino E, Friberg J, Gleicher N. Transcervical balloon tuboplasty. *Fertil Steril.* 1986;46:963–966.

26. Neuwirth R. Hysteroscopy. In: Friedman EA, ed. *Major Problems in Obstetrics and Gynecology.* Vol. 8. Philadelphia: Saunders; 1975:1–116.

27. Neuwirth RS, Amin HK. Excision of submucous fibroids with hysteroscopic control. *Am J Obstet Gynecol.* 1976;126:95–99.

28. Neuwirth RS. A new technique for and additional experience with hysteroscopic resection of submucous fibroids. *Am J Obstet Gynecol.* 1978;131:91–94.

29. Lomano JM. Photocoagulation of the endometrium with the Nd:YAG laser for the treatment of menorrhagia: a report of ten cases. *J Reprod Med.* 1986;31:148–150.

# 17

# Operative Hysteroscopic Procedures

*Richard E. Blackwell*

## CHAPTER OUTLINE

Although the operative cystoscope was modified for intrauterine surgery in 1927, it was not until 1970 that Edstrom and Fernstrom used dextran as the distending medium permitting hysteroscopists to perform complex transcervical surgery. The union of the modern operative hysteroscope with appropriate distending medium has made possible the precise localization of various intrauterine pathologies and their treatment with a variety of operative techniques, including sharp dissection, electrocautery, and laser.

The following will be discussed: the operative hysteroscopic treatment of patients with abnormal uterine bleeding, an abnormal uterine contour on hysterosalpingography, suspected Asherman's, requiring removal of an intrauterine foreign body, or evaluation of a suspected uterine perforation. In addition to these indications, operative hysteroscopy is used for the resection of uterine septae (Chapter 19), ablation of the endometrium (Chapter 18) and transcervical recanalization of the fallopian tubes (Chapter 20), as discussed elsewhere.

## Indications and Patient Selection

### Abnormal Uterine Bleeding

In the past, patients with abnormal uterine bleeding unresponsive to hormonal manipulation underwent dilation and curettage (D&C) to rule out malignancy and as a treatment. Unfortunately, this blind technique resulted in failure to render a diagnosis or provide treatment in a significant number of cases.[1] Removal of intrauterine polyps or submucous fibroids often requires direct visualization. The diagnosis of adenomyosis, although requiring a myometrial biopsy for confirmation, is made with greater assurance after a negative hysteroscopic examination.

## An Abnormal Uterine Contour on Hysterogram

In couples with reproductive failure the hysterosalpingogram (HSG) defines the size and structure of the uterine cavity, patency of the fallopian tubes, and often suggests the presence of adhesions or other pathology. When properly performed under fluoroscopic control small polyps, fibroids, and intrauterine adhesions may be diagnosed with considerable precision. In addition, congenital uterine malformations and tubal occlusion may be detected. In patients with a normal HSG there is probably little indication for hysteroscopy. Alternatively, most intrauterine filling defects are best investigated and treated by transcervical hysteroscopic surgery.

## Suspected Asherman's Syndrome

The patient with secondary amenorrhea who has a history of intrauterine trauma should undergo evaluation to rule out Asherman's syndrome. However, Asherman's syndrome presents most frequently with infertility or habitual pregnancy loss, and not amenorrhea. Asherman's syndrome (partial or complete obliteration of the endometrial cavity by synechiae) almost always occurs in the presence of uterine trauma or manipulation associated with infection and/or hypoestrogenemia, such as after D&C for miscarriage, removal of infected IUD, or retained products of conception. Patients with a negative history for such events should be investigated for hypo- or hypergonadotropism, resulting in the development of hypoestrogenemia and amenorrhea.

In the patient with suspected Asherman's syndrome an HSG should be attempted before hysteroscopy in order to define the lesion clearly. Often, however, there will be fusion of the lower uterine segment making performance of the procedure impossible on an outpatient basis.

## Suspected Intrauterine Foreign Body

The operative hysteroscope is extremely useful in the location of a lost IUD. Most frequently, these are buried in either the anterior or posterior fundal wall, in a uterus that is either markedly ante- or retroflexed. In addition, other intrauterine foreign bodies may be located and removed hysteroscopically. Further, patients who undergo a spontaneous abortion and develop secondary amenorrhea may be found to have retained products of conception, even 6 months after the miscarriage. Removal of the retained tissue generally results in restoration of menstruation.

## Evaluation of the Perforated Uterus

Some surgeons consider perforation of the uterus to be a contraindication to hysteroscopy, whereas others have suggested that this technique permits confirmation of the surgical accident and assessment of damage. Once a perforation is confirmed, tamponade of the uterine cavity or laparoscopy with electrocautery of the injury can be used to control bleeding. In rare occasions hysteroscopy and transcervical cauterization has been used to locate and coagulate intrauterine bleeding after transabdominal myomectomy.

# Equipment

Operative hysteroscopy can be performed using three distending media: carbon dioxide ($CO_2$), 5% dextrose in water ($D_5W$) and 32% dextran-70 (Hyskon). Electrolyte solutions (e.g., normal saline or lactate Ringer's solution) generally should not be used for operative work since these media will be electrically conductive. Each of these respective media have their proponents. The author usually prefers to use Hyskon. Dextran-70 has an excellent index of refraction, is immiscible with blood, is highly suitable for operative procedures, and is relatively safe.[2] It should be noted, however, that both pulmonary edema and anaphylactic reactions have been reported with the use of Hyskon, although no anaphylactic episodes have been seen at our institution during the past 20 years. Dextran-70 has the disadvantage of damaging operative instruments if the medium is allowed to dry on their surfaces or various orifices. Therefore, instruments should be cleaned in very hot water immediately after the procedures using Hyskon.

Operative hysteroscopes contain single or multiple channels that allow insertion of either rigid or flexible grasping forceps, biopsy forceps, scissors, coagulating electrodes, and laser fibers. Operative hysteroscopes may consist of a fore-oblique diagnostic hysteroscope (generally 4 mm in diameter) with a 6- to 7-mm operative sheath with operative ports for flexible operative 7 Fr instruments (see Fig. 16.1), or a dorsal fixed instrument tip resembling a cystoscope. Alternatively, the author prefers a 7-mm operating hysteroscope with an offset right-angle eyepiece and a 10° field of vision (Richard Wolf Corp, Rosemont, IL). This endoscope contains a single operative channel allowing the introduction of rigid 3-mm operative instruments (see Fig. 16.2). These are generally insulated for use as unipolar electrosurgical tips. The smaller 7 Fr flexible instruments used with some operative hysteroscopes are less powerful (see Fig. 16.3), and may increase the operative time and the amount of Hyskon, glycine, sorbitol, $D_5W$, or 5% mannitol required to complete the procedure.

Pediatric or adult urological resectoscopes have been modified for use in the resection of intrauterine fibroids, septae, and endometrial ablation. These are generally used in conjunction with a distending medium, such as Hyskon or $CO_2$, and an electrosurgical generator set at 60 to 120 W. The depth of burn with these instruments is usually not greater than 2 mm. Modification of these rectoscopes using a roller ball can be employed to ablate the endometrium (see Chapter 18).

Many types of fiber-transmitted lasers, including Argon, Nd:YAG and KTP, have been employed through the operative hysteroscope.[3] In my opinion none of these lasers is as efficient or user-friendly as the more conventional equipment described above. For additional discussion of hysteroscopic instrumentation, refer to Chapter 16.

# Specific Techniques

Operative hysteroscopy is best performed during the early to midfollicular phase because of the reduced risk of unsuspected pregnancy, reduced endometrial thickening, and clearest view of the tubal ostium. Furthermore, a corpus luteum will generally be absent if simultaneous operative laparoscopy is required.

## Resection of an Endometrial Polyp

Endometrial polyps are simple to remove via operative hysteroscopy. Once located with the diagnostic hysteroscope, polyp forceps can be used to extract them rapidly, after which a repeat hysteroscopy will confirm the absence of any additional lesions. Occasionally, difficult to extract polyps are removed after transection of their stalk with operative scissors. Little or no bleeding occurs with resection of these polyps.

## Removal of Submucous Myomas

Various types of fibroids may be treated with the operative hysteroscope.[4] The simplest to deal with is the pedunculated fibroid that protrudes into the uterine cavity, attached only to the endometrial wall via a thin stalk. These lesions, once identified, can frequently be grasped with polyp forceps, crushed, and removed in small pieces. This type of myomectomy usually progresses rapidly and twisting the stalk will minimize blood loss.

Some fibroids partially protrude into the cavity, the sessile submucous type. A few of these lesions may be extracted with polyp forceps producing a defect that may or may not require hemostasis with either transhysteroscopic electrocautery or the placement of a distended Foley catheter balloon. More commonly, these lesions are approached with the resectoscope, which is used to "shave" the myoma to the endometrial base.[5] This technique can be carried out alone or in combination with laparoscopy. See Chapter 13 for additional discussion of resectoscopic myomectomies. Postoperatively, a Silastic balloon catheter is placed within the uterine cavity and conjugated estrogens 1.25 mg twice daily are administered for a month to facilitate endometrial regeneration.

Three months of preoperative administration of GnRH analog suppression may result in a 40% to 50% reduction in myoma size and a decrease in tumor vascularity,[6] facilitating hysteroscopic removal. Furthermore, because GnRH analog suppression produces an even more marked reduction in uterine wall thickness, an intramural fibroid may become entirely submucosal.

## Removal of Intrauterine Synechiae and Adhesions

Intrauterine adhesions are perhaps the most common lesions encountered by the operative hysteroscopist.[7] Once diagnosed by HSG, a blind D&C can often be carried out to break up minimal intrauterine adhesions, followed by reinvestigation with radiography. More substantial adhesive disease is best treated with hysteroscopy. Some adhesions disappear during dilation of the cervix, and other times they can be simply lysed with operative scissors (Fig. 17.1). However, on occasion extensive intrauterine dissection is required to restore the normal uterine contour (Fig. 17.2). In severe Asherman's syndrome careful creation of a neouterine space with Hanks dilators under direct laparoscopic vision, followed by hysteroscopic dissection of both lower uterine segment and fundus, is required. Only in patients with extensive dissection and denudation of the endometrial lining are IUDs or balloon catheters inserted into the uterine cavity postoperatively, to prevent approximation of the opposing walls. As with the resection of uterine fibroids, 2.5 mg of conjugated estrogens are administered daily for 1 month. It is also suggested that with extensive intrauterine manipulation broad spectrum oral antibiotics be employed for 5 to 7 days.

## Removal of a Retained IUD

The most common foreign body that gynecologists are asked to remove from the uterine cavity is a retained IUD. Anteflexion or marked retroflexion of the uterus generally

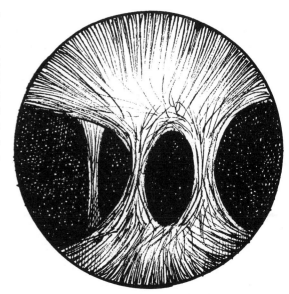

FIGURE 17.1. Extensive intrauterine adhesions obliterating the uterine cavity.

make the cavity more difficult to explore blindly. The location of the lost IUD may be established by transvaginal sonography or an HSG. Once localized, extraction is performed using an IUD hook or other appropriate instrument. In general, those IUDs that cannot be retrieved in the office with either a Novak curette, an IUD hook, or office hysteroscopy require operative hysteroscopy.

At hysteroscopy the IUD will generally be found embedded in the anterior or posterior uterine wall near the fundus. Most IUDs may be extracted by simply locating them with a diagnostic hysteroscope and subsequently removing them with a sharp serrated curette (e.g., Novak), using slow, sustained traction. If this maneuver fails to remove the IUD, polyp forceps may be inserted into the uterine cavity, after removal of the hysteroscope, and the object grasped and extracted. However, occasionally the IUD will break in two with this maneuver. Finally, adhesions covering the IUD may have to be lysed initially with operative scissors (Fig. 17.3). Occasionally an IUD will perforate the uterine wall and extend under the serosa. The IUD can be pulled back through the uterine wall with hysteroscopic biopsy forceps or may be extracted transabdo-

FIGURE 17.2. **A:** Hysterosalpinogram of patient with Asherman's syndrome following a D&C for placenta accreta. Note thin sliver of endometrial cavity.

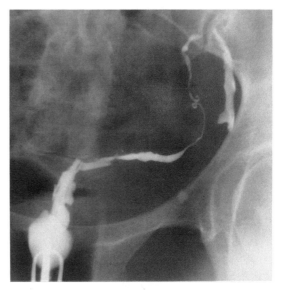

**A**

**B:** Same patient after hysteroscopic resection of intrauterine adhesions. Both fallopian tubes are now visualized. Although a small amount of residual synechiae are observed, these were not treated. The patient subsequently conceived and delivered at term. (courtesy of Dr. Ricardo Azziz).

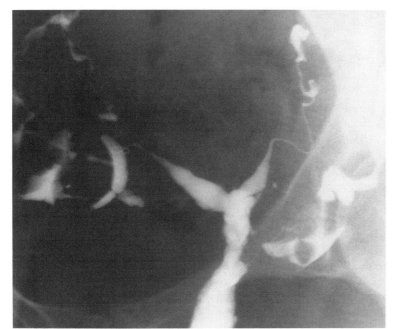

**B**

minally with the laparoscope. Infrequently an IUD will be so firmly lodged in the myometrium that the device must be cut in two with rigid operative scissors and each half extracted with combined laparoscopy/hysteroscopy. Any bleeding may be coagulated via laparoscopy, with the bipolar cautery forceps inserted into the perforation tract.

## Results

Hysteroscopy has proven to be highly useful in the diagnosis and treatment of abnormal uterine bleeding. When diagnostic hysteroscopy was compared to blind D&C in 342 patients, it was noted that both techniques gave similar results in 271, whereas in 60 patients hystero-

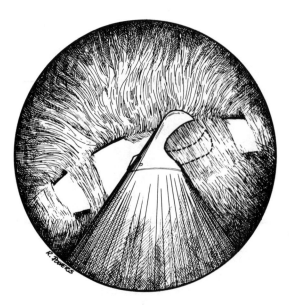

FIGURE 17.3. Hysteroscopic lysis of intrauterine adhesions with the rigid 3-mm scissors.

scopy and in 11 D&C was diagnostic.[8] Review of the literature for gestational outcome after the hysteroscopic treatment of intrauterine adhesions is equally favorable.[9] Blind interruption of adhesions in 69 patients collected from the literature resulted in a 40% term pregnancy rate. Alternatively, 62 patients treated hysteroscopically at the University of South California demonstrated an 87% pregnancy rate. The results for hysteroscopic myomectomy have been slightly less favorable. Review of the literature suggests approximately an 83.9% return to normal menses after resection of the fibroids and a 19% (21 of 94 patients) term pregnancy rate.[10] It is a rare exception when IUDs cannot be extracted either hysteroscopically or by combined hysteroscopic/laparoscopic technique.

## References

1. Gimpleson RJ. Panoramic hysteroscopy with directed biopsies versus dilatation and curettage for accurate diagnosis. *J Reprod Med.* 1989; 29:575–578.
2. Carson SA, Hubert GD, Schriock ED, et al. Hyperglycemia and hyponatremia during operative hysteroscopy with 5% dextrose in water distension. *Fertil Steril.* 1989;51:341–343.
3. Baggish MS, Baltoyannis P. New techniques for laser ablation of the endometrium in high-risk patients. *Am J Obstet Gynecol.* 1988;159:287–292.
4. DeCherney AH, Polan ML. Hysteroscopic management of intrauterine lesions and intractable uterine bleeding. *Obstet Gynecol.* 1983; 61:391–397.
5. Neuwirth RS. Hysteroscopic management of symptomatic submucous fibroids. *Obstet Gynecol.* 1983;62:509–511.
6. Friedman AJ, Barbieri RL, Doubilet PM, et al. A randomized, double-blind trial of gonadotropin-releasing hormone agonist (leuprolide) with or without medroxyprogesterone acetate in the treatment of leiomyomata uteri. *Fertil Steril.* 1988;49:404–409.
7. March CM, Israel R, March AD. Hysteroscopic management of intrauterine adhesions. *Am J Obstet Gynecol.* 1978;130:653–657.
8. Gimpelson RJ, Rappold HO. A comparative study between panoramic hysteroscopy with directed biopsies and dilatation and curettage. *Am J Obstet Gynecol.* 1988;158:489–492.
9. March CM, Israel R. Gestational outcome following hysteroscopic lysis of adhesions. *Fertil Steril.* 1981;36:455–459.
10. Derman SG, Rehnstrom J, Neuwirth R. The long-term effectiveness of hysteroscopic treatment of menorrhagia and leiomyomas. *Obstet Gynecol.* 1991;77:591–594.

# 18

## Endometrial Ablation

*JAMES F. DANIELL*

Abnormal uterine bleeding is a major health problem in women today. In the past, when hormonal therapy failed, this was treated primarily by hysterectomy. Over the last decade, hysteroscopic techniques of endometrial destruction have been developed that now allow some of these women with bothersome bleeding to avoid a hysterectomy or the need for hormonal therapy while controlling their abnormal bleeding. This chapter reviews the recent techniques for destroying the endometrium, including the Nd:YAG laser and the resectoscope, using both the wire loop electrode and the more recent roller ball electrode.

Radiotherapy has been used in the past to produce premature menopause with cessation of menses in women. Unfortunately, this also destroyed ovarian function and often had serious sequelae. Sclerosing agents have been investigated for intrauterine instillation to destroy the endometrium, but these have not met with success in large trials. Failure of therapy and/or accidental intraperitoneal spill with catastrophic consequences severely limits the use of these therapies. Goldrath and colleagues initially reported use of the Nd:YAG laser for destruction of the endometrium.[1] The laser energy was introduced via a flexible fiber simplifying hysteroscopic delivery. Over the last decade, this technique has been shown to be efficacious and of benefit to most women who meet the proper criteria for having the procedure performed.[2-6]

More recently, a modified urological resectoscope using a wire loop electrode or a roller ball electrode has allowed cautery to be used as an alternative to laser for destroying the endometrium.[7-11] The advantages of both laser and cautery are that the patient can avoid major surgery, maintain ovarian function, and can have permanent reduction and hopefully elimination of menstrual bleeding after appropriately applied energy.

## Indications

The indications for endometrial ablation are very clear today. They include significant menorrhagia that is bothersome to the patient and failure of the patient to respond to standard therapy, including hormone manipulation and dilatation and curettage (D&C). In addition, the patient should have a cavity free of pathology such as fibroids or polyps that may be inducing the abnormal bleeding. The patient should be through with childbearing and have a benign endometrium with no hyperplasia or premalignant lesions.

## Patient Selection and Preoperative Preparation

Careful preoperative counseling and selection of patients is critically important, both for proper fulfillment of expectations and understanding of the outcome by the patient. This counseling should include a discussion of the fact that the procedure may not eliminate bleeding, but hopefully will reduce the bleeding significantly and thereby reduce the patient's symptomatology. Patients who have intrauterine pathology, however, might opt for more definitive therapy such as hysterectomy because of the potential for recurrence of fibroids and/or polyps. The patient should be warned about the possibility of pregnancy, since the procedure does not sterilize. Incidental laparoscopic tubal sterilization should be offered to patients who are at risk for pregnancy.

The patient should be aware that preoperative suppression of the endometrium is critical for successful destruction of the endometrium down to the basalis. This can be accomplished with either medroxyprogesterone acetate (Provera or depo-Provera), gonadotropin-releasing hormone (GnRH) analogs (Lupron or Synarel), or by danazol (Danocrine) admin-

istration. All of these drugs should be administered for a minimum of 1 month preoperatively, and probably postoperatively as well in the younger patient.

Preoperative screening of the endometrial cavity should be done with an endometrial biopsy, preferably combined with an office hysteroscopy. This allows the elimination of any missed diagnoses that might occur from a blind D&C. We have found polyps and submucosal fibroids in patients having had multiple D&Cs and a purportedly "normal uterine cavity." It is important to note, however, that at endometrial ablation, small fibroids can be resected and removed, and polyps can also be removed for diagnostic purposes. Proper diagnosis and treatment may eliminate the metromenorrhagia without an ablative procedure.

Thus, our preoperative evaluation includes counseling, office hysteroscopy, and directed endometrial biopsy. Suppression of the endometrium to produce a hypoestrogenic state and a thin endometrium is begun. In patients who are anemic, preoperative suppression allows time for correction of the anemia by inducing a temporary amenorrhea.

Patients with known uterine fibroids should be counseled about the potential for persistent growth of fibroids with possible pain leading to the need for hysterectomy, even though abnormal bleeding may be controlled. In addition, patients with significant pain associated with bleeding may have adenomyosis or other pelvic pathology that could later lead to a hysterectomy. Patients need to understand this before hysteroscopic endometrial ablation. Certainly a concomitant laparoscopy can be offered to obtain a more definitive diagnosis. Laparoscopic treatment of endometriosis and transection of the uterosacral ligaments may be offered to patients with dysmenorrhea should pathology be found. If indicated, subserosal fibroids can be removed through the laparoscope at the time of the anesthesia for the hysteroscopic resection.

Patients with medical problems should be seen by the appropriate consultants and anesthesiologist preoperatively. Patients at high risk for complication at hysterectomy are commonly referred for endometrial ablation

FIGURE 18.1. Operating room set-up for operative hysteroscopy.

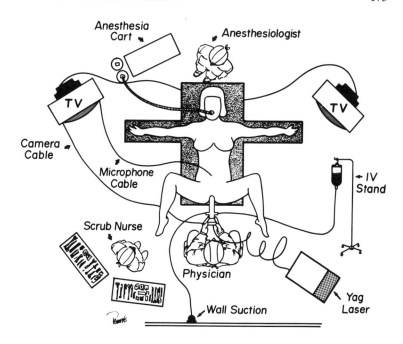

and can benefit most from this procedure. Appropriate medical and anesthetic consultation can minimize the risks. Fluid overload secondary to absorption of the distending media used during the hysteroscopic ablation is a significant risk. Other potential risks include uterine perforation with bowel injury.

## Instrumentation

The prerequisites for hysteroscopic endometrial ablation include adequate training of the physician in both diagnostic and operative hysteroscopy and a good understanding of laser physics (if the Nd:Yag laser is to be used) or electrosurgery (if the resectoscope is the chosen method). Appropriate informed consent should be well documented.

A typical operating room set-up is seen in Figure 18.1. Certainly a laser safety officer and laser-certified operating room circulating personnel should maintain the Nd:YAG laser and insure that proper safety precautions for protecting the eyes of the operator and others in the room are being followed. Fluid monitoring and fluid infusion rates are critical, and should be well understood and controlled by the circulating nurse in the operating room.

Instrumentation includes a good light source, a video camera, either with a direct coupler or beam splitter, depending on the preference of the operator, and a fluid infusion system. Our distention media of choice is glycine (1.5% solution), so that either cautery or laser can be used. Hyskon (32% Dextran-70) can be used, particularly if bleeding is a problem. If Hyskon is used, volumes greater than 300 cc should not be instilled except in rare circumstances and only after consultation with the anesthesiologist. Careful monitoring of the patient's circulatory and pulmonary status during the anesthesia is an important safety measure.

For endometrial ablation with the Nd:YAG laser, a three-channel hysteroscope is best, with 25° optics (Fig. 18.2). This allows constant infusion of the distending media and constant drainage of fluid. A third channel is used to introduce the 600-$\mu$m Nd:YAG fiber. With the Nd:YAG laser, an eye filter should be used at all times to protect the operator. Concomitant laparoscopy is probably a wise option when beginning endometrial ablation procedures, but is not routinely performed unless patients have an indication for laparoscopy or desire an elective sterilization procedure.

Bladder drainage is mandatory in all cases,

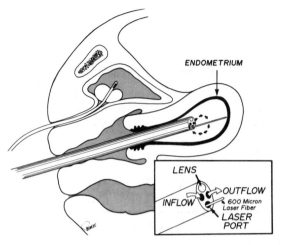

FIGURE 18.2. Endometrial ablation using the Nd:Yag laser is best performed with a three-channel hysteroscope with a 25° optic.

estimate the volume absorbed by the patient before continuing with the case. Intravenous diuretics can be given after consultation with the anesthesiologist, either electively before surgery or intraoperatively if fluid absorption is high. Central venous pressure monitoring lines can be used as indicated, based on the recommendations of the anesthesiologist or internal medicine consultants.

# Technique

## Nd:YAG Laser Technique

Under direct hysteroscopic view the 600-$\mu$m Nd:YAG fiber is used to photocoagulate around each tubal ostia. After this, the fiber is used to photocoagulate the intrauterine wall, being careful to treat each contiguous area adequately. We use a combination of airbrushing, a no-touch technique in which the fiber is held just off the uterine wall (Fig. 18.4), combined with gentle touching of the fiber to the uterine wall (stippling or pointillism). Finally, furrowing is accomplished by dragging the fiber away from the fundus in consecutive grooves along the lateral, anterior, and posterior uterine walls (Fig. 18.4). Under continuous high flow

and a system for accurately capturing all the fluid used for uterine cavity distention must be used (Fig. 18.3). We use 3-L containers of glycine and have a continuous flow with both the Nd:YAG laser and the resectoscope. At the end of 3 liters of infusion we measure the volume that has been recovered from the inflow port and the catch basin, then accurately

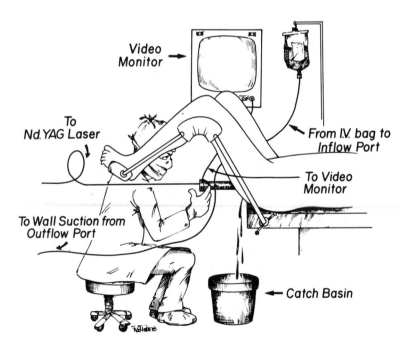

FIGURE 18.3. Operating room set-up for accurately capturing all the fluid used for uterine cavity distention during operative hysteroscopy.

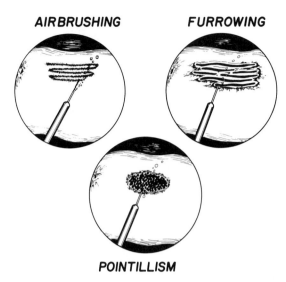

**AIRBRUSHING**   **FURROWING**

**POINTILLISM**

FIGURE 18.4. Nd:YAG laser techniques used to photocoagulate the intrauterine walls.

of media, all endometrial surfaces are treated under direct vision.

We prefer glycine as a distention media and reserve the use of Hyskon for cases in which bleeding becomes a problem. If visibility is obscured because of bleeding, the intrauterine pressure can be raised by temporarily blocking off the outflow of the glycine or by increasing pressure on the infusion bag. The goal is to have the intrauterine pressure of glycine equal the vascular pressure of the myometrium, so that blood flow is stopped in the basalis layer of the endometrium. In cases in which bleeding becomes a significant problem, we will stop the infusion with the glycine and gently instill one ampule of pitressin diluted with 20 cc of saline into the uterine cavity and infuse this into the cavity temporarily for a minute to allow absorption into the endometrium. This temporarily constricts the uterine vessels. After this, immediate coagulation of visible bleeders with the Nd:YAG laser usually effectively controls bothersome bleeding. One should avoid digging deep furrows into the uterine wall and lasering deeply along the cervical sidewalls. Deep penetration may lacerate the cervical branch of the uterine artery. After treating all contiguous areas, the hysteroscope is removed.

The total volume absorbed and the amount of energy used for the procedure is calculated and recorded.

## Wire Loop or Roller Ball Resectoscopic Technique

The set-up and technique for resectoscope is similar. The only difference is that the cervix usually has to be dilated a bit more because of the larger diameter of the resectoscope. It is important to use a continuous flow resectoscope that has both an inflow port and an outflow port. This allows continuous circulation of the distending media. Most urological resectoscopes do not have this feature, but endoscope manufacturers have now developed special hysteroscopic resectoscopes that have inflow of the distending media around the optics of the system and outflow on the outer channel of the hysteroscope. This allows continuous inflow of clean distending media in front of the lens and outflow of media from the uterine cavity.

If the wire loop is being used, it is mandatory to have a laparoscope in the abdominal cavity to visualize the external uterine surface since it is difficult to judge depth of penetration accurately with the wire loop electrode. If the roller ball is used, a laparoscopy is not routinely performed. The ball electrode does not penetrate deeply into the endometrium, and merely rolls along the surface of the endometrium.

The author prefers the roller ball technique. A power setting of 100 W on cutting current adequately treats the endometrium to the basalis and spares the myometrium. Ablation is begun by gently pushing the ball electrode into each cornua. This is the most dangerous part of the procedure, because too much upward pressure can lead to perforation or transmural bowel injury. Electrical energy can pass through the cornua of the uterus and damage a piece of bowel that is impinging on the outer surface of the uterine wall. The anterior uterine wall is treated next, because bubbling can occur with use of electrical current. These bubbles can be removed from the cavity by occasionally pushing the scope up against the fundus so that the bubbles will pass out through the outflow ports on the outside of the hystero-

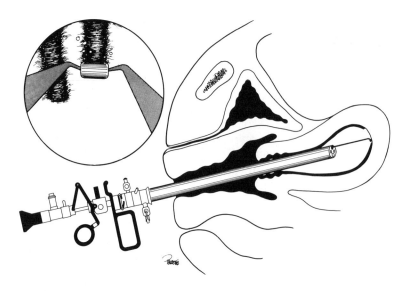

FIGURE 18.5. The roller ball technique consists of gently rolling the ball along the wall of the endometrial cavity and treating each contiguous area to the point of blanching the endometrium and thus achieving ablation down to the basalis.

scope. Since the outflow ports are at least 1 cm back from the tip of the scope, when the hysteroscope is pulled back into the cervical canal, obstruction of the outflow channels may occur and reduce visibility. Intermittently pushing the scope forward to allow circulation is helpful. This is usually only a problem with a small uterine cavity or when treating the lower portions of the cavity. The ball electrode is rolled gently along the wall of the endometrial cavity, treating each contiguous area so that there is blanching and ablation of the endometrium down to the basalis (Fig. 18.5). This can be visually determined by the whiteness that occurs. The ball electrode must be cleaned occasionally to remove tissue debris. A clean electrode will transmit energy more effectively. If bleeding is encountered, the same techniques previously described for Nd:YAG laser are used. If intrauterine pathology is encountered, a polypectomy or myomectomy may be performed.

## Alternative Techniques

The two techniques for endometrial ablation that have acquired the most acceptance are the Nd:YAG laser ablation and the roller ball electrode. The other alternative technique is the resectoscope wire electrode. The problem with

this technique, in our opinion, is that it must be performed concomitant with laparoscopy. Increased bleeding can be a risk because of inadvertently getting too deep into the myometrium. Because of this, only skilled hysteroscopists should use the wire electrode, and then almost certainly only under laparoscopic visualization. At present, it is unclear which technique has the greatest advantage for long-term control of metromenorrhagia. The Nd:YAG laser technique has a greater length of patient follow-up time, as it has been used for at least a decade. In the author's practice, endometrial ablation was begun in 1983 and the Nd:YAG laser was used exclusively until the late fall of 1988. Between the fall of 1988 and the next year, we used a combination of both Nd:YAG laser and resectoscope, using the Nd:YAG laser initially around the ostia and fundus while using the roller ball electrode for the lateral sidewalls. Beginning in 1990, we have used the roller ball exclusively for this procedure.

Our reasons for changing from endometrial ablation with the Nd:YAG laser to the resectoscope include the following:

1. Our operating time for endometrial ablation with the Nd:YAG laser averaged 45 min. At present, our operating time with the roller ball is approximately 15 min in

TABLE 18.1.  Results of Nd:YAG Laser Ablation: West Side Hospital, June 1984 to December 1988[a]

| Age (yr) | # Patients | Results | | | | | |
|---|---|---|---|---|---|---|---|
| | | Good (amenorrhea) | | Fair (light flow) | | Poor (persistent AUB)[b] | |
| 16–35 | 23 | 10 | (43%) | 3 | (12%) | 10 | (43%) |
| 36–45 | 68 | 31 | (46%) | 29 | (43%) | 8 | (11%) |
| 46–76 | 53 | 40 | (75%) | 9 | (17%) | 4 | ( 8%) |
| Total | 144 | 81 | (56%) | 41 | (28%) | 22 | (16%) |

144 over a 54-month study period, or 2.7 cases/month.
[a] Minimum 3-month follow-up.
[b] AUB: Abnormal uterine bleeding.

women with normal uterine cavities. This is a 200% reduction in patient anesthesia time.

2. The risk to the operator is less with cautery than with the Nd:YAG laser. There is no risk to the surgeon's eyes with cautery, whereas that risk always exists with Nd:YAG laser endometrial ablation.

3. The use of the fiber is more tedious and can lead to more bleeding problems, because the fiber digs into the wall of the endometrium, and larger vessels can be entered accidentally but are not occluded. The ball electrode does not have this problem because it rolls along the surface of the endometrium without trauma so that a uniform depth of destruction is obtained.

4. The Nd:YAG laser fiber is 600 $\mu$m whereas the ball electrode that we routinely use is 4 mm in diameter. This gives us a much greater surface area contact, which accounts for the rapidity with which we can accomplish this procedure of endometrial destruction using the ball electrode.

5. There is major difference in the cost of the equipment. A Nd:YAG laser costs approximately $100,000, whereas the equipment for endometrial ablation with the resectoscope is no more than $6,000.

Unfortunately, neither technique is taught in most residency programs, so interested gynecologists who have no experience in hysteroscopy for endometrial ablation must take special training. This is now easily available, as many workshops are occurring in various sites around the United States today that offer training both in endometrial ablation with the Nd:YAG laser and with the resectoscope. Usually these are held at different courses, but more recently, both techniques are being taught at some facilities.

## Results

Results for endometrial ablation with the Nd:YAG laser now span a decade with several reports including large numbers of cases. The initial success rate reported by Goldrath and colleagues[1] was as high as 90% although other investigators have not been able to confirm this and probably reflects the fact that Goldrath used greater power densities and more vigorous application of Nd:YAG laser energy.

Endometrial ablation using the resectoscope has a shorter history, and because of that, not as many reports have been published. Those that have appeared note similar success rates to that obtained with Nd:YAG endometrial ablation. Our personal results are listed in Table 18.1 for endometrial ablation with the Nd:YAG laser alone. Table 18.2 shows our early results with the resectoscope only. Note that the results are very similar for all techniques and are age-related.

Long-term results are not yet available for endometrial ablation with the resectoscope. However, long-term results with the Nd:YAG laser have demonstrated only a few reported cases of recurrence of bleeding after initial

TABLE 18.2. Results of Resectoscope Endometrial Ablation: West Side Hospital, January 1990 to June 1991[a]

| Age (yr) | # Patients | Good (amenorrhea) | | Fair (light flow) | | Poor (persistent AUB)[b] | |
|---|---|---|---|---|---|---|---|
| | | | | Results | | | |
| 14–35 | 4 | 2 | (50%) | 1 | (25%) | 1 | (25%) |
| 36–45 | 30 | 16 | (53%) | 11 | (37%) | 3 | (10%) |
| 46–60 | 6 | 5 | (83%) | 1 | (17%) | 0 | |
| Total | 40 | 23 | (58%) | 13 | (32%) | 4 | (10%) |

[a] Minimum 3-month follow-up.
[b] AUB: Abnormal uterine bleeding.

amenorrhea. In our practice, we have had three patients who developed recurrence of bleeding after more than a year of amenorrhea, suggesting some dormant endometrial tissue that slowly became reactivated. All of these patients were under 40 years of age, and subsequent office hysteroscopy and biopsy revealed small reddish areas of viable normal endometrium.

## Safety of Endometrial Ablation

The safety of endometrial ablation has been well documented. There is only one report noting bowel complications related to Nd:YAG laser endometrial ablation.[12] No reports of bowel complications resulting from endometrial ablation with the resectoscope have been recorded, but these will most likely appear as more surgeons attempt the procedure. Either Nd:YAG laser or electrocautery can be dangerous if not used appropriately and proper safety precautions are not followed. The operator must at all times be able to visualize either the tip of the fiber, roller ball, or wire electrode. Working in less than good visibility is risky, and working without proper training or equipment should not occur.

Credentialing processes should include the standard three phases of training:

1. obtain privileges for the basic hysteroscopy procedures
2. after adequate training in hysteroscopy, attend a course that offers hands-on training in use of the type of energy one wishes to

use for endometrial ablation, either laser or electrocautery
3. complete a preceptorship with an acknowledged expert in the procedure.

In our opinion, no one should attempt the procedure until these three steps are completed. One must obtain some hands-on experience in the operating room, both observing and participating in a case, under the direction of an experienced hysteroscopist. Certainly, expertise with the Nd:YAG laser does not imply expertise with the roller ball, and vice versa. Each technique has subtle differences, and adequate training and hands-on experience are necessary before attempting this procedure on patients.

## Conclusions

With the advent of the much simpler, less expensive, and rapid technique of roller ball endometrial ablation, many surgeons who were discouraged from this procedure because of concern with the use of the Nd:YAG laser or its costs will now begin to explore its use. Basically, there are two groups of patients requesting endometrial ablation:

1. Patients with menorrhagia refractory to hormonal therapy, and in whom the risk of hysterectomy is unacceptable due to surgical or medical problems
2. Those who have read or heard about the procedure, and seek it out because it is new technology. These patients often have

minimal menorrhagia, and often are not good candidates for the procedure.

There is great risk for abuse of the procedure, particularly as it becomes simpler to perform with the roller ball electrode. Some physicians are already promoting the procedure with television ads and local media publicity. The goal of all health care providers should be to provide quality health care while minimizing patient costs and risks. Certainly, endometrial ablation in the properly selected and counseled patient meets this goal. It may alleviate a bothersome problem through a simple and rapid outpatient procedure that, if properly performed, can be safe and effective. As more gynecologists become competent in hysteroscopy and become familiar with these techniques, there will be a tremendous increase in the number of women undergoing endometrial ablation. Twenty-five percent of the hysterectomies performed in North America today are for metromenorrhagia only, with benign endometrium. Most of these patients in the next decade could become candidates for a simple outpatient procedure that could replace the more complicated, expensive, and risky hysterectomy. However, proper education of both patients and physicians is critical so that all can benefit from this new technology.

## References

1. Goldrath MH, Fuller TA, Segal S. Laser photovaporization of the endometrium for the treatment of menorrhagia. *Am J Obstet Gynecol.* 1981;140:14–18.

2. Lomano JM. Photocoagulation of the endometrium with the Nd:YAG laser for the treatment of menorrhagia: a report of ten cases. *J Reprod Med.* 1986;31:148–151.

3. Daniell J, Tosh R, Meisels S. Photodynamic ablation of the endometrium with the Nd:YAG laser hysteroscopically as a treatment of menorrhagia. *Colposc Gynecol Laser Surg.* 1988:2:43–47.

4. Loffer RD. Hysteroscopic endometrial ablation with the Nd:YAG laser using a non-touch technique. *Obstet Gynecol.* 1987;69:67–69.

5. Gimpelson RJ. Hysteroscopic Nd:YAG laser ablation of the endometrium. *J Reprod Med.* 1988;33:872–875.

6. Lomano JM. Dragging technique versus blanching technique for endometrial ablation with the Nd:YAG laser in the treatment of chronic menorrhagia. *Am J Obstet Gynecol.* 1988;159:152–156.

7. Baggish MS, Baltoyannis P. New techniques for laser ablation of the endometrium in high-risk patient. *Am J Obstet Gynecol.* 1988;159:287–289.

8. Townsend DE, Richart RM. A new technique for ablating the endometrium. *Contemp Ob/Gyn.* 1989;33:90–94.

9. Vancaillie TG. Electrocoagulation of the endometrium with the ball-end resectoscope. *Obstet Gynecol.* 1989;74:425–429.

10. McLucas B. The resectoscope in gynecologic surgery. *Female Patient.* 1990;15:85–89.

11. DeCherney A, Diamond MP, Eavy G, Polan ML. Endometrial ablation for intractable uterine bleeding: hysteroscopic resection. *Obstet Gynecol.* 1987;70:668–671.

12. Perry CP, Daniell JF, Gimpelson RJ. Bowel injury from Nd:YAG endometrial ablation. *J Gynecol Surg.* 1990;6:199–203.

# 19

# Hysteroscopic Treatment of Congenital Uterine Anomalies

*J. Benjamin Younger*

Congenital anomalies of the Mullerian system is estimated to occur in approximately 0.1% to 1.5% of women in the general population. Of women with preterm fetal wastage the incidence of Mullerian anomalies is estimated to vary between 1% and 12%. Approximately 90% of these anomalies involve the uterus.[1] These malformations are often noted incidentally; in other cases the diagnosis is made during the work-up of infertility or repeated fetal wastage.

There are three general types of Mullerian anomalies: mullerian agenesis, disorders of vertical fusion (e.g., transverse vaginal septa), and abnormalities of lateral fusion. Pregnancy wastage has been associated with disorders of lateral fusion involving the uterus, which are either asymmetric or symmetric. Symmetric anomalies of lateral fusion include the didelphic, bicornuate, and septate uteri. The septate uterus is thought to occur when the Mulle-rian ducts fuse and canalize properly, but the midline septum does not resolve. The appearance of the septum is highly variable. It can be broad- or narrow-based, thin or thick. It can protrude from the fundus downward only a short way, or descend all the way through the cervix, giving the appearance of a "double cervix." Most commonly, the septum terminates near the level of the internal cervical os.

Septate uteri are associated with a higher incidence of fetal wastage than either the bicornuate or didelphic types, as high as 85% in some reports.[1] Even patients in whom the anomaly was detected incidentally previously had demonstrated the lowest previous pregnancy rate (78%), compared to patients with other uterine malformations. Various theories have been proposed to explain the increased fetal loss. The septum may be less vascular and more fibrous than normal myometrium, impeding proper implantation. This may also cause the endometrium covering the septum to be less responsive to hormonal stimuli. Finally, the septum may impede proper placental growth. Of all Mullerian anomalies the septate uterus is the only one amenable to operative hysteroscopic treatment.

The 1980s have seen the abandonment of the previous transabdominal approach in favor of the transcervical route for correction of this disorder. This new approach is equally successful, highly cost effective, and of significantly less morbidity. It can be performed in an outpatient setting and obviates the need for subsequent delivery by cesarean section. Finally, it does not carry the risk of postoperative pelvic adhesions (as do abdominal procedures), which may impede subsequent fertility. The transcervical route for removal of a uterine septum is not new. In 1882 Schroder performed the transvaginal division of a septum in a patient with a history of pregnancy wastage. He blindly introduced two long stomach clamps into the uterine cavity, placing one anteriorly and the other posteriorly, across the septum. The septum between the clamps was then divided with scissors. The clamps were left in place for 24 hr and then removed with minimal bleeding. Postoperatively the patient conceived within 1 month and carried a normal pregnancy. Although number of other investigators subsequently reported removing uterine septi in a similar fashion. However, for the majority of the 20th century the standard approach was by transabdominal surgery, employing either the Jones or the Tompkins metroplasty technique. However, it is rare indeed that these transabdominal procedures are required today.

## Patient Selection and Diagnosis

Most septa are discovered during work-up for a history of recurrent miscarriages, premature deliveries, or malpresentations. All patients complaining of habitual losses *must* undergo a full evaluation and be treated appropriately. Rock and Jones decreased the abortion rate from 76% to 12% in women with a "double

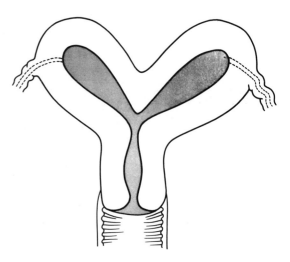

FIGURE 19.1. Depicted is a bicornuate uterus, whose HSG appearance is similar to the septate uterus (see Fig. 19.2). Laparoscopic examination of the uterine fundus is usually necessary to differentiate the two types of uterine malformations. Hysteroscopic surgery of a bicornuate uterus would quickly lead to fundal perforation, without correcting the defect.

uterus" by treating coexisting factors only.[2] Occasionally a septum is detected as part of an infertility evaluation at the time of a hysterosalpingogram (HSG). A septate uterus itself rarely causes difficulty in conceiving, and patients who complain of infertility should undergo a complete evaluation for other factors affecting fertility, before undertaking corrective surgery. Occasionally a septum is noted at the time of delivery, particularly at cesarean section or at dilatation and curettage (D&C) after incomplete abortion. Even less frequently, a particularly lengthy septum is noted on observing the cervix during pelvic exam, or is detected in conjunction with a vaginal septum. Importantly, the mere presence of a uterine septum in the absence of reproductive tract complaints does not warrant surgical intervention.

The most important study in detecting these uterine malformations is the HSG. The difference between a bicornuate (Fig. 19.1) and a septate uterus (Fig. 19.2) is in the shape of the fundus, and not whether the uterine division protrudes through the cervical os (Fig. 19.3).

Unfortunately, the HSG alone cannot differentiate a septate from a bicornuate uterus. A difference must be established since only the septate uterus that is amenable to hysteroscopic treatment. Generally, direct visualization of the uterine fundus in patients with a "double uterus" by either laparoscopy or, rarely, laparotomy is used to distinguish between the two anomalies. Occasionally sonographic or radiologic studies may be able to establish the diagnosis preoperatively.

## Preoperative Evaluation

In patients with a suspected septate uterus laparoscopic confirmation of the anomaly is generally preferable, since the septum may be treated hysteroscopically at the time the diagnosis is being made. A preoperative HSG should always be obtained, even in those in-

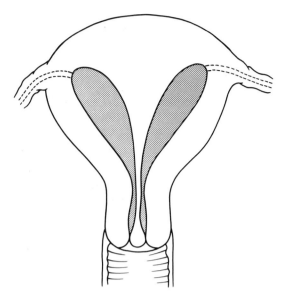

FIGURE 19.3. Complete septate uterus. The septum is thin and extends completely to the external cervical os.

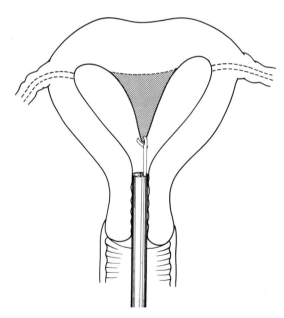

FIGURE 19.2. Depicted is a typical subseptate uterus. The uterine fundus viewed laparoscopically is broad and may have an external "notch" giving it a slight bicornuate appearance. The septum is thin in its lower portion and widens near the fundus. This type of septi is easy to visualize and divide hysteroscopically. The hysteroscope is kept in the lower uterus to increase the field of vision, and the scissors are advanced as the division progresses.

stances in which the septum has been diagnosed by prior hysteroscopy/laparoscopy, and should be available to the operator during surgery. A preoperative HSG provides a clear depiction of the length and thickness of the septum, particularly important since hysteroscopy is associated with a somewhat impaired depth perception. The HSG is particularly useful when one uterine cavity is much smaller, or when the septum extends all the way through the cervix. Finally, the HSG provides a permanent record of the anomaly, in addition to having a baseline with which to assess adequacy of surgery.

As some of patients with Mullerian anomalies also have congenital anomalies of the urinary tract, a preoperative IVP (intravenous pyelogram) is recommended. Candidates for corrective surgery should be in good general health and exhibit no coagulopathy. They should discontinue aspirin or other nonsteroidal antiinflammatory drugs at least 2 weeks before surgery. Patients undergoing this operation should have the desire to conceive and have a reproductively healthy male partner. There should be no other insurmountable or untreated cause, of infertility present.

# Instrumentation

The following description of the technique of operative hysteroscopic metroplasty focuses on the use of scissors, but either lasers or resectoscopes can be used to accomplish this division. The author prefers to use 3-mm rigid scissors, through a large right-angle operating hysteroscope with 170° field of vision (WOLF 8931.31). These scissors do a better job of dividing the thicker septum encountered at the uterine fundus and in puncturing or cutting a hole in a complete septum (see below) when necessary. The smaller 7 Fr flexible scissors may be used for the division of thinner septa.

There are several choices for distending media for operative hysteroscopy (see Chapter 16). This surgeon prefers Hyskon (32% dextran-70, Pharmacia Laboratories, Piscataway, NJ) because it is not miscible with blood and has a good refractive index, providing excellent visualization. However, this medium has some drawbacks (see Chapters 16 and 21). It may make handling of instrument difficult, and it is imperative that all equipment that comes in contact with Hyskon be cleaned in hot soapy water immediately after use. The use of Hyskon in gynecology has been associated with bleeding coagulopathy,[3] adult respiratory distress syndrome,[3] pulmonary edema,[4] and allergic reactions including anaphylactic shock.[5] Most adverse reactions have been associated with prolonged operating time and the use of large volumes of medium. It is recommended that the total volume of Hyskon used be kept under 300 cc per patient, regardless of operating time. Instruments that generate heat (e.g., resectoscopes and lasers) cannot be used with dextran-70 as it will tend to caramelize.

Carbon dioxide ($CO_2$) is also quite popular, particularly in Europe, but visualization in the presence of bleeding may be inadequate. Fortunately, most septa are thin and relatively avascular. $CO_2$ is the appropriate distending media when employing the $CO_2$ laser because its beam will not penetrate liquid. However, a significant complication of $CO_2$ distention is rapid intravenous absorption, which can lead to air embolization and death, particularly when used to cool laser fibers (see Chapter 21). Liquids less viscous than Hyskon can also be used (see Chapter 16) because they provide reasonably good visualization and are easier to handle and administer. Solutions containing dextrose do not mix with blood quite as easily as those without. Larger volumes can be absorbed, and hyperglycemia and hyponatremia have been reported using 5% dextrose in water.[6]

# Technique

The operation should be scheduled for a time shortly after the patient completes her normal menstrual flow, when there is minimum risk of pregnancy and endometrial visualization is optimum. In many instances the distinction between a bicornuate uterus and a septate uterus has not clearly been made preoperatively. A laparoscopy, along with the HSG, will establish the diagnosis and identify other pathology of the reproductive tract. Once the diagnosis of a septate uterus is confirmed, the laparoscope is left in place to monitor the hysteroscopic operation and to reduce the risk of perforation. A speculum is then inserted into the vagina and the cervix exposed and grasped with a tenaculum. The cervix should be dilated only enough to allow the insertion of the hysteroscope into the cavity, maintaining a tight fit around the instrument shaft, for good containment of the distending media. If there is not a snug fit, a double-tooth tenaculum or two single-tooth tenaculums, one on each side of the cervix, may be used. Alternatively, a purse string suture may be placed around the cervix to snug it around the hysteroscope and to serve for traction.

It is extremely important to maintain traction on the cervix throughout the procedure, keeping the long axis of the uterus parallel to the patient's sacrum. A flexed uterus is more likely to be perforated, and to reduce the visibility with rigid telescopes. Once the hysteroscope is placed within the uterus a full inspection of the cavities is performed, visualizing the tubal ostia for proper orientation. The inferior margin of the septum is then identified and divided transversely in the midline, using rigid scissors (Fig. 19.2). Successive bites of the septum are progressively taken upward. There is no need to resect the septum or remove any tissue. Once the septum is divided in its midportion, the cut fibromuscular tissue retracts into the contiguous uterine wall.

Septal tissue is generally quite fibrous and avascular. However, as division approaches the fundal area the septum becomes thicker and more vascular. Incision of the septum should be carried out until normal myometrial tissue is identified, generally by its increased vascularity. However, with the liquid distention media being injected under pressure, the vascularity of the tissue may not be immediately apparent. It is wise to reduce the distention pressure periodically, observing the bleeding of the incised tissue. Once the incised tissue is noted to be relatively well vascularized, division is discontinued.

Throughout the procedure the intensity of the laparoscopic illumination is occasionally reduced, allowing the observer to judge the thickness of the uterine fundus as the operation progresses. Although laparoscopic observation will not guarantee against perforation, it allows early recognition of this complication, reducing the risk of additional injury to surrounding organs.

The hysteroscope should not be inserted too far beyond the internal cervical os, since the surgeon should attempt to maintain both cornual areas in view. The hysteroscope should remain relatively fixed just beyond the internal os, extending only the cutting scissors. A difficult anomaly to treat is the broad-based septum, because it is difficult to keep both cornua visualized while maintaining good depth of field perspective. Increased bleeding and uterine perforation are more likely to occur in this situation.

If the cervix appears "double," due to the length of the septum (Fig. 19.3), one can cut through the cervical portion of the septum using Metzenbaum scissors. However, there is some concern that this may later lead to an incompetent cervix and, if this division is performed, one should consider placing a cerclage in a subsequent pregnancy. The preferred technique is to insert the operative hysteroscope

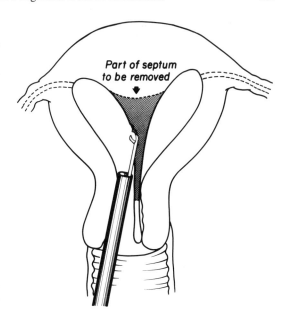

FIGURE 19.4. Hysteroscopic treatment of a complete septate uterus. The septum involves the upper cervix and the lower margin is difficult to see. However, at laparoscopy both tubes and a normal fundus are visualized. An opening is made in the septum near the level of the cervical internal os and division proceeds as usual.

into one of the uterine cavities, preferably the larger one, cutting a hole through the septum near the level of the internal cervical os (Fig. 19.4). Once this has been accomplished, one can proceed to divide the upper portion of the septum, leaving the lower cervical portion of the septum intact. On occasion, a small opening may be already present in the septum, near the level of the internal os, and division can proceed upward from that point.

A different situation occurs when the septum is long but does not extend to the external os. With this abnormality, the surgeon may have some difficulty identifying the lower septum margin and in having enough working room in front of the hysteroscope to allow the use of the scissors. Since the lower cervix is often patulous there may also be difficulty in being able to maintain adequate distention media pressure. In this situation, Metzenbaum scissors can be used to cut the lower portion of the septum blindly. The hysteroscope is then reinserted and the operation proceeds as usual.

Occasionally a repeat hysteroscopic procedure may need to be performed for incomplete septum resection, or because the metroplasty was prematurely terminated due to uterine perforation. Although this is an inconvenience, it is preferable always to incise the septum under good surgical control to avoid serious uterine perforations, particularly in patients with exceedingly wide septa.

## Complications

The primary complications of hysteroscopic metroplasty are perforation, bleeding, infection, and those complications related directly to the distending medium employed. The use of large volumes and prolonged operating time are major predisposing factors to the development of complications relating to the distention medium.

Uterine perforations generally occur in the fundal area and present little problem with blood loss. In these instances specific bleeding points at the perforation site can be cauterized with laparoscopic bipolar cautery. An alternate technique is to inject a 5- to 10-ml dilute solution of pitressin (20 mU in 30 cc 0.9% saline) into the uterine fundus, using a long spinal needle placed through the anterior abdominal wall under direct laparoscopic visualization. Hemostasis is usually rapidly apparent and usually, in the author's experience, no further therapy is necessary. Nevertheless, observation alone generally suffices for fundal perforations. Alternatively, if the perforation occurs laterally or in the region of the cornua or utero-ovarian ligament, brisk bleeding is likely and laparotomy for repair is usually required.

Although excessive bleeding from the septum division site is a concern, there is little need for hysteroscopic electrocautery. When excessive bleeding does occur, packing of the uterus or insertion of a balloon catheter to tamponade the uterine cavity is recommended. However, in the author's experience this is rarely necessary. Occasionally, the above technique for the myometrial injection of pitressin can be used.

Although the operative field is certainly not sterile, infection does not appear to be a major problem with hysteroscopic metroplasties. Nevertheless, little data is available on the use of antibiotic prophylaxis. The author prefers the administration of a single perioperative dose of a broad spectrum antibiotic, similar to that employed in a routine vaginal hysterectomy.

## Postoperative Care and Follow-up

In general, patients undergoing hysteroscopic metroplasty require little in the way of postoperative care. Although the postoperative administration of supplemental estrogen has been mentioned, there are no data to support its use. If the operation is timed in the early follicular phase of the menstrual cycle, the physiologic preovulatory rise in estrogen levels would make the addition of supplemental estrogen unnecessary.

Some have advocated the placement of an IUD or other device to separate the uterine walls after surgery. Again, there are no data to support this maneuver and, in theory, could increase the risk of postoperative infection. In contrast to the situation noted in Asherman's syndrome (see Chapter 17), the endometrial cavity in patients with a septate uterus has abundant healthy endometrium.

A repeat HSG should be obtained some 3 months after the procedure and compared to the original radiographs (Fig. 19.5). Many times the contour of the uterus may be less than perfect. This is particularly true when the surgeon has dealt with a relatively thick septum or a uterus with a broad fundus. Minor prominences giving the impression of a short septum or an arcuate fundus do not require additional surgical intervention. If intrauterine adhesions are detected, they are easily taken care of at a repeat hysteroscopy.

As has been previously mentioned, patients can and do get pregnant rather quickly after this operation. There is no need to prevent pregnancy for a period of time as there is when one has performed a Jones or Tompkins abdominal metroplasty. Furthermore, there is no need for a subsequent cesarean section.

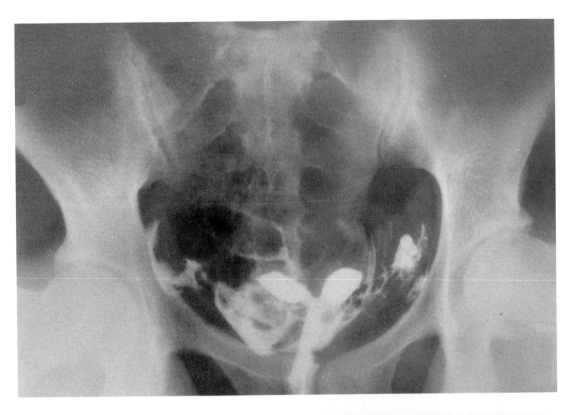

FIGURE 19.5. Preoperative **(top)** and postoperative **(bottom)** HSGs in a patient with recurrent abortions and a septate uterus, treated by hysteroscopic metroplasty.

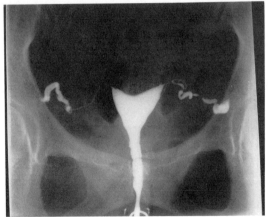

# Results

Hassiakos and Zourlas[7] have reviewed the literature concerning transcervical division of uterine septum. It is apparent that the results of hysteroscopic metroplasty are excellent, either equal or superior to that obtained by transabdominal approaches. In patients com-plaining of recurrent fetal wastage who desire a child, more than 85% have become pregnant, with 75% resulting in term live births. When the surgery is performed for the diagnosis of primary infertility the results are not nearly as good, since only one third of patients subse-quently became pregnant, two thirds of those delivering a term live born. Fewer than 5% of patients in the collected series required a repeat hysteroscopic procedure because of incomplete removal of the septum. Of those patients with an incompetent cervix, more than half had a preoperative history compatible with this disorder, which usually leads to the placement of a prophylactic cerclage.

# References

1. Rock JA, Sclaff WD. The obstetrical consequences of uterovaginal anomalies. *Fertil Steril.* 1985;43:681–692.
2. Rock JA, Jones HW Jr. The clinical management of the double uterus. *Fertil Steril.* 1977;28:798–806.
3. Jedeikin R, Olsfanger D, Kessler, I. Disseminated intravascular coagulopathy and adult respiratory distress syndrome: life-threatening complications of hysteroscopy. *Am J Obstet Gynecol.* 1990;162:44–45.
4. Leake JF, Murphy AA, Zacur HA. Noncardiogenic pulmonary edema: a complication of operative hysteroscopy. *Fertil Steril.* 1987;48:497–499.
5. Trimbos-Kempers TC, Veering BT. Anaphylactic shock from intracavitary 32% dextran-70* during hysteroscopy. *Fertil Steril.* 1989;51:1053–1054.
6. Carson SA, Hubert GD, Schriock ED, et al. Hyperglycemia and hyponatremia during operative hysteroscopy with 5% dextrose in water distention. *Fertil Steril.* 1989;51:341–343.
7. Hassiakos DK, Zourlas PA. Transcervical division of uterine septa. *Obstet Gynecol Surv.* 1990;45:165–173.

# 20

# Transcervical Tubal Cannulation, Tuboplasty, and Falloposcopy

*Eugene Katz*

## Etiology and Diagnosis of Proximal Tubal Occlusion

### Etiology of Proximal Tubal Occlusion

Tubal disease is the cause of 25% to 30% of female infertility, of which approximately 20% is due to occlusions located at the uterotubal junction.[1,2] Moreover, until recently one fifth of laparotomies performed for tubal occlusion were done in connection with this last entity.

The sequelae of salpingitis and salpingitis isthmic nodosa (SIN) appear to be responsible for the majority of proximal tubal occlusions. For instance, chronic salpingitis can be found in 40% to 60% of tubes being repaired for proximal occlusions.[3] More recently, chronic inflammation or its fibrotic sequelae were described in 60% of excised occluded proximal tubes.[4] SIN is present in 20% to 70% of such tubes[5] and intramural endometriosis appears to play a role in proximal obstructions in 14%

of cases.[4] In fact, remissions of proximal obstructions have been reported after danazol therapy.[6] Crystallized tubal secretions can also lead to proximal obstruction.[7] This finding may explain the high false positive occlusion rate for hysterosalpingograms (HSG) and provides the rationale for attempting to dislodge such plugs mechanically by cannulating the tubal lumen.

### Diagnosis of Proximal Tubal Obstruction

The initial diagnosis of tubal obstructions is commonly made by HSG. Unfortunately, HSGs carry a false positive rate of 15% to 40%.[8] It is therefore important to complement HSG with chromotubation during laparoscopy. In addition, it is not uncommon to find a normal proximal tube at the time of surgery, despite prior diagnosis of proximal tubal occlusion with both HSG and laparoscopy.[9–11]

Several pharmacological agents have been used to assist the passage of contrast media through the presumable spasmodic uterotubal junction during laparoscopy or HSG. Unfortunately, terbutaline,[12] glucagon,[13] and isoxuprine[14] have not been clearly shown to be effective in alleviating such spasm.[15]

# Transuterine Tubal Cannulation and Tuboplasty

Interest in transcervical/transuterine tubal sterilization stimulated research in the direct cannulation of the fallopian tube. Interestingly, Smith in 1849 attempted to pass whale bone sounds into the oviducts to treat infertility, the same year that other researchers reported a method of sterilization by applying silver nitrate to the cornual regions. More recently, Corfman and Taylor[16] described a balloon-tipped metal cannula to inject fluid directly into the tubes. The catheter was introduced into the uterine cavity and aimed at the uterine cornua before injection. Later, catheterization of the tubal ostia under hysteroscopic visualization was accomplished in an effort to occlude the fallopian tubes for contraception.[17] Platia and Krudy reported the use of fluoroscopically guided wires to recannulize proximal obstructed tubes.[18] The idea was further developed by Thurmond and colleagues[19] and by Confino and colleagues.[20] The latter introduced the idea of the balloon dilatation technique much like angioplasties for coronary artery disease.[20]

## Fluoroscopically Guided Tubal Cannulation

All forms of fluoroscopically guided procedures require an undistorted uterine cavity in order to reach the cornual portion of the tubes with the catheters.

### Wire Catheterization System

#### Instruments and Technique

The wire catheterization system as described by Thurmond et al.[21] includes a "hysterocath,"

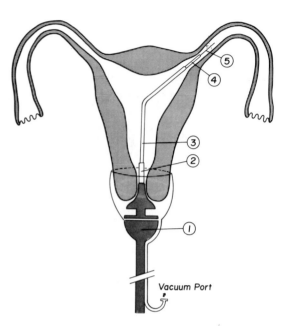

FIGURE 20.1. Wire catheterization system in place. 1, Hysterocath; 2, 9-Fr catheter; 3, 5.5-Fr catheter; 4, 3-Fr catheter; 5, guidewire.

three coaxial catheters, three guidewires, and a Tuhoy-Borst adapter (Cook Ob/Gyn, Bloomington, IN). The hysterocath consists of a central 25 cm long, soft plastic shaft with a central conduit 5 mm wide tapering to 2.5 mm at its acorn-shaped tip (Fig. 20.1). This plastic tube traverses a 2.5 cm long semiopaque soft plastic cup. When the sliding shaft is placed into the external os, the cup is slid over the cervix. Cups are available in three sizes (25, 30, and 35 mm) and include a side plastic conduit that attaches to a hand vacuum pump to keep the hysterocath in place.[22]

The procedure is performed under intravenous sedation and paracervical block. An HSG is initially performed through the hysterocath in order to confirm the diagnosis of proximal tubal obstruction. A 32-cm 9-Fr Teflon catheter is introduced though the hysterocath shaft and is placed under fluoroscopic control within the lower third of the uterine cavity. A 50 cm long 5.5-Fr polyethylene catheter with a 3-cm tip curved to a 45° angle is introduced next. A 0.035-in diameter curved safe-T-J guidewire is placed inside the 5-Fr catheter before insertion, and both catheter and guidewire are introduced through the 9-Fr catheter and directed toward the uterine cornua. Before final wedging the curved wire is replaced by a 0.035-in straight guidewire. The wire is then removed and a "selective HSG" is performed by injecting contrast media directly into the tubal cornua.

If the obstruction persists, a 3-Fr Teflon catheter with a 0.015 in diameter cope-mandril wireguide with platinum tip is advanced through the 5.5-Fr catheter into the fallopian tube (Fig. 20.1). The tube is then probed with back and forth movements of the guidewire. When accomplished, the wire is removed and contrast media is injected through the 3-Fr catheter. Additional cannulation equipment can be used if a second distal isthmic obstruction is encountered, which consists of an even smaller catheter tapering from 3 Fr to 2.2 Fr with a guidewire also tapering from 0.016 to 0.013 in. This equipment is used in a fashion similar to the 3-Fr catheter and wire described above.

## Results

Thurmond and colleagues[19] reported 100 consecutive patients with uni- or bilateral proximal tubal obstruction diagnosed by a single HSG. In this study the procedure succeeded in opening at least one tube in 86% of the patients, with a 5% incidence of uncomplicated tubal perforations. Only 20 patients presented with bilateral proximal obstruction and no other known contributing factors to their infertility. In 19 (95%) patients of this selected group wire catheterization succeeded in opening at least one tube. Twenty four of 39 (89%) tubes were opened. Nine pregnancies (45%) occurred within 6 months. Only eight nonpregnant patients returned for a 2- to 8-month follow-up HSG. In four cases (50%) reocclusion took place bilaterally and in two (25%) unilaterally.

## Transcervical Balloon Tuboplasty

### Instruments and Technique

The transcervical balloon tuboplasty (TBT) system (Bard Reproductive Systems, Billerica, MA) consists of an HSG or introducing cathe-ter, an angle guiding or "selective salpingography" catheter with a radiopaque tip, a balloon tuboplasty catheter, a wire-guide, an inflation device, and a Tuhoy-Borst adapter (Fig. 20.2). The HSG introducing catheter has a central lumen with a side lumen that allows the injection of contrast media. In addition, two inflation cuffs are connected to balloons proximal and distal to the cervical os (Fig. 20.2).

The procedure can be done under intravenous sedation or under general anesthesia with the patient in the lithotomy position. After cleansing of the cervix with Betadine, the anterior lip of the cervix is grasped with a single-toothed tenaculum. The HSG catheter is then introduced into the lower uterine segment and the distal balloon inflated with 5 ml of normal saline. The balloon is wedged against the internal os and the proximal balloon is then inflated. This stabilizes the catheter and seals the cavity. The presence of a proximal tubal obstruction is confirmed by injecting contrast media though the central lumen of the HSG catheter. A 2.5-mm diameter guiding catheter is then introduced through the central lumen of the HSG catheter and directed toward the tubal ostium. This catheter has a preshaped curve that allows the operator to position it at the cornua with little difficulty. A "selective HSG" is performed by injecting contrast media directly into the tube through the guiding catheter. If the obstruction is confirmed a balloon tuboplasty is performed.

The balloon tuboplasty catheter has a 1 mm thick shaft with a central lumen. A second lumen is connected to a small balloon that surrounds the distal portion of the catheter. The balloon is available in different diameters (2 and 3 mm) and in different lengths (Fig. 20.3). The longer but thinner variety is used in early isthmic segments, whereas the larger and shorter versions are recommended for obstructions of the cornual portions of the tube. Proximally the second lumen is connected to an inflation device with a manometer to avoid overinflation and rupture of the balloon (Fig. 20.4). Contrast media and a 0.6-mm guidewire are introduced through the central lumen of the balloon tuboplasty catheter. Proximally, the guidewire is introduced through the straight lumen of a

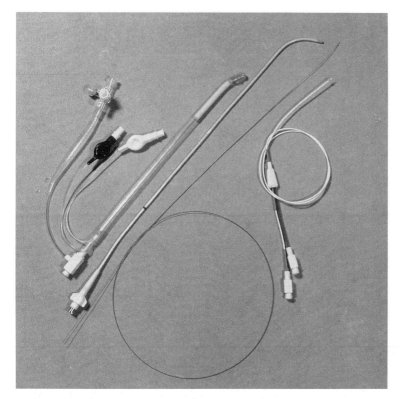

FIGURE 20.2. Components of the balloon tuboplasty system. **Left** to **right**: Introducing catheter, guiding catheter, guidewire, and balloon tuboplasty catheter. *Not shown*: inflation device and Tuhoy-Borst Y-connector.

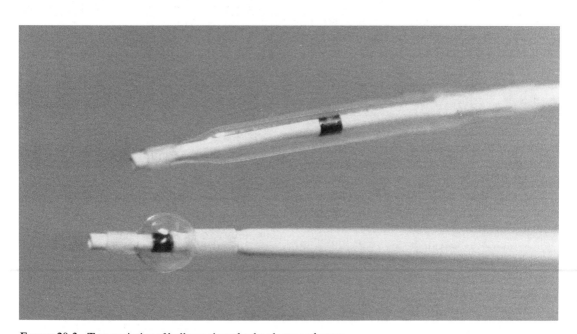

FIGURE 20.3. Two varieties of balloon-tipped tuboplasty catheters.

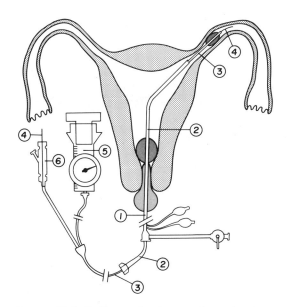

FIGURE 20.4. Balloon tuboplasty catheter in place. 1, Introducing catheter; 2, guiding catheter; 3, balloon tuboplasty catheter; 4, guidewire; 5, inflation device; 6, Tuhoy-Borst Y connector.

Tuhoy-Borst Y connector, whose side lumen is used for injecting contrast media.

Before insertion the balloon is purged of air and primed gently with either saline or contrast medium. The balloon is then connected to the manometer and vacuum is applied. A syringe with contrast medium is attached to the side arm of the Tuhoy-Borst Y connector and a soft-tipped guidewire loaded through the central lumen of the balloon catheter until the guidewire tip extends 1 to 2 mm beyond the balloon. The guidewire is then locked into position by securing the Tuhoy-Borst connector. The entire assembly is then introduced through the guiding catheter already in the cornual portion of the uterus (Fig. 20.4). The balloon catheter is advanced to the obstructed area. Often, the catheter negotiates the tubal lumen without difficulty. If an obstruction is encountered, the balloon catheter is inflated to 4 to 5 atm. Medium is then injected through the straight arm of the Y connector. When the obstruction is in the tubal isthmus, the guidewire can be advanced into the strictured area, the TBT catheter tracked over the guidewire, and the balloon inflated. Advancement and ballooning can be repeated until recanalization is achieved.

### Results

Among all the fluoroscopically and hysteroscopically guided tubal cannulation procedures, the TBT has been the most systematically studied. In a multicenter evaluation of the TBT system, 77 women underwent this procedure.[23] All had been previously diagnosed with bilateral tubal occlusion by both an HSG and laparoscopic chromotubation. In 92% of the patients at least one tube was recannulized. Among 64 patients with no other factors for infertility, a 34% pregnancy rate was reported after a median follow-up of 12 months. This represents a 38% pregnancy rate for those patients whose tubes were successfully recannulized. Although one ectopic pregnancy occurred, it was located distal to the site of the initial obstruction.

## Hysteroscopically Guided Tubal Cannulation

### Instruments and Technique

The procedure described by Novy and colleagues[24] uses $CO_2$ as the distending media for the rigid hysteroscope and concomitant laparoscopy (Cook Ob/Gyn, Bloomington, IN). A 30 cm long 5.5-Fr clear Teflon catheter with a metal obturator is introduced into the uterine cavity through the operating channel of the hysteroscope. A Y adaptor ending in Luerlok hubs is attached to its proximal end. The straight arm is used to inject dye or irrigation fluid, and is sealed with a screw cap when not in use. The other arm has an adjustable O-ring through which a 3-Fr catheter will be introduced (Fig. 20.5). This 3-Fr catheter is tapered to 2.5 Fr at its distal 3 cm.

A Teflon-coated stainless steel guidewire, 0.018 in in diameter with a flexible blunt tip, is placed into the lumen of the 3-Fr catheter. The 5.5-Fr catheter is placed at the tubal ostia under hysteroscopic visualization. The 3-Fr catheter and guidewire are introduced next, with the wire protruding slightly from the catheter tip. If resistance is met the catheter is

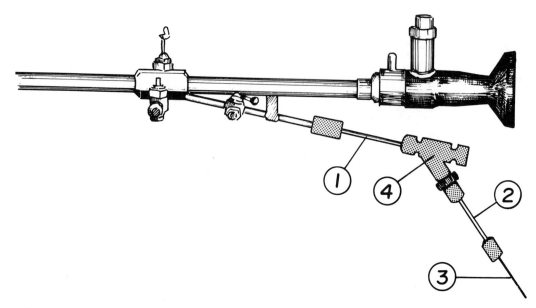

FIGURE 20.5. Wire catheterization system introduced through an operating hysteroscope. 1, 5.5-Fr catheter; 2, 3-Fr catheter; 3, guidewire; 4, Y connector.

advanced over the guidewire, the wire removed, and dye (methylene blue or indigo carmine) injected. Visualization of dye or the catheter tip through the fimbriated end of the tube by laparoscopy signals a successful cannulation. The procedure can also be performed using a flexible hysteroscope.

### Results

Novy and colleagues reported the successful cannulation of 11 of 12 tubes in 10 patients.[24] Five patients presented with bilateral proximal occlusion and three had a unilateral obstruction with an absent contralateral tube. The pregnancy rate in patients with bilateral proximal obstruction has not been reported to date.

Multiple studies have demonstrated that traditional tubal surgery for proximal tubal obstruction carries a pregnancy rate that at best does not exceed 40%. In addition, such surgery requires a lengthier hospitalization and recovery time. It is therefore anticipated that some of these proximal tubal surgeries will soon be replaced by transcervical tubal cannulation. Transcervical tubal cannulation should be offered to patients with proximal tubal obstruction before attempting laparotomy repair or in vitro fertilization.

## Falloposcopy

New instrumentation is currently being developed to visually explore the lumen of the fallopian tubes. The system as described by Kerin and colleagues[25] consists of a 30 cm long operating hysteroscopy with an outside diameter of (OD) of 3.3 mm, with an accessory operating channel (1.8 mm internal diameter). The proximal 25 cm of the hysteroscope is semirigid, and the distal 5 cm is flexible and steerable (Olympus Corp., Lake Success, NY). The falloposcope is a miniature fiberoptic endoscope with an OD of 0.5 mm, which is guided into the lumen of the fallopian tube through the operating channel of the flexible hysteroscope.

The flexible hysteroscope is introduced into the uterine cavity and directed toward the tubal ostia. A Teflon-coated, floppy, stainless steel, platinum tipped, tapered guidewire (similar to that described for hysteroscopic cannulation) is introduced through the operating channel of the hysteroscope into the fallopian tube for about 15 cm or until resistance is met. A 1.2- to 1.3-mm OD Teflon catheter is then introduced over the entirety of the guidewire, and the wire subsequently removed. A

Tuhoy-Borst Y connector is placed at the proximal end of the catheter and the fallo-scope is introduced through one arm of the connector into the catheter. The other arm of the connector is used to irrigate and minimally distend the tube, thus facilitating visualization.

The system is still under study and its diagnostic value remains to be defined.

# References

1. Musich JR, Behrman SJ. Surgical management of tubal obstruction of the uterotubal junction. *Fertil Steril.* 1983;40:423–441.
2. Holst N, Abyholm T, Borgerson A. Hysterosalpingography in the evaluation of infertility. *Acta Radiol.* 1983;24:253–257.
3. Grant A. Infertility surgery of the oviduct. *Fertil Steril.* 1971;22:496–503.
4. Fortier KJ, Haney AF. The pathologic spectrum of utero tubal junction obstruction. *Obstet Gynecol.* 1985;65:93–98.
5. Hellman LM. Tubal plastic operations. *J Obstet Gynaecol Br Commonw.* 1956;68:852–860.
6. Ayers JW. Hormonal therapy for tubal occlusion: danazol and tubal endometriosis. *Fertil Steril.* 1982;38:748–750.
7. Sulak PJ, Letterie GS, Coddington CC, et al. Histology of proximal tubal occlusion. *Fertil Steril.* 1987;48:437–440.
8. World Health Organization. Comparative trial of tubal insufflation, hysterosalpingogram and laparoscopy with dye hydrotubation for assessment of tubal patency. *Fertil Steril.* 1986;46: 1101–1102.
9. Musich JR, Behrman SJ. Infertility laparoscopy in perspective: review of 500 cases. *J Obstet Gynecol.* 1982;143:293–303.
10. Hutchins CJ. Laparoscopy and hysterosalpingography in the assessment of tubal patency. *Obstet Gynecol.* 1977;49:327–328.
11. Okonofua FE, Essen UI, Nimalaraj T. Hysterosalpingography versus laparoscopy and tubal infertility: comparison based on findings at laparotomy. *Int J Gynecol Obstet.* 1989;28:143–147.
12. Thurmond AS, Novy, Rosch J. Terbutaline in diagnosis of interstitial fallopian tubal obstruction. *Invest Radiol.* 1988;23:209–210.
13. Winfield AC, Pittaway D, Maxson W, Daniel G, et al. Apparent cornual occlusion by hysterosalpingography: reversal by glucagon. *AJR.* 1982;139:525–527.
14. Page EP. Use of isoxuprine in uterosalpingography and uterotubal insufflation. *Am J Obstet Gynecol.* 1968;101:358–364.
15. Cooper JM, Rigberg HS, Houck R, et al. Incidence, significance and remission of tubal spasm during attempted hysteroscopic tubal sterilization. *J Reprod Med.* 1985;30:9–13.
16. Corfman PA, Taylor HC. An instrument for transcervical treatment of the oviducts and uterine cornua. *Obstet Gynecol.* 1966;27:880–884.
17. Siegler AM, Haulka J, Peretz A. Reversibility of female sterilization. *Fertil Steril.* 1985;43: 499–510.
18. Platia MP, Krudy AG. Transvaginal laparoscopic recanalization of approximately occluded oviduct. *Fertil Steril.* 1985;44:704–706.
19. Thurmond AS, Novy M, Uchida BT, et al. Fallopian tube obstruction: selective salpingography and recanalization. *Radiology.* 1987; 163:511–514.
20. Confino E, Friberg I, Gleicher N. Transcervical balloon tuboplasty. *Fertil Steril.* 1986;46:963–966.
21. Thurmond AS, Rosch J. Nonsurgical tube recanalization for treatment of infertility. *Radiology.* 1990;174:371–374.
22. Thurmond AS, Uchida BT, Rosch J. Device for hysterosalpingography for fallopian tube catheterization. *Radiology.* 1990;174:571–572.
23. Confino E, Tur-Kaspa I, DeCherney A, et al. Transcervical balloon tuboplasty. A multicenter study. *JAMA.* 1990;264:2079–2082.
24. Novy ML, Thurmond AS, Patton P, et al. Diagnosis of cornual obstruction by transcervical fallopian tube cannulation. *Fertil Steril.* 1988; 50:434–440.
25. Kerin J, Daykhovsky L, Segalowitz J, et al. Falloscopy: a microendoscopic technique for visual exploration of the human fallopian tube from the uterotubal ostium to the fimbria using a transvaginal approach. *Fertil Steril.* 1990;54: 390–400.

# 21

# Complications of Laparoscopic and Hysteroscopic Surgery

*Samuel Smith*

CHAPTER OUTLINE

This chapter describes the most common complications associated with laparoscopic and hysteroscopic surgery, with emphasis on prevention and management. The reference text by Borten[1] presents a comprehensive treatment of laparoscopic complications, and every gynecologic endoscopist is recommended to review that, or a similar treatise.

## Complications of Operative Laparoscopy

The First Annual Report of the Complications Committee of the American Association of Gynecological Laparoscopists (AAGL) reviewed 12,182 laparoscopies performed in 1972 (Table 21.1).[2] Eighty two major complications were reported for a rate of 6.8 per 1000 procedures. In addition, three deaths occurred (25.0 per 100,000 cases). The AAGL had a 24% response rate to its 1988 membership survey on operative laparoscopy (Table 21.2),[3] with 36,928 operative laparoscopies reported. Five hundred and sixty eight major complications (15.4 per 1000 procedures) and two deaths (5.4 per 100,000 cases) were noted. This complication rate may actually be an underestimation of the true complication rate since the 76% of AAGL members who failed to respond to the survey may be a source of ascertainment bias. The Carbon Dioxide Laser Laparoscopy Study

TABLE 21.1. AAGL 1973 report: 12,182 laparoscopies.

| Complication | Rate/1000 cases | |
|---|---|---|
| Major | | 6.8 |
| Anesthetic | | 0.7 |
| Laparotomy for surgical trauma | | 3.2 |
|    Mesosalpingeal bleeding | 1.9 | |
|    Gastrointestinal | 0.5 | |
| Electrocagulation injury | | 2.3 |
|    Gastrointestinal | 2.2 | |

From Hulka, et al. *J Reprod Med.* 1975;10:301–306.

TABLE 21.2. AAGL 1988 survey: 36,928 operative laparoscopies.

| Complication | Rate/1000 Cases[a] | |
|---|---|---|
| Major | | 15.4 |
| Laparotomy for surgical trauma | | 4.2 |
|    Hemorrhage | 2.1 | |
|    Bowel *or* urinary tract | 1.6 | |
| Brachial plexus or sciatic/peroneal | | |
|    nerve | | 0.5 |

[a]24% response rate.
From Peterson et al. *J Reprod Med.* 1990;35:590–591

Group consists of 10 surgeons experienced in the field of operative laparoscopy (Table 21.3). Their initial report reviewed the complications experienced in 821 consecutive cases performed by the study group between January 1, 1983 and December, 1987.[4] Their major complication rate was 18.3 per 1000, similar to that in the AAGL's 1988 survey. From these reports it appears that major laparoscopic complications are more common today, probably related to the greater diversity of operative endoscopic procedures being performed. That notwithstanding, one may conclude that complications requiring laparotomy occurred far less commonly with the experienced surgeons of the carbon dioxide Laser Laparoscopy Study Group, and more commonly among the general AAGL membership. The principles minimizing complications during operative laparoscopy are summarized in Table 21.4.

## Anesthetic Complications

Complications of anesthesia are rare during laparoscopy. The AAGL survey of 1975 noted

TABLE 21.3. Carbon dioxide laser laparoscopy study group: 821 cases.

| Complications | Rate/1000 cases |
|---|---|
| Major | 18.3 |
| Laparoscopically controlled | |
|    hemorrhage | 11.0 |
| Uterine perforation | 3.7 |
| Unintended laparotomy | 1.2 |

From Carbon dioxide laser laparoscopy study group. *J Gynecol Surg.* 1989;5:269–272.

nine anesthetic incidents and nine insufflation difficulties (1.4 per 1000).[2] More than 50% of anesthesia-related deaths are related to hypoventilation. In the past, failed intubation and esophageal intubation were major causes of anesthesia related death during laparoscopy.[5] Inadvertent endobronchial intubation resulting in ventilation of a single lung may also occur, as the hilum of the lung is displaced upward in the deep Trendelenburg position.[1] The use of short endotracheal tubes minimizes this risk.

The Trendelenburg position and the increased intraabdominal pressure used with laparoscopy is associated with an increased risk of regurgitation of gastric contents.[1] However, the Trendelenburg position also reduces the risk of aspiration of regurgitated material into the airway, because of the beneficial effect of gravity. Cuffed endotracheal tubes should be used on all laparoscopies to prevent aspiration pneumonitis.[1]

Excessive intraabdominal carbon dioxide ($CO_2$) insufflation producing intraperitoneal pressures exceeding 20 mm Hg may lead to adverse cardiorespiratory effects.[1] During tension pneumoperitoneum the anesthesiologist may observe an increased resistance to ventilation. The insufflation of $CO_2$ and Trendelenburg position should be reduced. Needless to say, intraperitoneal pressure should be frequently checked and abdominal tension should be monitored. Some newer insufflators will automatically cut off gas flow when intraabdominal pressure exceeds a designated pressure, generally 12 to 16 mm Hg.

TABLE 21.4. Guidelines for minimizing complications during operative laparoscopy.

During anesthesia:
  −Use cuffed endotracheal intubation
  −Use nasogastric drainage
  −Avoid overforceful mask ventilation
  −Use complete muscle paralysis

In positioning patient:
  −Place in frog-leg lithotomy position
  −Avoid excessive hip or knee flexion or extension
  −Avoid excessive pressure on inner thighs
  −Use good shoulder padding
  −Use knee and foot supporting stirrups
  −Empty and continuously drain bladder
  −Maintain arm on operator's side (usually the left) parallel alongside body
  −Avoid excessive Trendelenburg
  −Lower the operating table to the level of the operator's hips to maximize control during insertion of umbilical or
    auxiliary trocars.

In establishing pneumoperitoneum:
  −Percuss left upper quadrant to detect gastric distention
  −During Veress needle insertion:
    −Test spring mechanism before placement
    −Leave valve open
    −Direct toward hollow of sacrum
    −Advance only 2–3 mm after piercing the parietal peritoneum
    −Perform aspiration test
  −Do not insufflate $CO_2$ at more than 1 L/min initially
  −If no loss of dullness to percussion over the liver edge is observed after insufflation of at least 1 L of $CO_2$, suspect
    intraperitoneal or omental extravasation
  −Avoid overinsufflation of abdominal cavity; generally maintain intraabdominal pressure below 18 mm Hg

During laparoscopic insertion and withdrawal:
  −During trocar insertion:
    −Maintain patient horizontal
    −Extend index finger to within 3 cm of trocar tip to protect against sudden deep penetration
    −Use controlled twisting motion
    −Direct trocar tip toward sacrum hollow
    −Advance no more than 2 cm beyond parietal peritoneum
    −When withdrawing trocar sheath, replace laparoscope (not trocar) first, after emptying the abdominal cavity of
      excess $CO_2$

During auxiliary trocar insertion:
  −Transluminate for visualization of epigastric vessels
  −Identify at laparoscopy the inferior epigastrics lateral to the umbilical artery remnants and arising near the origin of
    the round ligaments
  −Place trocars as high above the symphysis as cosmetically possible, but never less than 3 cm
  −Insert under direct laparoscopic visualization
  −Direct downward, toward uterine fundus, not laterally

During endoscopic surgery:
  −Minimize use of unipolar electrocautery
  −Disconnect or turn off all electrosurgical or laser units when not in use, even temporarily
  −Identify ureters before any surgery of the pelvic sidewall
  −Mobilize the ovaries completely before performing a cystectomy
  −Minimize forceful blunt dissection, especially when adhesions involve bowel serosa
  −Use traction/countertraction to identify tissue planes
  −Spread jaws of scissors to develop tissue planes, in lieu of cut across the tissues
  −Avoid cautery of bowel serosa
  −Cauterize vessels before transection
  −Avoid scissor action ("crossed swords") between different instruments to minimize the risk of pinching or traumatiz-
    ing bowel or omentum
  −Do not cut any tissue before fully identifying the anatomy

Improper anesthetic techniques may contribute to the development of endoscopic complications. Complete muscle relaxation must be maintained at all times during operative laparoscopy procedures. Movement, retching, or coughing during the procedure increases the risk of laceration or thermal injury. Furthermore, increased intraabdominal pressure before closure of the umbilical incision may lead to herniation of small bowel. Excessive and forceful mask ventilation during a difficult intubation may lead to gastric distention and subsequent perforation. The left upper quadrant should always be percussed before Veress needle insertion and, if found to be tympanic, a nasogastric tube should be placed.

## Complications of Pneumoperitoneum and Insufflation

### Associated with the Insertion of the Veress Needle

The majority of laparoscopic complications (whether operative or diagnostic) occur during placement of the Veress needle or trocars.[5] Leaving the valve of the needle open during insertion allows room air to enter the abdominal cavity, encouraging the peritoneal contents to fall away from the needle tip. Moreover, once the needle is felt to penetrate the fascia and parietal peritoneum it is advanced only 2 to 3 mm more. In this manner the Veress needle tip has minimal opportunity to lacerate an omental or mesointestinal vessel, become buried within the omentum or loops of bowel, enter the retroperitoneal space, or completely transect an adherent loop of bowel. A variety of techniques are described to minimize the potential for incorrect needle placement, including listening for the "hissing" phenomenon, the aspiration test, the "hanging drop" method, and the readings of intraabdominal pressure.[6] The hissing phenomenon refers to the sound made by a Veress needle when properly positioned within the abdominal cavity, upon elevation of the abdominal wall. A drop of saline may also be placed in the needle hilt and the abdomen elevated, the so-called hanging drop test. The intraabdominal

pressure is usually less than 1 mm Hg. Generally, fluctuations in intraabdominal pressure can be detected on the insufflator manometer accompanying the patient's respirations.

The most important safety maneuver to determine adequate placement of the Veress needle is the aspiration test.[1,6] The hilt of the Veress needle is attached to a syringe and, as soon as the needle is felt to be within the peritoneal cavity, gently aspirated. Normally no fluid should be recovered. Second, a small amount of saline is injected and reaspirated. Recovery of fluid suggests that the saline has been injected into a closed space, usually within the abdominal wall, or subperitoneally. Initial recovery of blood indicates that there is either free blood in the peritoneal cavity or that the tip of the needle has entered a blood vessel. Carbon dioxide should not be insufflated before these two entities are differentiated. In the case of vascular injury, laparotomy must be immediately performed.

Aspiration of intestinal fluid suggests injury to the intestinal tract, generally the small bowel (whose contents are more liquid, green, and usually sterile, compared to the large intestine). If accidental puncture of the small or large bowel has occurred with the Veress needle, the needle can be removed and a new one inserted, with laparoscopy then performed in the usual manner.[1] The site of gastrointestinal injuries should then be identified as soon as possible. In most cases, an intestinal puncture with the Veress needle will heal spontaneously without complication. Close observation for 24 to 48 hr, however, is indicated to rule out peritonitis.[1]

If urine is aspirated through the Veress needle, the needle can be withdrawn, a new needle inserted, and laparoscopy performed. Bladder punctures generally heal spontaneously. An indwelling catheter is usually left in place for 1 to 3 days.[1]

Some authors have suggested leaving the Veress needle in place in the event of intestinal contents or urine being reaspirated, so that the site is easily identifiable when laparoscopy is performed through a second site. However, this may result in the extension of a simple puncture into a laceration.[1]

Several authors have recommended omitting the Veress needle, inserting the laparoscopic trocar directly into the abdominal cavity, without the aid of prior pneumoperitoneum. Several large series describe this technique as safe, even in obese patients or women who have had prior laparotomy.[7–11] For example, the risk of bowel injury in women with previous laparotomy was 1 per 416 procedures in one series.[9] This technique may receive wider use in the future as disposable, safety-shield laparoscopic trocars become increasingly available.

### Extraperitoneal Insufflation

Extraperitoneal insufflation of $CO_2$ usually occurs preperitoneally, in the abdominal wall, but may also occur retroperitoneally (i.e., beneath the posterior parietal peritoneum). Accumulation of gas extraperitoneally can technically complicate continuation of the laparoscopic procedure and results in patient morbidity. Once the Veress needle is felt to be in place, $CO_2$ should be insufflated at no more than 1 L per min. Intraabdominal pressures are generally below 10 mm Hg during insufflation. The loss of dullness to percussion over the liver area should be elicited, generally within 1 L of insufflation. If the change in tympany is not noted, extraperitoneal or omental insufflation should be suspected.

Subcutaneous emphysema results when the Veress needle fails to penetrate the rectus fascia. Crepitation can be felt in the abdominal wall as $CO_2$ extends upward toward the loose areolar tissue of the neck and/or downward to the inguinal region. If the error is recognized early, the Veress needle is removed and reinserted. If the error is recognized only after a large volume of gas has been insufflated, disconnecting the gas tubing from the Veress needle, without moving the needle, will allow much of the gas to escape. If the error is first identified by laparoscopic visualization, the gas tubing should be disconnected from the trocar sheath; withdrawing the laparoscope then allows the gas to escape. Postoperative patient discomfort will be reduced if the amount of subcutaneous emphysema is reduced by these techniques.[1]

Insufflation of gas below the rectus fascia but outside of the peritoneal cavity creates preperitoneal emphysema. This is less likely than subcutaneous emphysema to be identified before insertion of the laparoscopic trocar. The aspiration test is critical to detect preperitoneal location of the Veress needle tip. High insufflating pressures are usually not seen because the preperitoneal tissues offer little resistance to the gas. In addition, the expected loss of liver dullness to percussion occasionally can be seen.[1]

Preperitoneal insufflation is usually identified when the laparoscope is placed, and the peritoneum is merely displaced by the insufflated gas. Once diagnosed, an 18-gauge spinal needle or similar aspirating needle can be inserted into the preperitoneal space and the emphysema reduced under direct vision. Pressing on the abdominal wall seldom facilitates escape of the gas; it usually results in lateral extension of the gas. Attempts at penetration of the peritoneum through the emphysema are discouraged because of the risk of damage to intraabdominal structures.

Pneumoperitoneum after preperitoneal insufflation can be established through the intraumbilical insertion of needle and trocar, a site where all tissue layers are fused. Insertion of the Veress needle through the cul de sac may also be helpful. Occasionally, with the use of an operating laparoscope the ballooned out peritoneum can be incised under direct visualization. As intraperitoneal insufflation of gas occurs, the increasing intraabdominal pressure will slowly push the preperitoneal gas through the spinal needle or previously placed trocar.[1]

Retroperitoneal insufflation is uncommon. Small accumulations of retroperitoneal gas can be left in situ to reabsorb. Larger volumes should be aspirated under direct vision with an aspiration needle. Always consider that vascular damage may have also occurred.[1]

### Gas Embolism

Gas embolism is a clinically rare and potentially fatal event. Minor amounts of gas entering the circulatory system may be absorbed and excreted without clinical recognition. Accidental puncture of a blood vessel and direct insufflation into the vessel is the most likely explanation for fatal embolization, although a variety of theories have been described.[5] If gas embolization is suspected, a central venous line should be advanced into the right atrium or superior vena cava to try to aspirate gas from the cardiovascular system.[1]

## Complications of Trocar Insertion

Insertion of sharp trocars rarely causes injury to intraabdominal structures. Placement of the laparoscopic trocar is more likely than auxiliary trocars to produce intraabdominal injury, because it is so difficult to predict the presence of bowel or omental adhesions to the anterior abdominal wall. The Veress needle can be moved laterally during insufflation; observing a sudden rise in insufflation pressure suggests the needle tip is touching omentum, bowel, or adhesions.[6] Semm's probing test may also be used as a safety check before inserting the laparoscopic trocar.[6] Insertion of the umbilical trocar should be directed toward the hollow of the sacrum. The patient should be completely flat, so as to maximize the distance between the umbilicus and the aorta (see below). The auxiliary trocars should be inserted under direct visualization.

The laparoscopic and auxiliary trocars should be inserted with controlled, twisting motions that minimize the risk of uncontrolled deep intraabdominal penetration and injury. Conical tipped trocars were designed specifically for a twisting insertion, whereas pyramidal tips were designed for direct insertion, producing a self-closing X-shaped (flapped) opening in the fascia. However, both trocars can be inserted in a twisting fashion. An index finger extended over the trocar stem will limit the depth of penetration.[1] Trocars that are slightly dulled pose an important risk for injury. Dulled trocars require greater force to penetrate the abdominal wall than sharp trocars, and there is a greater likelihood of an uncontrolled thrust by the laparoscopist.[12] This principle applies to both the primary and auxiliary trocars. Disposable safety-shield trocars, recently marketed in various sizes, require less force to penetrate the abdominal wall than reusable trocars.[13] They appear to offer an added measure of safety to trocar insertion.

## Vascular Injuries

Vascular injuries account for 30% to 50% of surgical trauma at laparoscopy.[12] Mintz's 1977 survey of 100,000 laparoscopic procedures reported 34 injuries to major internal blood vessels (0.34 per 1000 cases).[14] The pneumoperitoneum needle accounts for about 36% of vascular injuries, and the primary and auxiliary trocars account for about 32% each.[12] Additional bleeding can occur during the course of operative laparoscopic procedures. However, this type of bleeding is usually amenable to laparoscopic management.[1]

### Superficial Epigastric Artery

The superficial epigastric artery is a branch of the femoral artery that courses between layers of abdominal wall fascia.[1] It is at greatest risk of injury during insertion of auxiliary trocars. Transillumination of the abdominal wall with the intraperitoneal laparoscopic light may identify the superficial epigastric artery and other large subcutaneous vessels, and guide the placement of auxiliary trocars.[1]

Injury to deep subcutaneous vessels may be managed by occlusive pressure or by clamping and ligating the vessel through a small skin incision. Overnight hospitalization is recommended if the injury is treated by pressure, since recognition of subcutaneous bleeding is frequently delayed.[1]

### Inferior Epigastric Vessels

The midline linea alba of the abdominal wall is relatively avascular. Lateral to the linea alba lie the rectus muscles, whose blood supply derives from the inferior and superior epigastric arteries, branches of the external iliac artery and internal mammary artery, respectively.[1] The inferior epigastric artery that lies between the rectus muscle and its posterior fascia is particularly prone to injury during placement of auxiliary trocars. With exception of thin patients, this vessel generally cannot be identified by transillumination of the abdominal wall.[1] Thus, the paramedian insertion of the auxiliary trocar is truly blind with regard to the inferior epigastric vessels unless they can be seen lateral to the ligaments of the obliterated umbilical arteries. Laceration of these vessels is usually preventable if an avascular midline site is selected for auxiliary trocar insertion.[1] Alternatively, trocar insertion sites lateral to the external edge of the rectus muscle, 6 to 7 cm lateral to the midline, are generally safe.[15] However, proceeding too far laterally increases the risk of injury to the external iliac vessels. If laceration of the inferior epigastric artery or vein is identified during laparoscopy, full thickness sutures should be placed above and below the trocar insertion site. These sutures should be laparoscopically directed so as to avoid trauma to intraabdominal structures.[1] A large urologic curved needle or, in the event the patient is overweight, a special needle for transabdominal suturing designed by Semm (WISAP USA, #7664) can be used.

Laceration of the inferior epigastric artery may be initially diagnosed postoperatively. Large preperitoneal hematomas can accumulate whose only symptom may be excessive incisional pain in the area of an auxiliary trocar. Palpation of a large unilateral paramedian mass on the abdominal wall or identification of a significant decline in hematocrit suggest the diagnosis. An ultrasound of the abdominal wall is diagnostic. After diagnosis, the wound should be explored, the hematoma drained, and the artery or vein ligated proximal and distal to the laceration.[1]

## Major Retroperitoneal Vessels

Injury to a major retroperitoneal vessel with massive hemorrhage is one of the most catastrophic complications of laparoscopy. The vessels generally involved are the aorta, vena cava, and right and left common iliac arteries and veins.[5] Every laparoscopist must be trained in the prevention, identification, and management of this complication.

The umbilicus is located directly over the lower end of the aorta in the dorsosupine patient. The lower end of the aorta rotates upward in the Trendelenburg position, bringing the common iliac vessels and their branches closer to the horizontal plane. Furthermore, the umbilicus will be displaced upward, particularly in obese patients. As a result, the distance between the umbilicus and the aorta is reduced, and there is an increased risk of injury to retroperitoneal vessels if the laparoscopist fails to adjust for these positional changes.[1] The Veress needle and umbilical trocar should be directed toward the hollow of the sacrum, away from the sacral promontory, above which the aorta bifurcates.[1] The insertion of the auxiliary trocars should be directed downward, toward the fundus of the uterus, and not toward the sacrum.

Although the majority of penetrating injuries to major retroperitoneal vessels occur during insertion of the Veress needle or laparoscopic trocar, the aorta can also be penetrated by the scalpel used to incise the intraumbilical or subumbilical region of the abdominal wall. In very thin patients the anterior abdominal wall may be within 2 to 3 cm of the aorta, and in all patients, regardless of size or weight, the umbilicus itself is only 1 to 2 cm thick.[1]

Major retroperitoneal vessel injury due to the Veress needle may be identified at the time it occurs by the aspiration test.[1] If diagnosis is made at this time, the Veress needle is left in place and laparotomy is performed through a midline inferior skin incision. Leaving the Veress needle in place serves to obstruct the hemorrhage somewhat and to guide the vascular surgeon to the injured vessel. Vascular injuries caused by the laparoscopic or auxiliary trocars are larger than those caused by the Veress needle, cause profuse hemorrhage and are usually due to improper technique. The auxiliary trocars usually produce common or external iliac vessel injury due to the instrument deviating from the midline at the time of insertion; this contrasts with the uncontrolled thrust usually associated with primary trocar injuries.[1]

Immediate midline laparotomy should be performed whenever vascular injury is suspected.[1] Upon entering the abdomen, the laparoscopist should compress the aorta below the level of the renal arteries. This will reduce hemorrhage until the vascular surgeon arrives.[1] On occasion, the diagnosis is delayed because retroperitoneal bleeding has occurred instead of intraperitoneal bleeding. Cardiovascular collapse in the absence of overt intraabdominal hemorrhage may be due to retroperitoneal bleeding or anesthetic complications. The retroperitoneal space should be inspected and thoroughly checked for concealed hemorrhage. Cardiovascular collapse in the recovery room should be treated as retroperitoneal hemorrhage and hypovolemic shock unless proven otherwise.[1]

### Mesosalpingeal and Meso-ovarian Bleeding

Mesosalpingeal and meso-ovarian hemorrhage is the most frequent vascular injury associated with operative laparoscopy. Injury to mesosalpingeal vessels usually results from dissection, laceration, or transection at the time of tubal surgery. These vessels may also be damaged by the Veress needle or various trocars.[1] Hemostasis can usually be obtained laparoscopically with bipolar electrocoagulation, microfibrillar collagen, endocoagulation, clip application, silicone band ligature (Falope ring) or various intraabdominal sutures (Endoloop) (see Chapter 4). Although bleeding from the mesosalpingeal vasculature may initially seem profuse, the application of pressure to the bleeding site with an atraumatic grasper (e.g., Kleppinger bipolar paddles or adhesion grasper [Storz Co.]) for 3 to 5 min may suffice. The adnexa should be observed closely for hematoma formation, especially before removal of the laparoscope. Frequently an additional auxiliary puncture site is useful to facilitate exposure and compression of the injury. The laparoscopist should avoid hemostatic techniques that might compromise ovarian circulation, and should certainly avoid the infundibulopelvic vessels. Laparotomy is seldom needed to secure hemostasis.[1,4]

### Miscellaneous Vascular Injuries

A variety of vascular injuries may complicate operative laparoscopy. Perforation of omental vessels is usually diagnosed by visualizing the lacerated vessels. Broad ligament and mesosalpingeal vessels may be damaged by overvigorous manipulation of the uterus or adnexa. Biopsy site hemorrhage can occur, regardless of the size of the biopsy. Hemorrhage can occur during adhesiolysis, ovarian cystectomy, and uterosacral ligament ablation. Laparoscopic myomectomy sites may also bleed.[1,6]

The laparoscopist must make every effort to avoid hemorrhage. Vascular adhesions should be endocoagulated, electrocoagulated, or sutured before adhesiolysis.[6] Uterosacral ligament or posterior broad ligament bleeding must be handled carefully because of the proximity of the ureter.[1] Coagulation of most bleeding sites can be achieved laparoscopically.

## Gastrointestinal Injuries

Clinically evident gastrointestinal tract injury is a serious complication, with an incidence of up to 3 per 1000 operative procedures. However, the true incidence is believed to be higher since many small, self-limited injuries may go undiagnosed.[1]

Gastrointestinal injuries are due to either lacerations or burns (electrocoagulation, laser).[1] Lacerating injuries can be produced at the time of insertion of the Veress needle, laparoscopic trocar, or auxiliary trocars. Previous abdominal surgery, bowel distention, inflammatory bowel disease, and unsuspected intraabdominal disease are risk factors. However, more than half of gastrointestinal injuries occur in patients without risk factors. Lacerating injuries are frequently diagnosed at the time of laparoscopy. In contrast, thermal injury is usually diagnosed postoperatively, after a seemingly uncomplicated laparoscopy.[1]

### Stomach Injury

Gastric distention is the major risk factor for perforating injury to the stomach. Distention may occur before anesthesia as a result of aerophagia in an anxious patient. More often, however, gastric distention has occurred during preoxygenation before induction of anesthesia. The lower edge of the stomach may extend below the umbilicus in up to 25% of horizontally positioned women.[1]

Gastric perforation by the Veress needle is suspected when gastric juice is obtained during the aspiration test. If the aspiration test is not performed and gas is insufflated, eructation or stomach borborygmi is very suspicious for intragastric location of the Veress needle. A nasogastric tube should be placed to decompress the stomach if gastric perforation is suspected. Removal and reinsertion of a new Veress needle is then performed. During laparoscopy, it is important to identify the site of gastric perforation and assess the extent of damage and bleeding. If there is no bleeding, the gastric musculature will usually seal off the perforation spontaneously. A nasogastric tube is left in place; it facilitates healing by minimizing stomach distention and leakage of gastrointestinal fluid into the peritoneal cavity.[1]

A sharp trocar injury to the stomach is usually larger than that caused by the Veress needle. Injuries less than 5 mm in diameter may be managed conservatively, since they are no larger than those produced by a gastrostomy tube. Larger lacerations require laparotomy and primary closure.[1]

### Small Bowel Injury

Perforation of the small intestine by the Veress needle can be recognized when greenish intestinal fluid is recovered during the aspiration test. Small intestinal fluid is almost always sterile. Through and through perforations of the intestine may occur if the bowel is adherent to the anterior abdominal wall at the site of Veress needle insertion; these may escape detection by the aspiration test. Perforations of the small intestine with the Veress needle usually heal spontaneously. The musculature of the bowel wall generally seals off the perforation and prevents intraperitoneal leakage of intestinal fluid.[1] The Veress needle should be removed; laparoscopy can be completed by insertion of a new needle at a different angle. Every effort should be made to identify the site of perforation. Although serious complications seldom follow a Veress needle perforation of the intestine, there may be a lacerated blood vessel in the bowel wall or mesentery. In this

case, the degree of bleeding or hematoma formation is ascertained. Evidence of active bleeding or continued enlargement of a hematoma require laparotomy to secure hemostasis. If bleeding is minimal or the hematoma is stable, hospitalization for observation is recommended. Even in the absence of vascular trauma, any patient who has sustained a small bowel perforation should be hospitalized for 24 to 48 hr of observation.[1]

On occasion, gas will be insufflated into the lumen of the bowel because the aspiration step was omitted.[1] Intraintestinal pressure may be similar to intraperitoneal opening pressure. Several liters of gas may be insufflated into the intestinal lumen without raising the insufflating pressure. The passage of gas from the rectum may signal intraluminal insufflation into large bowel. This obviously increases the risk of subsequent trocar injury to the intestine.[1] Uncommonly, the Veress needle partially penetrates the intestinal wall. This is of little consequence, unless the abnormal location is not recognized and gas is insufflated causing bullous distention of the intestinal wall. Insufflation pressure will rapidly rise in this event. Diagnosis of bullous distention requires hospitalization for observation, because the intestinal wall may rupture. However, the gas is usually reabsorbed without sequelae.[1]

Injuries caused by sharp trocars may be more serious.[1] Superficial lacerations limited to the intestinal serosa do not need repair if the site is hemostatic. Patients can be discharged without overnight hospitalization. Deeper lesions to the intestinal wall require careful evaluation. Lacerations that are narrower than the diameter of a Veress needle can be managed conservatively by observation, nothing by mouth, and prophylactic antibiotic coverage for anaerobes and enterobacteria. Larger lacerations of the intestinal wall or small lacerations that have spilled intestinal fluid into the peritoneal cavity require laparotomy for repair. Clean-edged lesions can be repaired in layers.[1,16] Ragged lacerations, or lacerated bowel that has been avulsed from the mesentery, require segmental bowel resection and reanastomosis.[1,16]

Gastrointestinal injuries during laparoscopic adhesiolysis may occur during blunt separation of bowel loops. This is more likely to occur in patients with endometriosis, pelvic inflammatory disease, or prior laparotomy. Sharp dissection is preferred over blunt dissection when adhesions are dense or tissue planes are obscured.[16]

Thermal injury usually results from electrocautery devices, although lasers can produce similar injuries.[1,16–18] Thermal injuries are usually not recognized or suspected at the time of surgery. Unsuspected injury can occur by inadvertent direct contact of a monopolar electrode to the bowel, intraperitoneal transmission of sparks from an active monopolar electrode across to a nearby loop of bowel, or electrical discharge from an operative laparoscope through which a unipolar instrument has been placed (see Chapter 4). Alternatively, heat may be transmitted from the cauterized organ to a neighbor.[16] Thermal damage can also occur if the bowel wall is directly electrocoagulated to achieve hemostasis during adhesiolysis or to fulgurate endometriosis. Lasers such as the KTP and Nd:YAG can produce thermal injury mimicking electrocautery lesions. Last, the heat from the laparoscope can cause injury if it is inadvertently allowed to rest on the bowel.

Patients with thermal bowel injuries may remain asymptomatic for up to 3 days postoperatively.[1,16] Vague complaints of abdominal discomfort are replaced by early signs of peritonitis: nausea, vomiting, anorexia, fever and abdominal pain. The time course of symptoms cannot be used to reliably distinguish thermal from lacerating injuries.[17,18] Bowel lacerations usually become symptomatic within 12 to 48 hr, but sometimes the onset of symptoms is delayed for more than a week. In contrast, thermal injuries can become symptomatic before 48 hr postoperatively. Gross and microscopic analysis of the area of injury, however, reliably differentiates the cause of intestinal trauma. Microscopically, thermal injury demonstrates an area of coagulative necrosis, absence of capillary ingrowth and fibromuscular coat reconstruction, and absence of white blood cell infiltration except at the borders of the lesions.[17,18] Grossly, bipolar thermal injuries demonstrate blanched serosa and minimal necrosis, in contrast to unipolar thermal and lacerating injuries that demonstrate large perforations and prominent exudate within 4 days of injury.[17,18]

The possibility of small bowel injury should be suspected when a patient complains of increasing abdominal pain or peritonitis symptoms after laparoscopy.[1,18] These patients should be readmitted for observation and conservative therapy including antibiotics. If the patient fails to respond within 24 hr, laparoscopy should be repeated or laparotomy performed to search for a perforation site.[1,18] If the area of thermal damage is superficial and 5 mm or less, expectant management is appropriate.[19] Larger or deeper thermal injuries are treated with wide resection and reanastomosis. The resection should extend 3 to 5 cm into healthy tissue on either side of the bowel injury because of the extensive coagulation necrosis and inflammatory reaction that occurs.[16]

## Large Bowel Injuries

Traumatic injury of the large intestine during insertion of the Veress needle is a rare event, but can be serious due to the bacterial growth present in large bowel contents. It may be recognized by the recovery of fecally stained fluid during the aspiration test. The Veress needle should be withdrawn and pneumoperitoneum established by another Veress needle. The perforated area must be identified at the time of laparoscopy. Peritoneal fluid should be aspirated for bacterial culture.[1] Even small amounts of fecal contamination into the peritoneal cavity is serious. Perforating colonic injuries are usually treated by layered primary closure, copious peritoneal lavage, and broad spectrum antibiotic coverage.[1,16]

Injuries to the large bowel caused by a trocar are more serious than Veress needle injuries, and require laparotomy. Small 1- to 2-cm lacerations may be treated by primary closure.[1,16] More significant trauma to the ascending colon is generally managed by resection of the lacerated segment of bowel. Primary anastomosis can be performed, but more commonly the anastomosis follows a period of fecal diversion by ileostomy.[1] Major injuries to the descending colon, sigmoid colon, or rectum are usually treated by proximal diverting colostomy, resection of the injured segment of bowel, and delayed reanastomosis.[1,16] A proximal colostomy is generally indicated if the injury is large, the blood supply to the damaged bowel is compromised, the closure is under tension, or the bowel was inadequately prepared. Adjunctive measures involve copious peritoneal lavage, closed suction drainage, nasogastric suction, and antibiotic coverage.[16]

Thermal injuries and lacerations to the colon can occur during difficult adhesiolysis or during attempts to secure hemostasis. Thermal injuries are generally diagnosed postoperatively in patients presenting with peritonitis. Primary closure of the defect is generally not recommended since the area of damage extends lateral to the visible trauma. Resection, proximal colostomy, and delayed reanastomosis are usually indicated.[16]

### Small Bowel Incarceration

Incarceration of small bowel through a laparoscopic, usually the umbilical, incision is a very rare event, less than 1 occurrence per 5000 cases.[20] However, asymptomatic herniation or pinching of small bowel may be more common. Nausea, vomiting, anorexia, and abdominal distention generally begin 3 to 7 days postoperatively, but onset of symptoms has been observed in the immediate postoperative period.[21] The umbilical region becomes indurated and tender. Abdominal x rays demonstrate multiple air–fluid levels, dilated small bowel loops, and absence of air in the rectum. Laparotomy, resection of the nonviable intestinal segment, and primary anastomosis is the usual treatment. Expectant management in cases of symptomatic incarceration of intestine or omentum is inappropriate since spontaneous resolution seldom occurs. Delaying laparotomy increases the risk that the herniated bowel segment will be nonviable and require resection.[1,21]

Several authors have suggested that this complication can be eliminated by using 5- to 8-mm diameter trocars, instead of 11- to 12-mm trocars. However, maximum visualization and illumination are usually required for operative laparoscopy, best achieved with use of a 10- to 11-mm straight laparoscope. The "Z" track method for the insertion of the umbilical trocar has been recommended to prevent this complication. Closing the fascia with interrupted sutures may also reduce the risk of herniation. Most importantly, the laparoscope (not the trocar) should always be reinserted before removing its sleeve. Excess $CO_2$ should be allowed to escape, or be suctioned out under direct visualization, before removal of the umbilical sleeve plus laparoscope, and abdominal pressure (including the patient's coughing or heaving) should be minimized during removal.[1,21]

### Postoperative Ileus

Adynamic ileus may occur after laparoscopic lysis of bowel adhesions. Abdominal distention, nausea, vomiting, and constipation typically occur within the first 48 hr after surgery. Pain, fever, and peritoneal signs are minimal. Bowel sounds will be minimal to absent and a flat-plate x ray may be helpful. Treatment is conservative. Nasogastric suction removes swallowed air, prevents further gastric distention, and relieves nausea. Intravenous fluids are administered until intestinal function spontaneously recovers.[16]

### Open Laparoscopy

Open laparoscopy has been suggested as a useful technique to reduce the risk of intestinal injury. However, bowel injuries seem to occur with a similar frequency with both open and closed laparoscopy technique.[12] Despite this, open laparoscopy should be considered for patients who are at increased risk for bowel injury.

## Urinary Tract Injuries

The incidence of urinary tract injury during laparoscopy is approximately 1 to 2 per 1000 procedures.[3]

### Bladder Injury

Injury to the urinary bladder is most likely when the bladder has not been catheterized before or during laparoscopy and in women with distorted anatomy. Previous abdominal pelvic surgery may cause the bladder to be drawn upward, increasing the risk of bladder injury. However, the most common factor increasing the risk of bladder injury is a distended bladder. As little as 100 cc of urine exposes the bladder to an increased risk of trauma.[1] Therefore, the bladder should be catheterized before all laparoscopies, and an indwelling catheter is recommended for every operative laparoscopy.[1]

The bladder can be damaged by the Veress needle, sharp trocars, or any auxiliary instrument used during laparoscopic surgery. Veress needle injuries usually occur because the bladder was not emptied before surgery or because of a misdirected needle insertion. Short patients, children, and young teenagers have smaller umbilicopubic distances and small amounts of urine may raise the risk of bladder injury.[1] The aspiration test will usually yield urine if the bladder has been perforated. Insufflation of small amounts of gas will cause a rapid rise in insufflation pressure, suggesting that the needle is within a closed space, and gas may leak from the urethra. If the bladder has been perforated, the Veress needle is withdrawn and a new one inserted. The muscular bladder wall seals off this injury, facilitating spontaneous healing. Postoperative catheterization is maintained for 1 to 3 days. If gas has been insufflated into the bladder, it should be allowed to escape through the Veress needle before its being withdrawn. If the needle has already been removed, catheterization will usually deflate the bladder.[1]

Trocar injuries to the bladder occur as frequently as Veress needle injuries; about 50% of trocar injuries are due to the laparoscopic trocar and 50% are due to auxiliary trocars.[12] If the bladder has been raised and fixed due to prior surgery, the site of trauma is usually the attachment to the anterior abdominal wall. Trocar trauma to the bladder can also result from an uncontrolled thrust.[1] As with Veress needle injuries, a distended bladder is most at risk, but even a catheterized bladder can be injured if poor technique is used in placing the laparoscopic or auxiliary trocars. When the bladder lumen has been entered by a trocar, the size of the laceration generally dictates

therapy. Four to 5 days of continuous postoperative drainage is usually sufficient to allow 5-mm or smaller lacerations to heal. Larger lacerations will usually require primary closure in layers.[1] Closure of the bladder may be first attempted laparoscopically.

The bladder can also be damaged during the course of laparoscopic surgery. Blunt trauma may occur if excessive force is used to try to mobilize the bladder or adhesions. Adhesions between the bladder and the anterior uterine wall should be dissected sharply.[1] Electrocoagulating instruments and lasers can damage the bladder, and days may elapse before the onset of symptoms. The usual symptom is the inability to void spontaneously, and failure to obtain urine by catheterization. The bladder perforation may allow urine to extravasate into the peritoneal cavity or allow it to accumulate extraperitoneally in the space of Retzius. Large amounts of urine can accumulate in the peritoneal cavity or in the space of Retzius, asymptomatically. Suprapubic pain will eventually occur with extraperitoneal accumulations.[1] Retrograde cystograms confirm the diagnosis by visualizing the extravasation of contrast material. Transabdominal repair will usually be necessary for those injuries caused by laser or electrocoagulation instruments.[1]

## Urachal Cysts and Vesicourethral Diverticuli

Urachal cysts and vesicourethral diverticula may be perforated during laparoscopy with resultant hematoma formation, leakage of urine from incisions, or intraperitoneal spillage of urine. A voiding cystourethrogram and/or intravenous pyelogram (IVP) are usually diagnostic. Prolonged catheterization of the bladder may facilitate spontaneous healing of small punctures. Larger lacerations may require surgical resection of the urachal defect.[1,22]

## Ureteral Injury

The ureter is less commonly injured than the bladder.[1] Ureteral injury usually manifests symptoms within 5 days of surgery, but may be delayed for 2 to 3 weeks. Presenting symptoms usually include fever, peritonitis, pelvic mass, hematuria, and leukocytosis.[23] The ureter is most commonly injured 2 to 3 cm from the ureterovesical junction or at the pelvic brim. It is particularly susceptible to injury when cautery is used in the area of the uterosacral ligaments to control bleeding or fulgurate endometriosis. Ureteral damage localized to the pelvic brim is usually associated with laparoscopic sterilization procedures.[23] The technique of displacing the uterus in order to put the adnexa under tension stretches the infundibulopelvic ligament and displaces the ureter medially, closer to the site of cautery. In these instances, the cautery forcep probably inadvertently touches the pelvic side wall. The ureter is also susceptible to injury in difficult endometriosis cases, particularly those in which the ovary is adherent to the lateral pelvic side wall.[23] Hydrodissection has been recommended to protect retroperitoneal structures, but this is unlikely to protect the ureter since it remains attached to the medial leaf of peritoneum. It appears that a clear understanding of the course of the ureter within the pelvis is essential for the safe use of electrocautery or laser.[23]

Ureteral injury is usually diagnosed by an IVP. However, a repeat laparoscopy may be used to diagnose the injury. Since symptoms overlap with those of bowel injury, an IVP should be performed to eliminate ureteral injury from the differential diagnosis of bowel injury.[23]

Ureteral injuries will be treated surgically depending on the location and extent of injury. Uretero–ureteral reanastomosis, ureteroneocystostomy, and transverse ureteroureterostomy are usually required; however, placement of a ureteral stent may suffice in some situations.[23]

## Infectious Complications

Laparoscopy is considered a clean-contaminated operation. Although breaks in aseptic technique are unavoidable during operative laparoscopy, infectious morbidity is rare and may range from mild superficial incisional infection to life-threatening peritonitis.[1]

Wound infections occur in 0.8% to 1.3% of cases. Mild infections develop within 48 to 72 hr after the procedure. Erythema occurs early and may be replaced by suppuration. Sutures should be removed and the wound cleaned. Antibiotic coverage for *Staphylococcus aureus* and hemolytic streptococcus should be initiated, and the wound allowed to heal by secondary intention.[1]

Flare-up of clinically silent or chronic salpingitis may lead to pelvic inflammatory disease and peritonitis. Pelvic infection, however, rarely occurs as a result of laparoscopy, unless inadvertent gastrointestinal injury has occurred.[1]

Transcervical chromotubation may carry vaginal organisms into the peritoneal cavity; however, the level of contamination is low.[24] Dye should not be injected transcervically if active pelvic infection is present or suspected. If tubal patency needs to be assessed in a patient with apparent chronic salpingitis, antibiotic prophylaxis should be administered.[24]

## Neurologic Complications

Nerve injury complicated 0.5 per 1000 operative laparoscopies in the AAGL's 1988 membership survey.[3] Brachial palsy has been observed in patients maintained in a steep Trendelenburg position for an extended period of time, and use of a shoulder brace appears to increase this risk. Ample padding, adducting the patient's arms to her side, and minimizing the duration of the procedure reduces the risk. Hyperextension of the arm must be avoided, and the surgeon and assistant should not lean on the extended arm.[1]

Sciatic and/or peroneal nerve injury may occur because the patient is in the lithotomy or semilithotomy position. Sciatic nerve injury has occurred after as little as 35 min in the semilithotomy position. Stretching of the nerve presumably causes the injury.[1] Sciatic nerve injury sustained during laparoscopy is usually self-limited. Motor and sensory deficits usually appear immediately after surgery, progress for several weeks, and resolve over the following 3 to 9 months.[1] Suggestions to prevent sciatic/peroneal nerve injury include the use of knee- and foot-supporting stirrups, raising and lowering both legs simultaneously to place them in stirrups while carefully extending the hip and knee joints, flexing the knees before flexing the hips, limiting external hip rotation, and avoiding undue pressure on the inner aspect of the thigh.[1]

# Complications of Operative Hysteroscopy

The AAGL's 1988 membership survey on operative hysteroscopy had a 19% response rate.[25] The most commonly reported complication was uterine perforation not requiring blood transfusion (13.0 per 1000 procedures). The overall major complication rate, excluding benign uterine perforations, was 8.6 per 1000 procedures.[25] Other common complications included hemorrhage requiring transfusion (1.0 per 1000 cases), hospitalization for longer than 72 hr (1.8 per 1000 cases), hospital readmission (1.5 per 1000 cases), and water intoxication or pulmonary edema from the distention media (3.4 per 1000 cases).

Performing the procedure in an individual who has an undiagnosed pregnancy is a possible adverse occurrence during hysteroscopy. This complication is best avoided by scheduling procedures before ovulation and asking the patient to practice contraception.

Thermal injury to the intestinal tract can also occur during operative hysteroscopy. Peritonitis developing postoperatively as a result of this type of injury is managed by laparotomy and bowel resection.[26]

## Related to Distention Media

The most widely used distention media for hysteroscopy are $CO_2$, 32% dextran-70 (Hyskon), 5% dextrose in water, and other non-electrolyte solutions such as glycine or sorbitol. Any of the aforementioned liquid media may be used for operative hysteroscopy, since visualization is satisfactory and they do not conduct electrical current.

Intravascular intravasation of Hyskon has been associated with anaphylaxis, dissemi-

nated intravascular coagulation, adult respiratory distress syndrome, and noncardiogenic pulmonary edema.[27–29] Limiting Hyskon infusions to less than 300 cc seems to reduce these risks, although anaphylaxis can still occur.[27–29] The risk of anaphylaxis can be reduced by the intravenous administration of dextran-1 (Promit) 1 to 2 minutes before infusion of Hyskon. Surgeons should remember that Hyskon is a plasma expander, and when it enters the vascular system it draws 6 times its volume of extracellular fluid into the patient's vascular space, thus predisposing her to pulmonary congestion.

The use of 5% dextrose in water for uterine distention has been associated with severe hypoglycemia and hyponatremia.[30] However, any hypotonic liquid distention media may cause dilutional hyponatremia. This condition occurs when the distention media is absorbed into open uterine venous sinuses and enters the general circulation. The length of the hysteroscopic procedure as well as the amount of raw uterine surface created are important factors predisposing to dilutional hyponatremia. Infusing chilled distention media, which promotes vasoconstriction, under low pressure through a cervix that is slightly overdilated to facilitate egress of the media are safety measures that may reduce the risk of dilutional hyponatremia. Fluid intake and output have to be monitored closely. Electrolytes should be checked postoperatively.

Fatal gas embolism has been reported in association with the use of $CO_2$ as the distention media for hysteroscopic laser procedures.[26,31] In fact, the Food and Drug Administration now discourages the use of $CO_2$ for uterine distention during hysteroscopic laser procedures.

## Related to Surgical Procedure

Cervical dilatation can be complicated by formation of false passages and tenaculum tears. Uterine perforation can occur during cervical dilatation, during the insertion of the hysteroscope, or during the operative portion of the procedure. If not immediately recognized, uterine perforation should he suspected if large volumes of media fail to distend the uterus. Perforations may be managed expectantly, although laparoscopic assessment is indicated if intraabdominal or broad ligament bleeding or intestinal damage is suspected. The management of uterine perforations is outlined below.

Trauma to intraabdominal organs can occur even in the absence of uterine perforation. For example, the Nd:YAG laser has caused thermal intestinal injury during the course of endometrial ablation procedures. Clearly, laser energy can be transmitted through an intact uterine wall to adjacent loops of intestine or bladder.

Last, acute pelvic infection may occur after operative hysteroscopy. This is a very uncommon occurrence unless the procedure is performed in a patient with an unrecognized infection. If a patient develops peritonitis after a procedure in which thermal or laser energy was used, the surgeon should also consider the possibility of intestinal damage.

## Uterine Perforations

Uterine perforation may complicate all endoscopic surgery and can occur during the insertion of uterine manipulators, uterine manipulation per se, or hysteroscopic surgery. If a uterine perforation is suspected the procedure is discontinued. If there is the possibility of bowel or other organ damage then a laparoscopy is performed. Alternatively, it may be elected to observe the patient. Generally, damage to the integrity of the uterine cavity prevents continuation of the hysteroscopic procedure due to leakage of gas or dextran. If the intrauterine procedure must be continued a concomitant laparoscopy is performed.

Anterior wall, posterior wall, and fundal perforations do not usually bleed much, and bipolar electrocoagulation of the bleeding site generally achieves hemostasis. Perforations in the cornual region tend to bleed more vigorously. Electrocoagulation can usually obtain hemostasis, but extensive tubal destruction can

result. Microfibrillar collagen (Aviten) may also be used to secure hemostasis in this area. If this fails and the patient desires preservation of fertility, laparotomy and suturing of the injured site is indicated. Perforations of the lateral uterine wall are usually concealed between the layers of the broad ligament, and may become evident only when a hematoma distends the two leaves of the broad ligament. If a broad ligament hematoma is observed, the area is carefully dissected and the ureter identified before ligation of the uterine artery.[1]

Uterine perforations are best avoided by gentle insertion of the hysteroscope under direct vision. If laparoscopy is to be performed concomitantly, abdominal access should be established first. Laparoscopy during difficult hysteroscopic procedures decreases the incidence of uterine perforations and prevents additional damage should this occur. Fortunately, perforation sites are usually small and heal without remote adverse consequences.

## Certification in Operative Endoscopy

Currently, there are no uniform certification criteria that must be fulfilled before a physician performing operative laparoscopy. Each hospital creates their own criteria for credentialling. It is intuitively obvious, therefore, that physician experience may vary dramatically at the time certification is obtained. Some physicians may have hardly any experience at all the first time they "solo" in operative laparoscopy whereas others may have undergone extensive teaching and supervision.

The author believes that without nationally accepted credentialing criteria, it is the responsibility of each department of gynecology and obstetrics to assure that their physicians have adequate training before certification. A formal didactic course, hands-on laboratory experience, preceptorship with an expert in the field, and a number of supervised cases should be completed before certification (see Chapter 22). After certification, case lists, operative reports, and video documentation should be maintained for intermittent peer review. This allows for continued evaluation of a physician's surgical indications and quality of results. The author believes that strict surveillance serves the best interest of the patient, the surgeon, the hospital, and the academic community.

# References

1. Borten M. *Laparoscopic Complications: Prevention and Management.* Philadelphia: BC Decker Inc; 1980.
2. Hulka JF, Soderstrom RM, Corson SL, et al. Complications Committee of the American Association of Gynecological Laparoscopists: First Annual Report. *J Reprod Med* 1975;10:301–306.
3. Peterson HB, Hulka JF, Phillips JM. American Association of Gynecologic Laparoscopists' 1988 membership survey on operative laparoscopy. *J Reprod Med.* 1990;35:590–591.
4. Carbon Dioxide Laser Laparoscopy Study Group. Initial Report of the Carbon Dioxide Laser Laparoscopy Study Group: Complications. *J Gynecol Surg.* 1989;5:269–272.
5. Ohlgisser M, Sorokin Y, Heifetz, M. Gynecologic laparoscopy: a review article. *Obstet Gynecol Surv.* 1985;40:385–396.
6. Semm K. *Operative Manual for Endoscopic Abdominal Surgery.* Chicago: Year Book Medical Publishers; 1987.
7. Dingfelder JR. Direct laparoscope insertion without prior pneumoperitoneum. *J Reprod Med.* 1978;21:45–47.
8. Poindexter AN, Ritter M, Fahim A, et al. Trocar introduction performed during laparoscopy of the obese patient. *Surg Gynecol Obstet.* 1987;165:57–59.
9. Kaali SG, Bartfai G. Direct insertion of the laparoscopic trocar after an earlier laparotomy. *J Reprod Med.* 1988;33:739–740.
10. Byron JW, Fujiyoshi CA, Miyazawa K. Evaluation of the direct trocar insertion technique at laparoscopy. *Obstet Gynecol.* 1989;74:423–425.
11. Copeland C, Wing R, Hulka JF. Direct trocar insertion at laparoscopy: an evaluation. *Obstet Gynecol.* 1983;62:655–659.
12. Yuzpe AA. Pneumoperitoneum needle and trocar injuries in laparoscopy: a survey on possible contributing factors and prevention. *J Reprod Med.* 1990;35:485–490.
13. Corson SL, Batzer FR, Gocial B, et al. Measurement of the force necessary for laparo-

14. Mintz M. Risks and prophylaxis in laparoscopy: a survey of 100,000 cases. *J Reprod Med.* 1977;18:269–272.
15. Pring DW. Inferior epigastric hemorrhage, an avoidable complication of laparoscopic clip sterilization. *Br J Obstet Gynaecol.* 1983;90:480–482.
16. Alvarez RD. Gastrointestinal complications in gynecologic surgery: a review for the general gynecologist. *Obstet Gynecol.* 1988;72:533–540.
17. Levy BS, Soderstrom RM, Dail DH. Bowel injuries during laparoscopy: gross anatomy and histology. *J Reprod Med.* 1985;30:168–172.
18. Soderstrom RM, Levy BS. Bowel injuries during laparoscopy: causes and medicolegal questions. *Contemp Obstet Gynecol.* 1986;31:41–45.
19. Thompson BH, Wheeless CR. Gastrointestinal complications of laparoscopy sterilization. *Obstet Gynecol.* 1973;41:669–676.
20. Cunanan RG, Courey NG, Lippes J. Complications of laparoscopic tubal sterilization. *Obstet Gynecol.* 1980;55:501–506.
21. Thomas AG, McLymont F, Moshipur J. Incarcerated hernia after laparoscopic sterilization: a case report. *J Reprod Med.* 1990;35:639–640.
22. McLucas B, March C. Urachal sinus perforation during laparoscopy: a case report. *J Reprod Med.* 1990;35:573–574.
23. Grainger DA, Soderstrom RM, Schiff SF, et al. Ureteral injuries at laparoscopy: insights into diagnosis, management, and prevention. *Obstet Gynecol.* 1990;75:839–843.
24. Pyper RJD, Ahmet Z, Houang ET. Bacteriological contamination during laparoscopy with dye injection. *Br J Obstet Gynaecol.* 1988;95:367–371.
25. Peterson HB, Hulka JF, Phillips JM. American Association of Gynecologic Laparoscopists' 1988 membership survey on operative hysteroscopy. *J Reprod Med.* 1990;35:590–591.
26. Siegler AM, Valle RF. Therapeutic hysteroscopic procedures. *Fertil Steril* 1988;50:685–701.
27. Jedeikin R, Olsfanger D, Kessler I. Disseminated intravascular coagulopathy and adult respiratory distress syndrome: life threatening complications of hysteroscopy. *Am J Obstet Gynecol.* 1990;162:44–45.
28. Leake JF, Murphy AA, Zacur HA. Noncardiogenic pulmonary edema: a complication of operative hysteroscopy. *Fertil Steril* 1987;48:497–499.
29. McLucas B. Hyskon complications in hysteros-

copic surgery. *Obstet Gynecol Rev*. 1991;46: 196–200.

30. Carson SA, Hubert GD, Schriock ED, et al. Hyperglycemia and hyponatremia during operative hysteroscopy with 5% dextrose in water dis-

tention. *Fertil Steril*. 1989;51:341–343.

31. Brundin J, Thomasson K. Cardiac gas embolism during carbon dioxide hysteroscopy: Risk and management. *Eur J Obstet Gynecol Reprod Biol*. 1989;33:241–245.

# 22

# Training and Certification in Operative Endoscopy

*Ricardo Azziz*

The preceding chapters have dealt with the fundamentals and advanced techniques of endoscopic surgery, enumerating risks, complications, and outcome. However, the process by which a physician becomes trained and certified in these techniques is less clear. Proper training and certification are important to assure the highest quality of health care, maximizing success and minimizing morbidity. Furthermore, documentation of appropriate skills is essential for the medicolegal protection of the parent institution, the operating room personnel, and the surgeon. While complications are an accepted risk of endoscopic or any surgery, corroboration of a surgeon's training and skill in these techniques will minimize his or her liability in face of an eventuality. Following, a sequential program to assure proper training of surgeons in the area of operative endoscopy is outlined.

Aspiring operative endoscopists must first demonstrate knowledge and appropriate skills in the performance of diagnostic laparoscopy and hysteroscopy. For younger physicians these techniques may have been incorporated into their residency training. For other physi-cians these skills have been acquired through a process similar to that outlined below.

## Training/Certification

The training/certification process can be divided into three phases: didactic, observational or preceptorship, and tutorial phases (Table 22.1).

## Didactic

During this portion of a surgeon's training he/she will review the theoretical aspects of the surgery, including physical principles, patient selection, preoperative evaluation and preparation, surgical technique, alternative treatments, outcome, and morbidity. Generally, attending one or two training courses, complemented by review of an appropriate text, suffices. Nevertheless, there is a tendency for surgeons today to attend a myriad of such courses without further progression in their training, effectively halting their learning process.

As part of the didactic sessions, the surgeon

TABLE 22.1. Training/certification of endoscopic surgeons.

| Phase | Objectives |
| --- | --- |
| Didactic | Acquire theoretical knowledge concerning patient selection, preoperative evaluation and preparation, physics, surgical technique, alternative treatments, success, and morbidity of endoscopic procedures. Observe pretaped surgical procedures. Includes laboratory training to acquire specific skills such as laser use, endoscopic suturing, roller ball and resectoscopic ablation, etc., via the use of pelvic trainers and organ and/or live animal models |
| Observational | Observe between 10 and 20 live surgical cases, via video monitor, for each specific skill desired. Cannot be substituted by viewing pretaped surgical procedures. |
| Tutorial | Perform at least 10 to 20 cases for each specific skill desired under direct supervision of an expert endoscopist. The trainee must perform the majority of the procedure, and be responsible for patient selection and postoperative management |

TABLE 22.2. Suggested skill levels for the training and certification of operative laparoscopy.

| | |
| --- | --- |
| Level 1: | To include the ablation/removal of mild to moderate endometriosis, including endometriomas <3 cm in diameter, salpingo-ovariolysis of mild to moderate adhesions, and the treatment of ectopic regnancies |
| Level 2: | To include the resection of moderate to severe endometriosis, excluding extensive cul de sac dissection; resection of ovarian and paraovarian cysts, including edometriomas; oophorectomy $\pm$ salpingectomy; neosalpingostomy and fimbrioplasty; lysis of moderate to severe peritubal, ovarian, and abdominal adhesions; uterosacral oblation; and removal of select pedunculated subserosal fibroids |
| Level 3: | To include the performance of other more risky, innovative, or experimental procedures including appendectomies, presacral neurectomies, intramural myomectomies, hysterectomies, node sampling, etc |

will develop skills needed for the performance of operative endoscopy. Generally, the techniques acquired are fairly narrow and specific. Some do not involve the use of animal models, including learning to suture intraabdominally with a pelvic trainer and developing a familiarity with laser beam characteristics. To learn other procedures animal organ models may be used, such as the pig uterus for training in endometrial ablation and other hysteroscopic procedures. These models have the disadvantage that intraoperative bleeding does not occur and hemostatic skills are not tested. The use of live animal models is rarely used, unless the surgeon is developing or learning a particularly high-risk procedure.

Most operative endoscopy courses today combine didactic with laboratory training. However, the surgeon should not assume that 1 or 2 days of laboratory teaching suffices to develop a specific skill. As noted before, in general the skill acquired in the laboratory is generally very narrow, and requires continued practice.

## Observational (Preceptorship)

Having acquired didactic and laboratory knowledge, the surgeon now proceeds to observe live operative endoscopic procedures, generally via a video monitor. Viewing pretaped procedures is not an acceptable substitute, since the trainee must fully appreciate the placement and extraabdominal manipulation of the endoscopic instruments. Pretaped procedures can be a part of the didactic phase of training. While some training courses include live surgery observation, the period of time dedicated to this, by necessity, is relatively limited. The trainee should observe between 10 and 20 cases of a selected skill (see Tables 22.2 and 22.3). He/she may complete this portion of their training by spending a week or so observing the procedures of a busy endoscopist, or viewing cases once or twice weekly for approximately 1 to 2 months' time. This important portion of the training process is the one most frequently not fulfilled.

TABLE 22.3. Suggested skill levels for the training and certification of operative hysteroscopy.

| | |
|---|---|
| Level 1: | To include the removal of polypsy, small fibroids and lost IUDs; metroplasties; and lysis of mild to moderate synechiae |
| Level 2: | To include lysis of severe synechiae with obliteration of the uterine cavity, endometrial ablation, and removal of larger fibroids |

## Tutorial

Having observed 10 to 20 live cases, the physician is now ready to begin performing his own endoscopic surgery, under direct supervision. He/she should aim to perform at least 10 to 20 supervised cases at the specific skill desired. The supervising endoscopist should have proven expertise in the field and should allow the trainee to perform most or all of the surgery. To maximize objectivity the tutor should preferably belong to an outside institution. The trainee must be responsible for the preoperative patient selection and preparation and her postoperative management. Certification of competence must not be issued, for the sake of all involved, until the trainee readily demonstrates satisfactory endoscopic skills to the supervising surgeon.

The entire training/certification process can take as little as 2 to 3 months for each specific skill or set of skills being learned. The above training process has been readily incorporated into a number of reproductive endocrine/infertility fellowships and some residency training programs. However, barring these situations a surgeon may have to devise his/her own training program. Final certification is generally provided by the supervising endoscopist and/or the institution in which the surgery is to be performed. However, in the near future certification of competence may be required more broadly, and the process will become more uniform. Unfortunately, currently such training and certification depends on the surgeon's and the surgical institution's good will and desire for excellence.

# Index